Religious

AND

Ethical Factors

IN

Psychiatric Practice

The conference at which these papers were first presented was sponsored by The Park Ridge Center for the Study of Health, Faith, and Ethics.

The Park Ridge Center exists to study the deepest questions that confront people as they search for health and encounter illness. Its programs of research, publishing, and education explore dimensions of these fundamental human experiences that are frequently overlooked in an environment of specialization and technology. For this reason the Center gives special attention to the religious and secular expressions of faith that are present in all health care situations; it brings faith into conversation with more frequently heard medical, philosophical, and legal voices.

The Center is an independent, not-for-profit organization supported by grants, foundations, private and corporate contributors, and subscribing Associates. Additional information may be obtained by writing to The Park Ridge Center, 676 North St. Clair, Suite 450, Chicago, IL 60611.

Religious
AND
Ethical Factors
IN
Psychiatric Practice

Edited by

Don S. Browning, Ph.D.

Thomas Jobe, M.D.

Ian S. Evison, D.Min.

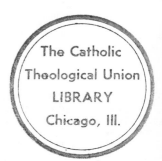

NELSON-HALL/ CHICAGO

In association with
The Park Ridge Center
for the Study of Health, Faith, and Ethics

Project Editor: Dorothy Anderson
Copy Editor: Carol Gorski
Designer: Sandi Lawrence
Compositor: Graphic Composition

LIBRARY OF CONGRESS CATALOGING-IN-PUBLICATION DATA
Religious and ethical factors in psychiatric practice / edited by Don S. Browning, Thomas Jobe, Ian S. Evison.
   p.   cm.
   Includes bibliographical references (p.   ).
   ISBN 0-8304-1225-5.—0-8304-1265-4 (pbk)
   1. Psychiatry and religion. 2. Psychiatry—Moral and ethical aspects. I. Browning, Don S. II. Jobe, Thomas. III. Evison, Ian S.
RC455.4.R4R45   1990
174'.2—dc20
                                                        89-14413
                                                        CIP

Copyright © 1990 by Nelson-Hall Inc.

Manufactured in the United States of America

10 9 8 7 6 5 4 3 2 1

TM The paper used in this book meets the minimum requirements of American National Standard for Information Sciences—Permanence of Paper for Printed Library Materials, ANSI Z39.48-1984.

CONTENTS

PART TWO: *Ethical Issues and Psychiatry*

PART THREE: *Religion and Psychiatric Practice*

PREFACE

Religious and Ethical Factors in Psychiatric Practice is a product of the research interests of the Park Ridge Center for the Study of Health, Faith, and Ethics, an interfaith research institute sponsored by the Lutheran General Health Care System. Over the last five years, the Center's research projects have resulted in several important publications interrelating health, ethics, and religion.

The project that culminated in these essays was begun by Kenneth Vaux, Ph.D., Professor of Ethics at the University of Illinois Medical Center, Chicago. Professor Vaux assembled the original team that commissioned these papers. Once a month for over three years the contributors to this volume met to read papers and discuss fundamental questions dealing with religious and ethical issues in psychiatric practice. I want to express my appreciation to Kenneth Vaux for bringing this group together and asking me to be its chair.

I also want to thank James Wind, Director of Research and Publications for the Park Ridge Center, for his continuing belief in this project. The support given by David Stein, Executive Administrator of the Center during the principal years of this project, was crucial for the health and well-being of our seminar. In addition, I am grateful to each of the contributors and to my co-editors, Thomas Jobe and Ian Evison, for making the chairing of the project such a delightful experience in collegiality.

Don S. Browning

CONTRIBUTORS

Douglas E. Anderson, M.D., is Assistant Professor of Neurosurgery at Loyola University Medical Center in Maywood, Illinois. His current area of primary research interest is microcerebrovascular disease processes.

Herbert Anderson, B.D., Ph.D., is Professor of Pastoral Care at Catholic Theological Union in Chicago. He has written *All Our Losses, All Our Griefs* and *The Family and Pastoral Care.*

Daniel J. Anzia, M.D., is Director of Psychiatric Residency and Scholar in Residence in the Section of Clinical Ethics at Lutheran General Hospital.

James B. Ashbrook, Ph.D., is Professor of Religion and Personality at Garrett-Evangelical Seminary and Advisory Member of the Graduate Faculty of Northwestern University. His most recent book is *The Brain and Belief: Faith in the Light of Brain Research* (Wyndham Hall Press).

Don S. Browning, B.D., Ph.D., is Alexander Campbell Professor of Religion and Psychological Studies at the Divinity School of the University of Chicago. His most recent book is *Religious Thought and the Modern Psychologies* (Fortress Press).

Prakash Desai, M.D., is Chief of Psychiatry at the West Side V.A. Medical Center and Associate Professor of Psychiatry at the University of Illinois at Chicago College of Medicine. Recent publications include *Health and Medicine in the Hindu Tradition* (Crossroad, 1989), and "Indian Medical Ethics," in the *Journal of Medicine and Philosophy* (August 1988).

Ian S. Evison, D.Min., is a Ph.D. student in practical theology at the Divinity School of the University of Chicago. He recently co-edited *The Education of the Practical Theologian: Responses to Joseph Hough and John Cobb's Christian Identity and Theological Education* (Scholars Press, 1989).

Donald M. Jacobson, M.D., is a private-practice psychiatrist and member of the College of the American Guild of Organists. Areas of specialty include mood disorders and multiple personality disorder.

Thomas H. Jobe, M.D., is Associate Professor of Clinical Medicine in the Department of Psychiatry of the University of Illinois at Chicago College of Medicine, Director of Outpatient Services, and Associate Residency Director. Recent articles include "The Devil in Restoration Science: The Glanville-Webster Witchcraft Debate," in *ISIS: An International Review Devoted to the History of Science* (1981), and "Moral Therapy and the Dynamics of the Treatment Cycle," *Journal of Operational Psychiatry* (1982).

Steven D. Kepnes, Ph.D., is Assistant Professor of Philosophy and Religion at Colgate University. He recently co-edited *The Challenge of Psychology to Faith*. He has also published articles in the journals *Judaism* and *Jewish Studies* and is currently working on a book on Buber's influence on psychology.

Marie McCarthy, Ph.D., is Associate Professor of Pastoral Care at Catholic Theological Union in Chicago. Recent publications include "Love, Justice, and Mutuality: The Foundations of Transformation," in *Economic Justice: Catholic Theological Union's Pastoral Commentary on the Bishop's Letter on the Economy* (Pastoral Press, 1988).

James P. Wind, Ph.D., was Director of Research and Publications at the Park Ridge Center for the Study of Health, Faith, and Ethics, where he edited *Second Opinion* and the series Health/Medicine and the Faith Traditions. He is now Program Director in Religion at Lilly Endowment, Inc. His book *Places of Worship: Exploring Their History* was published in 1990 by the American Association for State and Local History in Nashville.

Philip Woollcott, Jr., M.D., is Psychiatrist in Charge at the University of Illinois Hospital and Professor of Clinical Psychiatry at the University of Illinois at Chicago Medical Center. Recently he has published a number of papers on different forms of sudden psychological change including conversion; currently he is working on a theory of dissociated consciousness linked with these phenomena.

INTRODUCTION

Don S. Browning, Ph.D.
Ian S. Evison, D. Min.

Are psychiatry and religion competitive enterprises in our society? Do the premises of each of these cultural practices undercut those of the other? Or can psychiatry and religion complement each other? Recent research indicates that large portions of the American public believe psychiatry disparages all religion (Larson et al. 1986). If this is so, need it be? These are the basic questions that the essays in this volume seek to address.

These papers show the lines of congruence that one would expect from authors who met for three years to discuss common issues. Some lines of agreements we were aware of and expected; they had emerged in our conversation and took shape before our eyes. What is surprising, however, are the overlaps and implicit agreements that only became apparent during the final reading of the papers for the preparation of this introduction. We are convinced that these deeper unanticipated commonalities reflect a broader emerging consensus, not only within our group, but within the larger culture among those who work responsibly in the field of mental health and religion.

Hence, this introduction is not just a summary of papers that reflect our conversations; it is an analysis of possible deeper assumptive structures that may be emerging in some quarters of psychiatric and religious practice independently of the discussions that our group pursued.

In reviewing common themes in these papers, we do not mean to say that our authors agree on all matters. Differences will be apparent to the careful reader. But even though differences do exist, the following paragraphs of introduction are true to the overall direction of the papers in emphasizing the themes below.

1

The Need for a Public Philosophy for Psychiatry

At least half the articles in this volume directly call for the development of a public philosophy for psychiatry. Chapters that do not directly use this phrase still contribute indirectly to both the idea and the content of such a philosophy. Yet, what is meant by a public philosophy for psychiatry? And what purposes would it serve?

In the discussions from which these papers grew, we dealt primarily with the ways in which religious and ethical factors impinge on psychiatric practice. We gradually became convinced that many of the questions we pursued could not be answered on strictly scientific grounds. These questions seemed to require clarification of basic definitions, theories of human nature, and understandings of science, ethics, religion, and metaphysics.

What were the questions which brought us together and kept us in discussion for three years? Our questions were simple to state but proved difficult to answer. How does psychiatry relate to religion in the clinic, both to the religious commitments and experiences of the patient and to those of the therapist? How does psychiatry handle ethical issues at the various levels of its practice—the morality of its patients, the ethics of the psychiatric profession, and the relation of ideas of health care to the normative ethical models held forth to individuals by the wider culture? And finally, how does psychiatry relate to religious institutions and their healing traditions? How do psychiatrists and ministers distinguish between religious and psychological healing? Can pastoral counselors contribute to health? Do pastoral counselors have goals besides health guiding their work, such as salvation, self-transcendence, or righteousness? If so, what is the relation between health and these other goals? Do religious congregations have a contribution to make to mental health? If so, what form should it take? Should psychiatrists, ministers, priests, and rabbis cooperate, or should they see the respective types of healing that they promote as basically competitive and antagonistic?

The idea of a public philosophy for psychiatry arose as we gradually realized that to answer these questions we had to advance some basic definitions and address some fundamental issues which were logically philosophical. The idea of a public philosophy for psychiatry began to mean a philosophy that could be communicated to psychiatrists and to *the wider public*. Furthermore, this philosophy should define the special focus of psychiatry and relate this focus to a variety of other areas of social life such as law, politics, economics, ethics, social philosophy, and religion. For the purposes of our discussion in this book, we are primarily interested in a public philosophy that would clarify the relation of psychiatry to ethics and religion.

In the articles that follow, a number of authors call for and discuss the idea of a public philosophy for psychiatry. Don Browning's paper suggests that various Protestant theologians and philosophers of religion, from William James to Reinhold Niebuhr and Paul Ricoeur, directly contributed to such a public philosophy. In an effort to state the philosophical grounds for the Protestant spirituality they championed, James, Niebuhr, and Ricoeur used both American philosophical pragmatism and European existential phenomenology to express an appreciation for psychiatry and the special province of religion. Basically, they stated the philosophical grounds upon which psychiatry could avoid its latent and frequently manifest positivistic tendency to handle religion reductionistically.

Marie McCarthy also argues in her paper that a public philosophy for psychiatry is needed. She shows how, as mainline Protestants use pragmatism and existential phenomenology, so Karl Rahner uses transcendental Thomism to provide a doctrine of human experience large enough to include both the concern of psychiatry with biological and developmental conditionedness and the concern of theology with freedom, responsibility, and religious experience. Similarly, Ian Evison discusses the tension within psychiatry between value neutrality and social concern and uses the theological concept of *calling* to delimit psychiatry's responsibility as supporting "basic human functioning," a task which is both publicly defensible and practicable. Steven Kepnes draws on the Jewish thinkers Martin Buber and Mordechai Rotenberg to build an understanding of the role of psychiatry that affirms the hermeneutics of suspicion developed by Freud and Marx, but which also articulates the constructive role of history and tradition in human development. Finally, Daniel Anzia addresses the question of a public philosophy for psychiatry in advancing the idea that the concept of "competence" rather than health or autonomy ought to define the central goal of psychiatry.

History of the Psychiatry-and-Religion Relation

The essays in Part 1 touch on the history of the relation between psychiatry and religion. McCarthy, Kepnes, and Browning survey respectively the Catholic, Jewish, and Protestant responses to modern psychiatric practice. It is interesting to note that these histories are quite different: mainline Protestantism developed early a positive yet critical stance, Catholicism was far more skeptical, and Judaism almost completely silent, while at the same time providing the leaders of psychoanalytically oriented psychiatry. James Wind gives a more general view of the interaction between religion and psychiatry. Thomas Jobe develops a view of this interaction from the perspective of psychiatry. Collectively, these essays point to at least one truth: from the moment modern psychiatry emerged as a distinct profession, psychiatry and religion have overlapped and at times overtly competed. The reason for this is clear: both seek to heal forms of brokenness that stand on the ambiguous borderline between body and what is variously referred to as "psyche" or "spirit." As Wind and Jobe demonstrate, psychiatry has always had either positive or negative tacit relations with religion. The formulae governing the relations can be variable and surprising. Psychiatry in its more biological phases often enjoys positive relations with religion; a division of labor can emerge in which psychiatry deals with mental illness that is primarily biological in origin, while religion deals mainly with moral and spiritual problems in living. On the other hand, there are totally positivistic forms of biological psychiatry that tend to reduce all human problems to their biological foundations, thereby appearing to reject the relevance of religion to solving human problems. More psychological, and perhaps even spiritual, forms of psychiatry were advanced by A. T. Schofield, R. M. Bucke, and later Trigant N. Burrow that, according to Jobe, helped to prepare for the acceptance of psychoanalysis. According to authors such as Wallace (1983), Szasz (1987), and Browning (1987), one can now justifiably acknowledge the psychospiritual dimensions to both Freudian and Jungian forms of psychiatry. These more psychospiritual forms of psychiatry projected, in the name of science, religio-ethical views of life that sometimes functioned as genuine alternatives to classical Jewish and Christian visions. It was these forms of psychospiritual psychiatry that the Protestant, Catholic, and Jewish responses reviewed here were most concerned to critique and place in proper perspective.

Although the more biological and pharmacological psychiatries can appear at first glance to be the antithesis of the more psychospiritual psychiatries if they absolutize and overgeneralize their biological models, they too can function as quasi-religious (albeit mechanistic) metaphysical views of the meaning and possibilities of human existence. Yet it is possible to envision a psychiatry that would be friendly and supportive of the more classic formulations of the religious and ethical traditions of its culture. It might do this by refusing to absolutize its special foci on the biological and developmental dimensions of mental health. Such a psychiatry might even properly exercise a modest critical function with regard to those religious and ethical practices that seem to be destructive of mental health. But as the historical essays amply suggest, such a delicate and precise delineation between psychiatry and religion has been difficult to achieve and sustain.

A major point of these historical essays is to suggest that the issues between psychiatry and current forms of religious and ethical practice continue whether psychiatry is in its more biological or positivistic stages (the two should not be equated). The terms of the discussion will vary, but the need for philosophical clarification of their jurisdictions and relations will always exist. Thus, the call for a public philosophy for psychiatry should really be a call for continuing public conversations among representatives of a variety of perspectives. Each shift on the part of psychiatry, religion, or current ethical understandings will produce new tensions and possibilities. It is impossible to develop a static public philosophy for psychiatry that will serve for all time. But there is a great need for ongoing critical reflection and writing that will help clarify before the general public the special foci and possible complementarities between these areas of life. All of this should be done to strengthen the moral and institutional life undergirding our social and cultural existence.

Psychiatry's Need for a Philosophical Anthropology

Several of the authors call for a broader philosophical anthropology within which to locate the special concerns of psychiatry. The development of such an anthropology would be one significant dimension of a public philosophy for psychiatry. Two major strands in these papers fill out different dimensions of such an anthropology. The first strand is developed by McCarthy, Browning, Kepnes, Evison, and to some extent Anzia and calls for psychiatry to conceptualize the delicate and ambiguous way in which humans are conditioned by nature and history and yet also possess capacities for freedom, self-transcendence, and self-reflection. The second strand is developed by Jobe, Woollcott, and Desai, and involves a new effort to reconceptualize the model of the natural which undergirds psychiatry.

The first strand was elucidated by Reinhold Niebuhr, who wrote about the dialectical relation in humans between what he called "nature" and "spirit." Paul Tillich spoke of this ambiguity in humans as "finite freedom." Paul Ricoeur wrote about the dialectical relation between energetics (libido, instinct) and our capacity to identify with cultural "figures of the spirit." McCarthy tells us about Roman Catholic theologian Karl Rahner's non-Cartesian and nondualistic emphasis upon humans as unities of conditionedness and freedom. Evison presents another formulation of this duality in calling for psychiatry to direct itself to a goal of "basic human functioning." Even Anzia, from the perspective of psychiatry, while fully recognizing the biological conditionedness of humans, argues that to account for the category of health, psychiatry must have concepts of competence which, in turn, require assumptions about both human freedom and capacity for practical reason.

This dialectical relation between natural conditionedness on the one hand and degrees of freedom and self-reflection on the other, is an insight into human nature that can be derived from the theological anthropologies of Saint Paul, Saint Augustine, and Søren Kierkegaard, as well as from

Jewish scripture and *midrash*. However, as presented by Niebuhr, Tillich, Rahner, Ricoeur, and the authors of the early essays in this book, this image of the human can be abstracted from its theological heritage and supported by phenomenological description and philosophical reason. It then can be used by psychiatry to balance its image of the human and locate its special focus without obscuring the fuller dimensions of the human. As Douglas Anderson, Anzia, Woollcott, and Desai suggest, psychiatry may indeed be primarily interested in disturbances in the biological and developmental dimensions of human conditionedness. Yet McCarthy, Evison, Ashbrook, and Browning argue that religion and ethics basically are concerned with the orientation of our freedom and self-reflection concerning questions of moral value and deeper images of the ultimate context of life. It may well be that in some situations biological imbalance or developmental impediments can so seriously limit our freedom that we have little energy for the more distinctively human capacities of self-reflection and practical reason. In these situations, psychiatry is clearly the most directly relevant discipline. However, psychiatry, in its appeals to patients to become more involved in their therapy, its interest in gaining patient consent for chemical and surgical interventions, and its invitations to clients to take more responsibility for their lives, assumes at least limited capacities for the kind of freedom and self-transcendence that religion and theology feel are their special provinces.

The strategy recommended here is not designed to Christianize or Judaize psychiatry. The proposal is to use philosophical anthropology as common ground to relate psychiatry, theology, and ethics. Such a philosophical anthropology should be adequate to the special needs of each of these cultural pursuits and yet broad enough for each to locate its special concerns in relation to the others. As we suggested above, this philosophical anthropology would draw from the deep metaphors and fundamental symbolic and narrative expressions of the principal religious traditions informing a particular culture. The philosophical anthropology advocated by several of the papers may have been most distinctively stated by Saint Paul, who in turn was synthesizing the teachings of Jesus with various aspects of Jewish and Greek religion and philosophy.

The philosophical maneuver advocated here is akin to the hermeneutic phenomenology of Hans-Georg Gadamer and Paul Ricoeur (Gadamer 1982, 364–97; Ricoeur 1970, 37–58). Such a strategy presupposes that at their depth and at their best, our philosophical anthropologies arise from reflection on the fundamental symbols and narratives that form our religiocultural traditions. Ricoeur gave this point of view a striking formulation with his famous phrase, "the symbol gives rise to thought" (Ricoeur 1967, 347–57). The claim in this simple statement is staggering. It suggests that our philosophical thought about human nature is first of all nourished by the fundamental intuitions into reality found in the basic religious symbols of our culture. It further suggests that our so-called secular cultural disciplines are never quite as secular as we think. Our thinking starts from somewhere, and not from absolute objectivity. Our images of what it means to be human are formed first of all by our religiocultural traditions, and no matter how abstracted our thoughts may become from these traditions, they are still silently, subtly, and significantly formed by them. As Dennis Klein and David Bakan have argued in quite different ways, it is impossible to understand Freud's psychoanalytic formulations without also understanding the Jewish religiocultural heritage that shaped significant parts of his thinking (Klein 1981; Bakan 1958). Nevertheless, the philosophical anthropology that might emerge from a specific tradition can still be abstracted from the particular dogmas of that tradition. It can furthermore be embellished and amplified by dialogue with discoveries of the sciences, the insights of phenomenological description, and interaction with other religiocultural traditions. In this way, it can achieve the heuristic power to provide a larger and more balanced image of the human within which to locate the special interests of psychiatry, religion, and ethics.

The second strand of philosophical anthropology running through these papers involves a possible new model of nature undergirding psychiatry. Whereas the first strand attempts to state the dialectical relation between nature and self-transcendence, the second attempts to replace the individualism implicit in older psychiatric views of nature with a model that emphasizes the natural human need for community and relatedness.

A good case can be built that the biology of psychoanalysis and the value assumptions of Western society have interacted to give psychiatric practice an individualistic tone. Although psychoanalysis is no longer the dominant influence on contemporary psychiatry, its value commitments may still influence psychiatric practice. As Rieff (1966, 59), Kakar (1981, 10; 1982, 88), Browning (1973, 86–90; 1987) and others have claimed, these value commitments lean decidedly toward individualism. Sudhir Kakar writes that "the assumptions of Western psychotherapy are also the highest values of modern individualism" (Kakar 1982, 88). By psychotherapy, in this quotation, Kakar means psychoanalysis and its impact on psychiatry.

However, these value commitments may derive from something more than a chance coincidence between the personal values of Sigmund Freud and the values of Western capitalism. They may derive partly from the way Freud and his psychiatric followers tended to read the facts of human biology. Freud's theory of tension reduction seems to suggest a highly individualistic image of human biological need. In his early "Formulations Regarding the Two Principles in Mental Functioning" Freud portrayed human infants as first hallucinating the objects that could satisfy their wishes and only later reaching out from frustration to real human objects (Freud [1911] 1963, 22). Hence, object relations, in early Freudian theory, always have a transitory and secondary meaning; they are necessary not so much as ends in themselves but as means of satisfying needs that we would prefer to satisfy by ourselves.

In the chapter by Thomas Jobe and the one jointly authored by Philip Woollcott and Prakash Desai, we have a novel turn toward a biological model quite different from the one found in Freud and much of psychiatry influenced by him. These authors all acknowledge that psychiatry has special interests in the biological conditionedness of human beings. But the model of biological need that they find attractive not only is considerably different from Freud's individualistically oriented tension-reduction model, but also helps explain the peculiar form that human spiritual yearnings tend to take.

Both papers turn toward the phylobiology and the psychoanalysis of the American psychiatrist Trigant N. Burrow (1875–1950). Although Burrow was not a traditionally religious man, he developed a model of human biology that articulated well with Saint Augustine's view of the teleology of human desire as *caritas*. Burrow believed that each person has a fundamental need to relate positively to the human phylum or species. This need takes the form of a natural desire for "species solidarity," a desire, however, that is broken by the emergence of the human symbolic and defensive maneuvers that give rise to the "I persona." Woollcott and Desai take Burrow's concept into the study of mysticism. They hypothesize that this primordial species solidarity is split off from consciousness in normal Western socialization. The mystical experience dissolves the barriers that wall off this line of development and bring us back into contact with our natural sense of attachment to and love of the larger phylum of the human race.

This use of Burrow by Jobe, Woollcott, and Desai accomplishes several things. It launches a new model for psychiatry to conceptualize the natural and biological in humans. It is a model that emphasizes the human need for relations and community. Although contemporary British object relation theorists are also now going in the direction of emphasizing the fundamental need for relations as ends in themselves, they do this with only meager interest in articulating the biological basis of this need (Guntrip 1971, 45–68; Greenberg and Mitchell 1983, 3). Jobe, Woollcott, and Desai make explicit the biological basis of these needs. Their work stands as a vigorous hypothesis based at the moment mainly on historical and theoretical reflection on the nearly forgotten contributions of Burrow. Their work, however, points not only in the direction of British object relations theory but also in the direction of the work of John Bowlby (generally not considered a genuine object relations psychologist precisely because of his biological interests) (Bowlby 1969, 1973) and toward the intersection of sociobiological theory and psychiatry in the work of Frank Sulloway (1979) and Anthony Stevens (1982). However, in the work of Jobe, Woollcott, and Desai, this reconstructed biology also is used as an interpretive perspective that illuminates some of the psychobiological infrastructures of human spirituality.

From the perspective of the broader interest in developing a philosophical anthropology complex enough to locate both the special interests of psychiatry and those of ethics and religion, the work of Jobe, Woollcott, and Desai should be of as much interest to Jewish and Christian theologians as to the psychiatric community. If much of contemporary Jewish and Christian thought has moved toward an anthropology that advances a dialectical relation between nature and self-transcendence, the question still remains: which model of our human needs and tendencies will the religionists hold? Here their own religious traditions will be partially suggestive. Kepnes uses the story of the *Akedah,* or binding Isaac, as a framework for a model of growth built on the transformation and development, rather than the renouncing, of relationships. As Herbert Anderson points out in his chapter on the relation of psychiatry to the religious congregation, Western religious traditions have tended to assume a fundamental need for community in human beings. Although Western religious traditions have assumed this, models that clarify the biological grounds for this need for community should help religious leaders not only in their ministries but in cooperation with other contemporary practices such as psychiatry. All this suggests that a viable philosophical anthropology will not be developed solely out of philosophical hermeneutics. The framework of such an anthropology might be generated by this procedure, but the details of the view of the natural might come from more scientific models of the kind put forth by Jobe, Woollcott, and Desai.

Systems, Models, and Field Theory

Another theme running through several of these papers may be vitally important for a public philosophy of psychiatry. The chapter by Donald Jacobson is the most intentional in introducing a systems model for relating psychiatry and religion. But this is also a prominent aspect of Herbert Anderson's discussion of the role of the church in mental health, and Browning writes about the importance of field theory as an instrument for relating psychiatry to religion in the thought of James, Boisen, and Hiltner.

Systems theory has a long and complex history. We associate it with some of its more recent and prominent exponents such as Talcott Parsons

(1951), Ludwig von Bertalanffy (1968), and Roy Grinker in psychiatry (1953). But we often overlook its presence in philosophical pragmatism, especially in the writings of William James, where it is referred to most often with the metaphor of "field." As Browning points out in his essay, James, Boisen, and Hiltner overcame the temptations of theological and scientific positivism by accepting both religious experience and the determinisms studied by science as raw data, assuming that human consciousness and behavior can be influenced by a variety of fields. Human consciousness can conceivably be simultaneously influenced by chemical fields, biological fields, and spiritual forces. Eugene Fontinell reminds us of the suitability of describing James's theory of the self as "fields within fields" (Fontinell 1986). James influenced Boisen and Hiltner to solve the question of the relation of psychiatry and theology by refusing to absolutize either perspective and by assuming that each had something important to say about the total field of human action.

Although Jacobson makes little reference to this pragmatic tradition, systems theory is fundamental for guiding him as a working psychiatrist through the maze of issues pertaining to the clinical handling of patients who exhibit religious thinking and behavior. Jacobson is interested in how to evaluate religious experience and belief in the psychiatric setting. Does it contribute to or detract from mental health in a particular case? Jacobson believes that this is a serious clinical question; psychiatrists who fail to take the consequences of religion seriously and do not take adequate religious histories of their patients make a serious mistake. To understand the psychodynamic significance of religion, the psychiatrist must know more than the denominational affiliation of the patient. Jacobson advocates a longitudinal systems approach to the evaluation of religious experience and ideation. He writes:

> In our evaluation of religious experience, we will want to attempt to understand the origins of this experience, how it has evolved over time, whether or not it appears to be age and subculture appropriate and whether it has been stable or has demonstrated marked and perhaps pathological changes.

This list of criteria dealing with origins, time perspective, developmental appropriateness, cultural appropriateness, and stability virtually points to a variety of interlocking systems from which to view the efficacy of a patient's religious involvements. It acknowledges that events originating principally in one system can have both positive and negative consequences in other systems. Using this model, Jacobson can acknowledge, as would Douglas Anderson, the importance of events in our biological system for certain types of religious experiences. For instance, he describes how temporal lobe epilepsy, schizophrenia, and bipolar disorder can intensify our religious experience, reminding us that even our spirituality is affected by biological factors. On the other hand, he also acknowledges that mystical experiences sometimes have integrational consequences for more mundane psychological and emotional systems or levels of consciousness.

Some form of interactionalist model of the relation between body and mind seems to accompany systems theory. It suggests that certain systems of thought and experience can influence biological or bodily systems and that certain biological systems can affect states of consciousness. Although these papers neither address nor solve the intricacies of the mind-body problem, they do seem to assume this interactionalist or dialectical model. Douglas Anderson's recounting of the ethical struggles around psychosurgery suggests that theologians and religionists (and some psychiatrists as well) who resist the idea of surgical interventions into the brain, may want to attend more closely to the results of this approach in certain intractable mental illnesses. There may be ways of making use of some of the advances in psychosurgery without sacrificing normative images of the human as simultaneously self-transcending and conditioned by nature and the current state of our brains. The brain as biophysiological instrument may influence systems above it just as these psychospiritual systems may have consequences in turn on the brain and other bodily systems.

Herbert Anderson uses systems theory in clarifying the relation of psychiatric practice to religious communities. The question of the relation of psychiatry to religious communities raises the larger question of its relation to human community in general. Doesn't psychiatry necessarily assume viable human community performing the socializing, supportive, affirming, corrective, and norm-maintaining tasks that initially produce mental health? Doesn't this make psychiatry a subsystem of a larger human community that may itself exhibit varying degrees of health or unhealth? Anderson believes that religious congregations may be one of the few remaining expressions of community in advanced industrial nations that are sufficiently wholistic, continuous over time, face-to-face, and life cycle inclusive to give individuals the simultaneous sense of individual identity and social solidarity needed to live in mobile, highly differentiated, and quickly changing modern societies. As a subsystem of the larger society, psychiatry needs to be related to other systems that function as counterplayers complementing and supporting its own special functions.

James Ashbrook gives us a more intimate portrait of the way some actual psychiatrists relate to the religious communities through their cooperative work with individual pastors who represent religious communities in performing a specialized pastoral counseling ministry. Through a series of interviews that Ashbrook reports with psychiatrists who have working relations with pastoral counselors, we learn something about the actual motivations and exchanges that integrate these partnerships. As Ashbrook says, psychiatrists and pastoral counselors in these relations "complete each other's unconscious longing." By this he means that psychiatrists in these partnerships enjoyed contact with the larger world of values, meaning, and religious beliefs that the ministers presented. On the other hand, the pastoral counselors gained from being reminded about the role of biology and the body in shaping emotions. Although for Ashbrook psychiatrists and pastoral counselors function as two complementary subsystems of the larger society, he repudiates any "artificial division of professional responsibility" that would too simplistically partition either profession from the focus of the other. Ashbrook gives us something of a summary of the position of several of the chapters when he writes,

> The practice of medicine needs connections to something like the practice of ministry, and the practice of ministry needs the mechanisms of something like the practice of medicine. Every aspect of the human environment dissolves into human functioning and permeates the whole.

Such a position admits that although each has its special focus, there can be no rigid division of labor that categorically separates psychiatry from older religious modalities of healing.

Religion and the Phenomenological Stance

Several of the authors write about the importance of the phenomenological stance for the handling of religious issues by psychiatry. Phenomenology is an epistemological stance that brackets and temporarily sets aside questions about how something is caused or comes into being. A phenomenological attitude also suspends judgment about whether an object of study is actually real. Instead, phenomenology studies its objects from the perspective of their modes of appearance. Phenomenology is a method of study strongly associated with the European philosopher Edmund Husserl, who is commonly considered to be the founder of the phenomenological movement (Husserl 1970). But as Browning points out, William James developed within his pragmatic philosophy of religion his own brand of phenomenology. James criticized the tendency on the part of the medical materialists of his day to reduce religion to its origin in infancy, sexuality, or emotional pathology. On the one hand, he believed religious expressions should be first approached descriptively in terms of the full richness they have to those who experience them. On the other hand, he was interested in evaluating religion, not on the basis of genetic associations with pathology or infancy, but on the basis of its moral consequences for human life. On the whole, Protestant response to psychiatry, from Anton Boisen to Paul Tillich to Paul Ricoeur, has taken a similar phenomenological stance, although it has not always accepted James's pragmatic evaluation of religion. The phenomenological attitudes of Ricoeur and the Roman Catholic theologian Karl Rahner come more directly from Husserl and the European tradition than from the Jamesian American tradition.

Woollcott and Desai also invoke a phenomenological stance in their study of mystical experience. They are far more interested in describing the modes of appearance of mystical experiences than they are in tracing their genesis or determining the actual existence of the sacred realities that these experiences presuppose. They seem to agree with Jacobson's statement that it may be premature to "exclude the possibility of a spiritual dimension" in the absence of a totally satisfactory scientific explanation of religion. In the absence of such a model, Jacobson too basically takes a phenomenological attitude toward religious experience and belief, attempting to establish how they affect the various systems that converge on the selfhood of the patient.

Taking a phenomenological attitude toward religious experience and belief is probably the only defensible public stance for psychiatry as a profession. In reducing religious expressions to the emotional ambivalence of the oedipal conflict, Freud never fully understood the philosophical and metaphysical obligations that his position would entail if it were fully argued (Freud [1913] 1938). It is one thing to argue that some, or even all, religious experience contains some oedipal projections. It is another argument altogether to defend the positivist position that religious experience is "nothing but" these projections. Such a position would require complex metaphysical arguments of the kind that psychiatry as a profession would be wise to avoid. In view of the present state of our epistemological competence, the phenomenological stance is the most comfortable public position toward religion for psychiatry to take.

However, there is evidence that the general public does not see psychiatry taking such a stance. Studies made by Larson et al. suggest that the general public sees psychiatry on the whole taking a negative, if not completely reductionistic, attitude toward religion (Larson et al. 1986). This may be part of the reason why certain segments of the religious population are turning away from psychiatry toward either their own religious counselors (King 1978) or toward the therapeutic promises of various contemporary religious cults (Kilbourne and Richardson 1984). A phenomenological stance toward religion as a part of the public philosophy for psychiatry might help restore the confidence of the vast majority of the public that still, according to recent surveys, believes in a supreme being and that still participates, to varying degrees, in religious institutions (Larson et al. 1986). In view of the fact that psychiatry in Western nations must function in pluralistic societies and, in the case of the United States, must function with a legal separation of church and state, the phenomenological attitude has much to commend it both as a public stance and as a perspective guiding the work of individual psychiatric practitioners.

Pragmatism and a Public Philosophy for Psychiatry

The public philosophy for psychiatry that emerges in these papers has strong affinities with the American tradition of philosophical pragmatism. There are at least four themes that run through these chapters that are also consistent with major emphases in philosophical pragmatism. These are: (1) the respectful, phenomenological, and nonreductionistic handling of religious expressions, (2) a field or systems understanding of both epistemology and reality, (3) a broader understanding of the empirical than can be found in more experimental or positivistic understandings of science, and (4) an interest in testing the worth of religious claims in terms of their moral fruitfulness. We have already seen how both American pragmatism, particularly the thought of James, and the essays in this volume, exhibit features one and two, i.e., the phenomenological handing of religious expressions and field theory in epistemology and metaphysics. We will conclude with a brief discussion of the other pragmatic themes, dealing with a larger understanding of empirical and moral fruitfulness as a test of the value of religious claims and experiences.

First, all the papers setting forth elements of a philosophical anthropology that understands human existence as a dialectical relation between nature and spirit, or nature and self-transcendence, assume this larger understanding of the empirical and experiential. Such an anthropology may be derived in part from a hermeneutical appropriation of the dominant religious symbols of the West, but it is also held and defended because it is thought to be consistent with human experience itself. Experience in this large sense teaches humans to understand themselves as limited by the rhythms and pressures of nature, and yet able to think, make choices, and develop reflexive images of their own selves and behavior. If one has a narrowly positivistic view of experience, holding that the only things that are empirical are those that can be counted, measured, and experimentally repeated, then it will seem impossible to establish a philosophical anthropology that holds these two poles in tension. Other philosophical schools besides Jamesian pragmatism—such as existentialism and transcendental Thomism—have interest in more comprehensive models of the empirical, but this is certainly a part of pragmatism as well.

The concern to advance a moral evaluation of religion as a clinical strategy is even more typically a part of philosophical pragmatism. In chapter 1 Browning reviews in some detail James's mixture of moral with adaptive criteria in his evaluation of religion. The category of the moral is not limited to formal principles of universalization in James as it is in Kant (Kant [1785] 1959; Kant [1788] 1956). In James, the category of the moral brings health and adaptation values together with moral values of fairness and justice. Hence, James evaluates religion from the standpoint of how it meets various fundamental human needs. But he does so in such a way as to be concerned with how these satisfied needs fit justly and fairly with the needs of others.

Woollcott and Desai tip their hats toward the usefulness of pragmatic criteria in the clinical evaluation of mystical experience. They acknowledge that the moral consequences of mystical experience are part of the psychiatrist's evaluation of its authenticity and worth. Jacobson is less explicit about the category of the moral, but he is concerned to assess the "integrational" value of religious experiences, a concept that may serve to bring together both health values and values that reconcile conflicts between competing moral claims.

It is not our purpose to argue for the virtues of American pragmatism as a resource of psychiatry in developing a public philosophy of its work. Our goal is rather to use this philosophical tradition to illustrate what such a philosophy might look like. There are other resources and other issues besides the ones reviewed here. Even these papers, for all that they have accomplished, still leave to be investigated the various ways psychiatry should relate to wider issues in social philosophy. But if the idea of a public philosophy for psychiatry has merit, issues in social philosophy can be addressed in further conversations.

References

Bakan, David. 1958. *Sigmund Freud and the Jewish Mystical Tradition*. Princeton: D. Van Nostrand.

Bertalanffy, Ludwig von. 1968. *General Systems Theory: Foundations, Development, Application*. New York: G. Braziller.

Bowlby, John. 1969. *Attachment*. New York: Basic Books.

———. 1973. *Separation: Anxiety and Anger*. New York: Basic Books.

Browning, Don. 1973. *The Moral Context of Pastoral Care*. Philadelphia: Westminster Press.

———. 1975. *Generative Man: Psychoanalytic Perspectives*. New York: Dell.

———. 1987. *Religious Thought and the Modern Psychologies*. Philadelphia: Fortress Press.

Fontinell, Eugene. 1965. *Self, God, and Immortality*. Philadelphia: Temple University Press.

Freud, Sigmund. 1983. "Totem and Taboo." In *Basic Writings of Sigmund Freud,* (1913), ed. A. A. Brill. New York: Random House.

———. 1963. "Formulation Regarding the Two Principles in Mental Functioning" (1911) In *General Psychological Theory,* ed. Philip Rieff. New York: Collier Books.

Gadamer, Hans-Georg. 1982. *Truth and Method.* New York: Crossroad.

Greenberg, Jay and Stephen Mitchell. 1983. *Object Relations in Psychoanalytic Theory.* Cambridge: Harvard University Press.

Grinker, Roy. 1953. *Psychosomatic Research.* New York: Norton.

Guntrip, Harry. 1971. *Psychoanalytic Theory, Therapy, and the Self.* New York: Basic Books.

Husserl, Edmund. 1970. *The Crisis of European Sciences and Transcendental Phenomenology.* Evanston: Northwestern University Press.

Kakar, Sudhir. 1981. *The Inner World.* Delhi, India: Oxford University Press.

———. 1982. *Shamans, Mystics, and Doctors.* New York: Knopf.

Kant, Immanuel. 1959. *Foundations of the Metaphysics of Morals* (1785). New York: Bobbs-Merrill.

———. 1956. *Critique of Practical Reason* (1788). New York: Bobbs-Merrill.

Kilbourne, Brock and James Richardson. 1984. "Psychotherapy and New Religions in a Pluralistic Society." *American Psychologist* 39, 3 (March): 237–51.

King, Robert R. 1978. "Evangelical Christians and Professional Counseling: A Conflict of Values?" *Journal of Psychology and Theology.* 6, 4 (Fall): 276–81.

Klein, Dennis. 1985. *Jewish Origins of the Psychoanalytic Movement* (1981). Chicago: University of Chicago Press.

Larson, David B., et al. 1986. "Systematic Analysis of Research on Religious Variables in Four Major Psychiatric Journals." *American Journal of Psychiatry,* 143, 3 (March): 329–34.

Parsons, Talcott. 1951. *Toward a General Theory of Action.* New York: Harper and Row.

Ricoeur, Paul. 1970. *Freud and Philosophy.* New Haven: Yale University Press.

———. 1967. *The Symbolism of Evil.* New York: Harper and Row.

Rieff, Philip. 1966. *The Triumph of the Therapeutic.* New York: Harper and Row.

Stevens, Anthony. 1982. *A Natural History of the Self.* New York: Morrow.

Sulloway, Frank. 1979. *Freud: Biologist of the Mind.* New York: Basic Books.

Szasz, Thomas. 1987. *Insanity: The Idea and Its Consequences.* New York: Wiley.

Wallace, Edwin R. IV. 1983. "Reflection on the Relationship between Psychoanalysis and Christianity." *Pastoral Psychology,* 31, 4 (Summer): 215–43.

PART ONE

Historical Interactions

THE PROTESTANT RESPONSE TO PSYCHIATRY: CONTRIBUTIONS TO A PUBLIC PHILOSOPHY FOR PSYCHIATRY

Don S. Browning, Ph.D.

The response of the mainline Protestant churches to the emergence of psychiatry in the United States has been basically favorable. This was particularly true insofar as psychiatric practice in the twentieth century became increasingly influenced by the psychoanalytic theories of Sigmund Freud. The New England Protestant medical establishment, especially Morton Prince and James Jackson Putnam, supported Freud's ideas and communicated them to the general public (Holifield 1983, 193–95). But more than that, several important Protestant thinkers (philosophers of religion and theologians) were friendly to psychiatry in general and, for the most part, to psychoanalytic ideas in particular.

This was certainly true of William James, although James must be seen as a bridge figure whose career spanned all the way from medicine in his early years to psychology, ethics, philosophy, and finally the psychology and philosophy of religion in his later years (Allen 1967, 88–101). But later, more specifically Protestant theological thinkers such as Anton Boisen, Seward Hiltner, Paul Tillich, Reinhold Niebuhr, and Paul Ricoeur were hospitable to psychiatry, especially in its more psychoanalytic forms. All these thinkers were identified with the mainline Protestant churches, and all significantly influenced Protestant theological thinking. They were all either Americans or individuals with an extensive experience in American academic institutions, as was the case with Tillich and Ricoeur. Clearly, they represent the best and most responsible efforts of the Protestant community to grapple with psychiatry, especially as it was predominantly influenced during most of the twentieth century (except possibly in recent years) by psychoanalytic concepts and methods.

Their basically positive response to psychoanalytically oriented psychiatry was qualified in a variety of ways. They advanced powerful justifications for the role of psychiatry in social life. However, they also worked

19

to limit the role of psychiatry while, at the same time, extending its imagination to both understand and have empathy for the religious and ethical dimensions of life. In addition, they worked to control its occasional positivistic impulses from reductively intruding upon the wider religious and ethical practices of everyday social life. Hence, these thinkers tried to restrain psychiatry from following Freud's less philosophically defensible identification of all religion with obsessive-compulsive neurosis and most ethics with more or less arbitrary superego prohibitions (Freud [1907] 1963, 17–26).

In doing this, they contributed to a philosophy of psychiatry. By a philosophy of psychiatry, I mean a broad intellectual understanding of both its proper focus and its relationship to the wider aspects of social and cultural action. Every profession needs such a philosophy of its practice distinguishable from the body of knowledge (scientific, legal, or historical) that constitutes its special province of expertise. Since psychiatry is a social practice and not just a science, a philosophy of psychiatry would clarify the moral foundations of its practice, identify the kind of practice psychiatry is, and relate this practice to a variety of other practices that make up the larger context of social action. The philosophical foundations of any professional practice can never be elaborated solely by the members of the professional group in question, although, of course, they will contribute to that philosophy. But since psychiatry is a practice first and a science second, the generic features of this practice can be clarified by any one of a number of sources, many of which are outside the profession. The Protestant response to twentieth-century psychiatry constituted one of the sources contributing to the philosophical clarification of the foundations of its practice.

Although the Protestant response to psychiatry and its subsequent contribution to a philosophy of psychiatry is generally overlooked by psychiatry, I will argue that this contribution is important and needs to be acknowledged. Furthermore, Protestantism was quicker to develop critiques of psychiatry than either Catholicism or Judaism, although with the comparatively recent contributions of such Roman Catholic thinkers as William Meissner, Hans Küng, and others, this leadership can no longer be said to exist (Meissner 1984; Küng 1979). Furthermore, the Protestant responses, as well as many of the other religious responses, helped to clarify both the ethical foundations of psychiatry and the relation of psychiatry to religion. Understanding its relation to religious practice is a very significant part of the total task of establishing an adequate philosophical portrait for the practice of psychiatry. Of course, psychiatry must also understand its relation to other forms of practice such as medicine, law, education, and politics. Accounting for all of these practices would be part of the total task of a philosophy of psychiatry. But understanding its relation to religion would be one important part of that total philosophy of psychiatry for which I am calling. Much of the Protestant response to psychiatry properly can be understood not so much as trying to make professional psychiatry in some way religious as trying to help psychiatry understand its appropriate relation to religion.

I will concentrate primarily on the years from 1935 to 1985. But I will also discuss William James, not only for his contributions to a Protestant critique of psychiatry, but for his contributions to philosophical pragmatism, of which he was a major architect. James's work influenced much of the entire Protestant attempt to cope with the larger social meaning of psychiatry. The Protestant response to psychiatry never advanced its case on strictly scriptural or theological grounds. It developed its views always in conjunction with some larger philosophical stance that cleared space, in more neutral philosophical terms, for the possibility of the religious and ethical visions typical of Protestant Christian views of life. American philosophical pragmatism and Continental existential-phenomenology constituted the two principal philosophical sources. Pragmatism was important for James and Boisen, while existential-phenomenology was important for Tillich and Ricoeur. Niebuhr, on the other hand, had the virtue of borrowing from both of these schools although principally, I believe, from pragmatism.

There have been several recent attempts to provide a philosophy for psychiatry. All of these primarily have sought to give an account of the ethical dimensions of psychiatry. Many of them have addressed first the larger field of medicine and have included psychiatry as a dimension of medicine (Culver and Gert 1982; Pellegrino and Thomasma 1981; Hare 1981). There has been little effort in the recent literature to state philosophically the relation of psychiatry to religion. This latter issue will be the primary topic of this paper, although the relation of psychiatry to ethics will be an implicit secondary interest. My historical investigation into the various Protestant responses to psychiatric practice will move gradually toward a more constructive consideration of the question of what this response can contribute to a philosophy of psychiatry's relation to religion.

William James and the Medical Reduction of Religion

All of these Protestant thinkers acknowledged the legitimate role of psychiatry as an interpretive perspective on human behavior. More specifically, they acknowledged the neurological and biological conditioning of all human action, the importance of developmental factors in shaping adult behavior, the reality of neurotic or psychotic states, and even the neurotic or psychotic conditioning of some religious experience. But they also resisted the idea that neurobiological and developmental factors exhaustively accounted for all aspects of either religion or general human action. They criticized especially those forms of psychiatry dominated by scientific positivism or medical reductionism. These forms of psychiatry undercut not only the possibility of healthy forms of religion but the reality of human responsibility and what was variously called human fault, sin, or the divided self.

The first chapter of James's monumental *The Varieties of Religious Experience* (1903) has the title "Religion and Neurology." In the early pages of his investigation, James readily admits that many forms of religious experience seem to originate in pathological psychological states, developmental disorder, and even sexual conflicts (James [1903] 1950, 24–26). But he denies that the causal factors that shape the origins of any human experience can constitute the philosophical grounds upon which the value and truth of that experience can be judged (James [1907] 1950, 31). The view that a religious experience is "nothing but" its lowly origins in developmental conflict, neurological conditioning, or sexual disorder James calls "medical materialism" (James [1903] 1950, 29). To qualify such a materialistic or positivistic frame of mind with the word *medical* clearly suggests that James found this attitude widely prevalent in the psychiatric practice of his day.

In this and succeeding chapters of the *Varieties,* James sets forth, in answer to medical materialism, his pragmatic philosophy of religion. Even in this chapter, he makes his famous distinction between two types of philosophical judgments that can be brought to the analysis of religious experience—"existential" judgments and "spiritual" judgments. These rather quaint-sounding terms are designed to distinguish between judgments of facts and origins (existential judgments) and judgments of value and worth (spiritual judgments). The crux of his pragmatic philosophy of religion was that "neither judgment can be deduced immediately from the other. They proceed from diverse intellectual preoccupations" (James [1903] 1950, 23). More specifically, James insists that "existential facts by themselves are insufficient for determining the value of a religious experience, tradition, or teaching" (James [1903] 1950, 23).

James developed his own American brand of phenomenology and applied it to the interpretation of religious experience. In fact, recent studies have demonstrated that James influenced the phenomenological ideas of Edmund Husserl and through him the entire European existential-phenomenological philosophical movement (Edie 1970, 487; Linschoten 1968, 194). James's pragmatic approach to the evaluation of religion was built on a nonreductive phenomenological beginning point; he simply accepted phenomenologically the "objects" of religious experience (whether concrete personages or abstract ideas) and took at face value the thick sense of "reality" and "objective presence" that sometimes accompanies them (James [1903] 1950, 61). This did not mean that James overlooked the neurological or developmental conditionedness of religious experience, especially in its more pathological forms. James began with a careful description of the experience in all of its richness, and viewed causal explanations as an important but nonexhaustive perspective within this larger phenomenological description. In fact, it is the richness of James's description of religious experience that constitutes the essence of his psychology of religion in the *Varieties*. Close analysis reveals that James uses only a very few explanatory models in his psychological classic.

As we have seen, James acknowledged the conditioned nature, to varying degrees, of religious experiences. For this reason he could and did to some extent absorb into his system the dynamic explanation of religion associated with psychoanalysis and so widely used by contemporary psychiatric practice. But in contrast to Freud's tendency to depreciate religion because of the sexual or infantile aspects of its origins (Freud [1907] 1963, 17–24; Freud [1927] 1953, 92), James developed an elaborate three-fold test for the value or "spiritual truth" of religious experiences and ideas.

The three tests should interest psychiatry. James tell us that "immediate luminousness," "philosophical reasonableness," and "moral fruitfulness" rather than origins are criteria to be used to judge the value of religious experience (James [1903] 1950, 32). Immediate luminousness, James insists, should count for something in the evaluation of religion; if people claim that religious experience has changed them, enlightened them, or taught them truth, James believes that we should take this seriously as one small aspect of the total evaluative process. The general philosophical reasonableness of the experience also counts; does the experience make sense in light of commonly accepted views of knowledge and the world? Last, and most important, is the experience morally helpful? As James says, we should weigh "not its origin, but *the way in which it works on the whole*" (James [1903] 1950, 34). James pressed his Protestant ancestor Jonathan Edwards's *Treatise on Religious Affections* to his cause: "By their fruits ye shall know them, not by their roots ... The *roots* of man's virtue are inaccessible to us" (James [1903] 1950, 34).

James's final punch, however, is delivered against the medical materialists when he points out that they do not apply the argument by origins to scientific ideas. "In the natural sciences and industrial arts, it never occurs to any one to try to refute opinions by showing up their author's neurotic constitution" (James [1903] 1950, 32). James believes that consistency dictates that we should extend the same consideration to the products of religious experience.

Of the three criteria for the evaluation of religious experience and belief, moral fruitfulness is the most important to James and the most relevant to a philosophy of psychiatry. But what did James mean by *moral?* James's view of the moral is complex and a matter of debate (Browning 1980, 211–36; Levinson 1981, 89–94). On the whole, he saw ethics guiding the actualization of the fundamental psychobiological needs and interests that evolutionary history has bequeathed to humans. But, according to his model, humans have more psychobiological interests than can be actualized compatibly (James [1878] 1967, 52–53; James [1890] 1950, 2: 404). This was why, for James, ethics was necessary. Ethics orders the richness and conflicting superabundance of our psychobiological interests. Ethics serves these interests, but it also organizes them into hierarchies; some interests are rendered dominant and others subordinated and occasionally altogether sacrificed. Morality advances human interests and needs. It further organizes the natural order of our interests. The natural order of our interests, although present and necessary, is not sufficient for the complexity of civilized life. Therefore morality orders our natural interests to make them compatible with the needs and interests of others (James [1897] 1956, 205). When, for James, religious experience and belief are evaluated, the criteria are not origins but consequences; they are assessed principally from the perspective of moral helpfulness as defined in this way. Hence, for James, theistic or monistic, mystical or rational, extreme or average forms of religious experience are evaluated, not in terms of their origins (although these are in principle acknowledged as an aspect of a full understanding of them) but in how they fit into, support, and contribute to the whole moral pattern of a person's life.

James's pragmatism both assumes the existence of a moral capacity in humans and brings a moral perspective to the evaluation of religious experiences. Yet, in spite of this interest in the category of the moral, James is fully aware of the mass of determinisms that shape human life. In fact, on the whole, he sees the range of human freedom and moral responsibility as relatively small although indeed crucial. For James, freedom and the will grow out of, build on, yet guide the involuntary dimensions of life (James [1890] 1950, 2: 486–593). James holds an understanding of the reciprocal relation of the voluntary and involuntary not unlike that developed by Paul Ricoeur in his *Nature and Freedom* (Ricoeur 1966). Hence, the mass of determinisms affecting human life for James is soft rather than hard or exhaustive. It never completely eliminates freedom but does greatly limit it. Human freedom for James is a conditioned freedom. Furthermore, the range of conditioning can vary. Freedom is simply the capacity of our minds to keep our attention on one thing; it gives us the capacity to reinforce or accentuate with our attention some desires and influences more than others (James [1890] 1950, 2: 562–71). Such a view leaves enormous room for science in charting the determinisms that shape or incline our will even though these determinisms are soft and our attention can grab hold of them and direct them to a limited yet crucial degree. Humans do not have much freedom. But the limited amount that they do have makes all the difference in the world.

James's pragmatism was designed to accomplish a variety of tasks, one of which was to provide philosophical space for the claims of religion in general and his view of the Protestant experience in particular. A sampling of his actual moral evaluations will help illustrate the potential usefulness of Jamesian pragmatism for a philosophy of psychiatry. Monistic religious experience in which humans are identified with the divine and God with the world conveys security and warmth. Humans feel that they have a place in the world and that the world will be hospitable to their actions. But such monism tends to deemphasize the realities of human brokenness and particularity and lulls us into believing our moral action is unnecessary (James [1897] 1975, 123–25). Mystical experiences, if they are of the monistic variety, can do the same thing (James [1910] 1971, 739–59).

Thus James both appreciates a variety of religious experiences as contributing to moral adaptation and has a special fondness for more Protestant images of God. Yet he has in mind a particular version of the Protestant experience. He emphasizes a God immanent in and yet transcendent over human experience. God as immanent in experience is a source of warmth, support, and strength. Yet God as transcendent over human experience is not totally identified with the world. God is sufficiently distant to provide a sense of moral leverage on and expectation for human experience. Thus James proposes a limited theism (James [1910] 1971, 269), and what he in one place calls "pluralistic mysticism" (James [1910] 1971, 739–40). By this he means little more than to depict God as sufficiently related to, yet sufficiently differentiated from, human experience to place effective moral expectations on us, not unlike the way warm but differentiated parents place moral expectations on their children. But we should be reminded that, although James used his pragmatism to make a special apology for his vision of the Protestant experience, it can function to provide philosophical space for religion in general. Supplemented with the insights of dynamic psychology, it may also provide a philosophical framework for a nonreductive sympathy with and evaluation of religious experience for the purposes of clinical psychiatry.

It is the phenomenological beginning point of the pragmatic approach to religious experience that makes it nonreductive. James simply begins with the data of religion in all their thickness, their sense of divine presence, and their sense of ultimate seriousness. Although he is aware of the way our God-images partially are shaped, especially during the earlier years of our lives, by our parental and social experience, he does not understand this as profoundly as modern psychiatrists do. But he never assumes, like some modern psychiatrists, that these projections exhaust all religious experience. Instead, he looks at the consequences of religious experience measured by his own synthesis of evolutionary adaptive theory and his brand of moral responsibility. Religion is good when it furthers creative adaptation within the constraints of moral responsibility. From this perspective, some religion can indeed be seen as creative and some not. In his willingness to distinguish between good and bad religion, he shares a pervasive impulse in Christian experience in general and Protestant experience in particular. This is the tendency, which can be charted back to Jesus and Saint Paul, to distinguish between authentic religion and idolatrous or destructive religion. James advanced the resources of pragmatism to further this distinction.

Anton Boisen

Anton Boisen was a Protestant hospital chaplain and a founder of the clinical pastoral education movement in the United States. In his two major books, *Exploration of the Inner World* (1936) and *Religion in Crisis and Custom* (1945), he furthers the Protestant response to psychiatry that one finds in James. It is a distinctively Protestant response because it attempts to clear a place for a constructive appreciation in psychiatry for certain types of intense conversion experiences which have been, at least on the American scene, typical of Protestant evangelical experience stemming from eighteenth- and nineteenth-century revivalism. It also continues the pragmatic view of religion that originated with James; it recommends this view as an attitude that psychiatry itself should take toward religion. Although Boisen never expresses it this way, he is elaborating a philosophy of psychiatry that would give it grounds to take better account of the moral and religious aspects of psychiatric problems.

Against physicalistic or older Kraepelin approaches to mental illness, especially schizophrenia, Boisen argues for a more functional approach to mental illness. He sees mental problems as basically a result of breakdowns in people's relations to their social environments, due primarily to moral failures or deficiencies in the coherence and internal solidity of their philosophies of life (Boisen 1936, 220). Furthermore, he sees many psychotic episodes as basically creative attempts at "problem solving" designed to overcome a sense of personal failure in social life (Boisen 1936, 53). More specifically, he believes many of these episodes to be religious renewal experiences designed to reorient a person's values, relationships, and even ultimate commitments (Boisen 1936, ix). Boisen had his own psychotic break and spent a long period of recovery in the very hospital where he was the chaplain (Boisen 1936, 5). He felt it was a religious renewal experience for him and could also be that for at least some other patients if the psychiatric community were sufficiently sensitive to the meaning of these experiences. In the religious histories of such individuals as Saint Paul, Jeremiah, Ezekiel, George Fox, John Bunyan, and himself, Boisen thought he could identify many of the features of functional mental and emotional difficulties. But he also thought that he could identify creative religious problem solving and renewal that psychiatry should understand and be sympathetic toward.

Both James and Boisen attempted to create the philosophical grounds for a sympathetic understanding of mystical or conversion experiences typical of certain aspects of American Protestantism. Both of them gravitated toward a pragmatic philosophical stance. But Boisen took his message much more directly into the inner precincts of established psychiatry than James. Boisen's career spanned the years when psychoanalytic thought was beginning to influence psychiatry strongly. Yet both older and newer forms of more physiologically oriented psychiatry were also visible. Boisen believed that neither had the philosophical grounds to understand ways in which a sense of moral failure and religious renewal operates in some functional psychoses. The tendency of psychoanalysis to overemphasize sexual dimensions in the etiology of mental illness and to see religion as a defensive compromise between the need for protection from yet fear of parental figures, makes it unsuited to comprehend the more creative and renewing role of religion in human life (Boisen 1936, 105–108). More physiological approaches simply fail to recognize the functional nature of some mental illness. These approaches, then, cannot handle those aspects of mental illness that do entail value conflicts, personal failures, moral failures, and the dramatic attempts at renewal that some of the subsequent illnesses entail (Boisen 1936, 99–100). If judged by either of these schools of psychiatry, religious experiences of a Saint Paul, George Fox, or John Bunyan might be mishandled, undercut, or disastrously misunderstood, thereby undermining their creative reconstructive potential.

In effect, Boisen offers a new epistemological stance for psychiatry. On the one hand, he acknowledges that these renewal experiences can be seen as the work of nature (Boisen 1936, 54). On the other hand, he sees no scientific grounds to deny the possibility that behind these natural revitalization energies, there may be the gentle hand of a more divine source. Since this issue is basically metaphysical and cannot be solved on narrowly scientific grounds, Boisen approaches religion with a heuristic and undogmatic functionalism. He looks at religion in more than one way. Seen from one perspective, religion contributes to individual and social adaptation. Looked at from another, it renews life by aligning people with the central reality of the universe. The common factor relating the two perspectives is the shared emphasis on the renewal and revitalization of life. The two perspectives could be held together in his mind because neither was held positivistically. He saw neither the evolutionary-adaptive nor the theological perspective as the only possible interpretation of life.

Boisen seemed to sense that psychiatry, in its professional role, should take the functional or evolutionary-adaptive point of view. But it should do this undogmatically and nonpositivistically. His message is distinctively Jamesian; without reducing religion to strictly functional terms, it is useful to look heuristically at religion in terms of what it contributes to personal cohesion, revitalization, courage, identity, and moral clarity. He writes, "The test of the worth of any religion or of any ethical system would thus be the extent to which it enabled its adherents to survive in the struggle for existence, and to attain to the abundant life" (Boisen 1936, 212). Not just adaptation, but creative adaptation, and indeed, morally responsible adaptation—this is the heuristic philosophical stance that Boisen urges upon psychiatry.

In taking the large-minded view of adaptation, Boisen is holding a functionalism nearer to that of James than, for instance, that of Herbert Spencer. James, in contrast to Spencer, believed that humans have many interests. Survival is only one of several (James [1878] 1967, 40–68). James writes that humans always try to balance their interests in survival with all of their other aesthetic, moral, and religious interests. Hence, they not only attempt to live; they attempt, as Whitehead also said, to "live well" (Whitehead 1929, 29). Nonetheless, James's and Boisen's functionalism is a variation on the evolutionary-adaptive point of view, which they took undogmatically and nonpositivistically as one useful perspective from which to assess religious experience. It is a view that they suggest psychiatry take—undogmatically and nonpositivistically—as well.

Seward Hiltner

Boisen had distinctively practical motivations; he wanted to find a model that would permit psychiatrists and chaplains to work together in the back wards of mental hospitals. Seward Hiltner, his student and later a professor at both the Divinity School of the University of Chicago and at Princeton Theological Seminary, had equally practical interests. He wanted to find ways for ministers, including the chaplains, to work with a wide range of mental health professionals. He built on and yet extended the implicit perspectivalism of Boisen. In the end, Hiltner was probably the single most influential theologian in the American scene in the twentieth century working to overcome theological positivism among the American clergy. By theological positivism, I mean the view that holds that a theological perspective on human behavior is exhaustive and must therefore be intolerant of all other perspectives, including the medical and psychiatric viewpoints.

In taking this view, Hiltner did not divide human nature into various sectors or regions—such as body, psyche, and soul—and then assign various parts of the human respectively to the biomedical, psychological, or religious points of view. Hiltner developed a perspectivalism not unlike Boisen's but much more explicit and systematic. The minister and the psychiatrist can cooperate because they take different yet complementary perspectives on human behavior. Hiltner writes that a perspective

> suggests that there is a certain point of view in the subject who is performing the viewing or feeling or helping. But it implies also that this subject is not completely described by this slant or point of view. If he were not capable of other points of view as well, which need not be competitive, we should be speaking of him in entirety and not of an aspect of him. (Hiltner 1958, 18)

Hence, the psychiatrist and the minister have differing perspectives, but neither exhausts the reality of the people they try to help.

Hiltner believes that a perspective is formed primarily by the kinds of questions that a person brings to experience (Hiltner 1958, 55). The minister brings primarily theological questions to the helping relationship, asking such questions as how a person orients whatever freedom he or she enjoys to matters of ultimate origin and destiny. The psychiatrist, on the other hand, might ask how a patient's developmental history or brain chemistry limits personal freedom and self-direction. Neither perspective exhausts the reality of the patient. Furthermore, the two perspectives necessarily overlap and complement. The minister's task of orienting a person's freedom to more fundamental values is enhanced by the psychiatrist's capacity to increase individual agency by liberating it from debilitating developmental or biochemical deficits. On the other hand, the psychiatrist, in order to enhance a patient's self-direction, may need to make assumptions about the potentiality of human freedom and dignity not unlike certain religious views of the human typical of our inherited religious traditions. Hence, Hiltner tries to interrelate perspectives by using a field theory model of human behavior (Hiltner 1958, 99–100). Although the perspectives of the psychiatrist and the minister are distinguishable, their respective foci are different aspects of the total field of the human. Since their respective perspectives fall within this single field, the work of each necessarily has implications for the other.

Hiltner tried to develop strategies of professional cooperation and self-understanding between the church and the broad field of the medical disciplines. His interests included psychiatry but went beyond this specialty to the entire range of the secular helping disciplines. He tried to overcome the epistemological narrowness and positivism of both religion and the scientifically oriented helping professions, including psychiatry. His perspectivalism is more of a critical realism than a pure instrumentalism. He does not believe, like the instrumentalists, that our perspectives completely determine the realities we see. Hiltner thinks there are realities in the person (he generally called them "needs") that vaguely correspond to the respective interpretive perspectives of religion and medicine (Hiltner 1958, 101). Clinical and cultural cooperation between religion and psychiatry depend upon a commitment by their respective professional representatives to stay within their particular perspectives, eschewing positivism and appreciating the best products of their differing traditions of inquiry and help.

Reinhold Niebuhr

The remaining figures to be covered in this review—Reinhold Niebuhr, Paul Tillich, and Paul Ricoeur—were less interested in the clinical and more interested in the cultural encounter between religion and psychiatry. They grant the legitimacy and importance of psychiatry as a clinical discipline, but they are concerned about its influence on larger cultural images of human nature. All these Protestant religious thinkers tend to associate psychiatry with Freudian psychology. They respond to the Freudian ethos surrounding mid-twentieth-century psychiatry in two ways. On the one hand, they criticize the Freudian view of religion. On the other hand, however, they are even more concerned with the flattened image of the human that they believe psychoanalytic psychology implies.

Niebuhr appreciates yet criticizes Freud's image of human nature. He is sensitive to the way the Freudian view of the human permeates the wider culture beyond the clinic. He sees this image as having an ambiguous impact on modern self-understanding. It is particularly destructive, he writes, to the sense of individuality necessary for effective political action in modern democratic societies.

From one perspective, Niebuhr affirms what he calls the "realism" of the psychoanalytic view of human nature. Niebuhr's writing career began in the wake of World War I, embraced the Depression and World War II, and lasted even into the Korean conflict, the Cold War, and the beginning of the Vietnam debacle. These tragic times led him to become totally disillusioned with enlightenment and liberal optimism about the potentialities of human nature. Niebuhr believed that the Christian view sees human nature as having great capacities for creativity as well as enormous potential for destructiveness. Thus, the presupposition for the possibility of controlling human destructiveness is the frank admission of its existence as a pervasive feature of human nature. Furthermore, the Freudian pessimism about human nature is an ally in the reinterpretation of self-understanding.

To Niebuhr, Freud's theory of libido and his tension-reduction model of personality suggest that humans everywhere, even in the healthiest activity, are basically self-seeking (Niebuhr 1974, 270). Seeing the ego as sandwiched between the impulses of the id and the blind dictates of the superego undermines our confidence in all uncomplicated rationalism of either the Kantian or the Hegelian kind (Niebuhr 1974, 264).

These emphases in Freudian psychology, Niebuhr writes, balance the superficial optimisms of Enlightenment and liberal views of human nature, which ruled the American consciousness up to and even somewhat after World War I. In spite of his appreciation for Freud, Niebuhr feels he makes two mistakes that undercut his contributions to modern self-understanding. First, Freud identifies human self-seeking too completely with the natural in human personality, i.e. libido, sexuality, and impulse (Niebuhr 1974, 269). Nature becomes the problem in Freud. Niebuhr feels that in placing the blame on the biological, Freud fails to understand the subtle ways that human freedom and anxiety interpenetrate nature to produce the inordinate self-interest that fuels so much of human destructiveness (Niebuhr 1941, 42–43).

Second, Freud's structural view of the personality fails to find a place for what Niebuhr calls the "self." In noticing that the Freudian division of the personality into ego, superego, and id has no place for a self, Niebuhr is close, although not exactly identical, to the criticism of Freud that begins to be developed in Hartmann's concept of self-representation, Erikson's concept of identity, and Kohut's concept of the self (Hartmann 1964, 127–28; Erikson 1968, 208–9; Kohut 1971, xiii-xiv). Niebuhr believes Freud lacks an understanding of the self-reflective and self-representational self that is created and internalized in dialogue (interpersonal and historical) with surrounding selves (Niebuhr 1941, 42; Niebuhr 1955, 8–11). But Niebuhr emphasizes—more than Hartmann, Erikson, and Kohut—the capacities of this self to objectify itself and to exercise modest but effective degrees of freedom and responsibility over its directions. It is this self (which earlier Niebuhr calls "spirit") and its tendencies to yield to the terrors of anxiety, and not to our natural impulses as such, that is the source of the inordinate self-concern that is so fundamental to human social and political destructiveness.

Niebuhr uses the resources of American pragmatism to elaborate a philosophical version of the Pauline concept of original sin. This understanding of the human, he believes, will restore a realism to modern self-understanding that the Freudian anthropology hints at but grounds too simply on nature and impulse. In his imperial, two-volume *The Nature and Destiny of Man* (1941), Niebuhr combines the insights of Saint Paul, Saint Augustine, and Kierkegaard and argues for an image of the human as a dialectical unity between *nature* and *spirit*. Niebuhr describes these antinomies of human existence with almost poetic force when he writes,

> The obvious fact is that man is a child of nature, subject to its vicissitudes, compelled by its necessities, driven by its impulses, and confined within the brevity of the years which nature permits its varied organic forms, allowing them some, but not too much, latitude. The other less obvious fact is that man is a spirit who stands outside of nature, life, himself, his reason and the world. (Niebuhr 1941, 3)

By asserting that humans have a capacity to transcend themselves, he is not saying that humans can stand outside of nature completely, or that they have a relation with the supernatural. Here he is saying simply that humans have some capacity to look back at themselves as their own objects and exercise a limited freedom within the constraints of their conditionedness.

The concept of original sin, which Niebuhr uses to counter Freudian realism, arises from human freedom and anxiety. The capacity for self-transcendence gives all humans the ability to perceive the precariousness of their finitude and the indefiniteness of the possibilities their freedom permits. This situation evokes anxiety, an existential anxiety that is more fundamental than any particular interpersonal or social anxiety. As Niebuhr writes

> Man is anxious not only because his life is limited and dependent and yet not so limited that he does not know of his limitations. He is also anxious because he does not know the limits of his possibilities. (1941, 183)

Original sin, for Niebuhr, is the inevitable tendency of humans to try to secure their lives through inordinate self-regard in view of the anxiety of contingency and possibility. It is a pervasive and ubiquitous problem of human existence. It is the problem even of the healthy adult. It is the problem in human existence left over even if we have had the best mothers, the best fathers, the most secure and creative families that one can have. It is the problem left over when neurotic anxiety has been dissolved. We all face the contingencies of existence and the anxiety of indefinite possibility. And our natural healthy self-regard becomes inordinate in face of this anxiety. It is not the *nature* in human nature that makes us inordinately self-concerned, as Niebuhr felt Freud would have it; it is our mishandled existential anxiety that makes us so.

Niebuhr felt that a culturewide preoccupation with a psychoanalytic perspective on human behavior would overemphasize the importance of developmental and biological determinants in human behavior. It would blind us to more pervasive problems in living, undermine our sense of responsibility and individuality, and deprive us of certain perspectives necessary for the healthy self-criticism of our normal adult behavior. Psychiatry in general and psychoanalytic psychology in particular can tell us much about the developmental and biological conditionedness of life. However, if this perspective totally dominates modern human self-understanding, the deeper levels of both human creativity and destructiveness will be lost from sight. Lost as well will be a vision of the religious resources needed for humans to address the antinomies and brokenness of the human situation.

Niebuhr uses both existentialism and American pragmatism to support his efforts to limit the sphere of psychiatry's cultural influence. He wants to create cultural space for a sympathetic hearing for the Judaeo-Christian view of man. He uses the existentialism of Martin Buber to elaborate his dialogical understanding of the human self (Niebuhr 1955, 88). Pragmatism helps defend philosophically his doctrine of original sin. It is surprising to hear that Niebuhr calls the concept of original sin an "empirical" concept. When he uses *empirical* in this way, he is distinguishing it from more narrow understandings that limit the empirical to discrete ranges of experimentally testable data. This model of the empirical, taken over into psychiatry and the behavioral sciences from the natural sciences, functions to "obscure the facts about the self which can be known only through introspection and in dramatic encounter" (Niebuhr 1955, 129). The obvious facts that Niebuhr had in mind are the self's conditioned freedom, its anxiety, and its efforts to secure itself through inordinate concern. These features of the self fit the facts of experience when "experience" is used in that much broader sense that William James spells out in *The Principles of Psychology* (1890) and *Essays in Radical Empiricism* (1912). Original sin is basically a hypothesis that we need to make sense out of ordinary conflictual aspects of our political, social, and familial experience. Various behavioral sciences, including psychiatry, can obscure this dimension of the human if they dogmatize their naturalistic interests.

Paul Tillich

Niebuhr tries less to Christianize psychiatry and psychoanalysis than to offer a broader anthropological and philosophical context within which these disciplines could work and locate their own more specific concerns. A similar point can be made about the message of the great German-American theologian Paul Tillich. Although Tillich is far more positive in his response to psychoanalysis than Niebuhr, on the whole he also worked to restrict the cultural influence of psychoanalytically oriented psychiatry.

Tillich and Niebuhr were colleagues on the faculty of Union Theological Seminary. Although they were the best of friends during the 1930s and 1940s, their differing responses to psychoanalysis, as Richard Fox points out in his *Reinhold Niebuhr: A Biography* (1985), was one of many issues that strained their relations in the later years of their lives. Tillich's theology resonates far more positively with psychoanalysis than Niebuhr's. He speaks of intriguing analogies between psychotherapeutic acceptance and the Christian doctrines of forgiveness and justification by faith (Tillich 1960). He holds a doctrine of self-actualization that has affinities with the concept in neo-Freudian and humanistic psychologies (Tillich 1952, 18–20). He believes that Freud's description of the contradictions of human nature gives a very accurate picture of human experience under what Tillich calls the conditions of "estrangement" (Tillich 1959, 112–26).

But the idea that Tillich uncritically affirms psychoanalysis, in either its more Freudian or neo-Freudian forms, is not quite true. Tillich, like Niebuhr, distinguishes neurotic and existential guilt (Tillich 1952, 52–53). He believes that psychoanalysis and psychiatry make a legitimate contribution to the mitigation of various forms of pathological guilt. But Tillich, like Niebuhr, works hard to preserve the notion of real guilt; both thinkers are concerned to preserve at the wider public and cultural level ideas about human life as basically ethical, relatively free, and in this sense meaningful (Niebuhr 1955, 13; Tillich 1952, 52). Tillich makes a distinction similar to Niebuhr's between neurotic anxiety and existential anxiety. Tillich, however, relates anxiety more to the fear of finitude and death and less to indefinite possibility than Niebuhr does. He believes that psychiatry can help remove neurotic anxiety produced by pathological relations with parents or, perhaps, by chemical imbalances. But psychiatry alone cannot provide resources of meaning to relieve those deeper and more pervasive existential anxieties caused by the contingencies of life—illness, death, or indefinite possibility. If psychiatry either fails to recognize the reality of these anxieties or attempts to relieve them, it becomes either a positivistic scientism or a quasi religion dressed in the garb of scientific medicine.

Tillich does not claim that psychiatry needs directly or officially to have a religious foundation. But at the same time, it must recognize that when it makes either negative or positive judgments about the reality of religious ideas and symbols, it has moved out of the realm of science and into the realm of metaphysics. For instance, if psychiatry claims, with Freud, that all religion is a projection, then psychiatry must realize it has assumed responsibility for making judgments, not just about matters of psychological health and disease, but about the way the world really is. Tillich astutely observes that any theory that claims that religion is *only* a projection is also taking responsibility for judging whether or not there is a something behind the projection—a "screen" perhaps, upon which the projection is placed (Tillich 1951, 212). It is better, Tillich advises, for psychiatry to restrict itself and refrain from assuming responsibility for this judgment. Tillich, like James, thinks that psychiatry should take a more phenomenological approach to religion—as he recommended, in fact, for any discipline making a serious study of religion (Tillich 1950, 106–108). In urging this, Tillich, like James, is fully aware that humans project varying amounts of their own childhood and interpersonal experiences on whatever they claim is divine. But he believes that to insist that these projections exhaust religious experience in all respects entails metaphysical judgments that are difficult to argue and unnecessary for the purposes of a public philosophy undergirding a helping discipline such as psychiatry.

Whereas pragmatism informs the philosophical perspectives of James, Boisen, and to a considerable extent Niebuhr, Tillich's philosophical sources are a combination of European existentialism and certain aspects of Platonic and German idealism. Such a philosophical stance is a long way from the evolutionary-adaptive point of view that is common to both pragmatism and much of twentieth-century psychoanalysis and psychiatry. Both pragmatism and existentialism have room for a phenomenological attitude toward religion and at this level are equal. It is my conviction that pragmatism provides a more powerful philosophical stance for psychiatry to make appropriate contact with the world of religion and ethics. Much of contemporary psychiatry assesses human behavior from the perspective of how it contributes to the creative adaptation of the person involved. James, as we saw above, has a sophisticated way of combining adaptive and moral points of view for the philosophical testing of religious symbols, claims, and behavior. Pragmatism is closer to the implicit world view of much of psychiatry than European existentialism or Greek and German idealism. If psychiatry were to search for a larger philosophical framework within which to locate itself, at least from the perspective of handling questions of religion, the philosophical commitments of James might serve better than the commitments of Tillich. Of course, there is much to learn from Tillich on specific points.

Paul Ricoeur

Even though Ricoeur is a French Protestant philosopher of religion, since the late 1960s his career has been staged primarily in the United States. He has extensively influenced both theology and the philosophy of the social sciences. In his monumental *Freud and Philosophy* (1970), Ricoeur has made a valuable contribution to the philosophy of psychiatry in its effort to discover its appropriate public stance toward religion. Although Ricoeur is primarily addressing Freud and his interpretation of religion, Ricoeur's position is useful, I believe, to the broad field of psychiatry.

Ricoeur is concerned about the reductive view of religion found in Freud and the influence this has over much of psychoanalysis, psychiatry, and the wider culture shaped by these disciplines. The psychoanalytic view that religion is basically a public expression of obsessive-compulsive neurosis disregards the creative forms of religion (Freud [1907] 1963, 17–25). Ricoeur is fully aware that the symbolism of religion is rife with maternal and paternal figures and references to birth, death, and conflicts around aggression, dependency, and sexuality. Hence, he is quick to admit that human beings project their own developmental "archeology" into their religious symbolism. By *archeology,* Ricoeur means that fund of unconscious desires and energies that lie beneath consciousness and that we project on all our experiences, including our religious experiences (Ricoeur 1970, 439–52). The idea of the archeology of the subject is Ricoeur's way of acknowledging the partial truth of the psychoanalytic view of both culture and religion. All of our cultural and religious ideals and idealizations entail sublimations and restructurings of archaic childhood desires (Ricoeur 1970, 446).

The first and most proper task of psychoanalysis in confronting religious phenomena—either in the clinic or in the wider culture—is to "dispossess" the surface meanings of consciousness and uncover the developmental origins of the religious meanings in childhood desires and experiences (Ricoeur 1970, 439). But Ricoeur develops the novel argument that, even within Freud, uncovering the archaic substrates of religious meanings does not exhaust the total act of interpretation. Ricoeur detects in Freud a dialectic between archeological and teleological levels in the interpretation of religious meanings (Ricoeur 1970, 447–93). Although the teleological moment can be found in Freud, it is unthematized and implicit. Ricoeur uses Hegel to suggest ways in which the great religiocultural figures of a historical tradition (what he calls "figures of spirit") become objects of our desire and identification. Moses, Jesus, Mohammed, Luther, or Gandhi can become figures on whom we project our archeology—our infantile needs for dependency, gratification, and recognition. But just as our infantile needs color and to some extent distort our perceptions of these figures, so, through the mechanisms of identification and sublimation, our childhood archeologies are restructured, differentiated, amplified, and upgraded in their aims. In healthy expressions of religion, there is a "dialectic" between archeology and teleology; just as we project infantile meanings on our religious objects, so too do these objects, figures, and personages restructure the aims of our desires. Through attachment and identification with these figures, humans become adults by being led to "abandon" earlier attachments and to substitute more universal, ethically commanding, and generally adequate ideal figures (Ricoeur 1970, 463).

This subtle theory of the dialectical relation of archeology and teleology in religion both affirms the reality of the projection of infantile desires into religion and denies that they exhaust the meaning of religious experience. Like James and Tillich, Ricoeur takes these "figures of spirit" phenomenologically. He first of all describes them and attempts to discern the "mode of being-in-the-world" that they open up to those who are attracted to them. In healthy religion, archeology and teleology interact; real growth occurs as archeology is gradually abandoned, restructured, and developed under the influence of the teleological aspects of the religious symbol. However, just as this model gives us the hermeneutical tools to understand healthy and adult forms of religion, so too it helps explain its more childish or neurotic forms. Neurotic religion is precisely religion in which archeology dominates over teleology. The maturer dimensions of the religious experience or symbol are swamped by its more regressive archeology. But not all expressions of religion are like this, and it is important for psychiatry, both in the clinic and in the wider culture, to understand that fact.

There is little doubt that in developing this philosophical perspective on the psychoanalytic interpretation of religion, Ricoeur is attempting to clear philosophical space for his own form of Barthian and Reformed Christian spirituality. Ricoeur believes that we humans grow when confronted by sacred figures who both challenge us to become more than we are and give us grace and strength to match this challenge. However, like the prior figures we have reviewed, in clearing philosophical space for the plausibility of a particular form of religious experience, Ricoeur contributes to an emerging philosophy of psychiatry, especially to its clinical and public view of religion. None of these Protestant thinkers asks psychiatry or psychoanalysis to adopt his particular form of spirituality. But in attempting to make these forms of religion intelligible to both Christians and the wider public, these thinkers give psychiatry good reasons and philosophical resources for creating a more sophisticated attitude toward religion than that bequeathed by Freud.

Whether my slight preference for the resources of pragmatism over those of existentialism finally can be sustained is not a debate we need settle in this paper. That some form of philosophy is required for psychiatry to locate itself in the ethical, legal, political, and religious worlds within which it functions seems to be patently clearer as the years go by. These Protestant thinkers and the philosophical resources they employ give us suggestive pointers for a philosophy of psychiatry on the question of its relation to religion. In addition, the contributions of these thinkers should also enable psychiatry to take a friendly attitude toward the substance of the more classic forms of Protestant spirituality of the kind represented by these six irenic Protestant thinkers.

The long-term philosophical solutions to the problem of psychiatry's relation to religion will doubtless take time to develop. Pragmatism and existentialism are two positions that these thinkers reviewed here have employed. Ordinary language analysis is another philosophical tool frequently employed in recent years. In the end, however, some kind of perspectivalism will doubtless be used. Boisen and Hiltner, building on James, may have been pointing in the most fruitful direction. Some brand of pragmatism, with its evolutionary-adaptive and functionalist overtones, may be the best philosophical framework to accomplish the tasks of psychiatry. If it follows the pointers of James, it will also take a basically phenomenological attitude toward religious experience and examine the way it functions in human life to foster a morally responsible adaptive strategy.

Such a philosophical perspective will not serve all the needs of religion itself. Religions have their internal histories and their special ways of interpreting their experience of the sacred. For religion to be open to pragmatism as one useful perspective on religious experience does not mean that it must take only this perspective on the special events and truths that inform religious lives. A pragmatic point of view need not exhaust the meaning of religion either for religious bodies themselves or for a psychiatry that might use this perspective more directly to inform its work.

The point of this paper is that neither religion nor psychiatry should be used positivistically in the modern world. Religion need not fear either a pragmatic view of itself or psychiatry's use of this perspective. This can be true, however, only if both psychiatry and religion renounce their respective positivisms, which sometimes lead them into clinical and cultural conflict.

References

Allen, Gay W. 1967. *William James*. New York: Viking Press.

Boisen, Anton. 1936. *Exploration of the Inner World*. New York: Harper and Bros.

———. 1945. *Religion in Crisis and Custom*. New York: Harper and Bros.

Browning, Don. 1980. *Pluralism and Personality: William James and Some Contemporary Cultures of Psychology*. Lewisburg, PA: Bucknell University Press.

Culver, C. M., and Gert, B. 1982. *Philosophy in Medicine*. New York: Oxford University Press.

Edie, James. 1970. "Critical Studies: William James and Phenomenology." *Review of Metaphysics* 23 (March).

Erikson, Erik. 1968. *Identity, Youth and Crisis.* New York: Norton.

Fox, Richard. 1985. *Reinhold Niebuhr: A Biography.* New York: Pantheon.

Freud, Sigmund. 1907. "Obsessive Acts and Religious Practices." In *Character and Culture,* ed. Philip Rieff. New York: Collier, 1963.

———. 1911. *The Future of an Illusion.* New York: Liveright, 1953.

Hare, Richard. 1981. "The Philosophical Basis of Psychiatric Ethics." *Psychiatric Ethics.* New York: Oxford University Press.

Hartmann, Heinz. 1964. *Essays on Ego Psychology.* New York: International Universities Press.

Hiltner, Seward. 1958. *Preface to Pastoral Theology.* Nashville: Abingdon Press.

Holifield, E. Brooks. 1983. *A History of Pastoral Care.* Nashville: Abingdon Press.

James, William. 1878. "Remarks on Spencer's Definition of Mind as Correspondence." In *Collected Essays and Reviews.* New York: Russell and Russell, 1967.

———. 1890. *The Principles of Psychology,* vols. 1–2. New York: Dover, 1950.

———. 1897. *The Meaning of Truth.* Cambridge: Harvard University Press, 1975.

———. 1897. *The Will to Believe.* New York: Dover, 1956.

———. 1902. *The Varieties of Religious Experience.* New York: Bantam, 1950.

———. 1910. *A Pluralistic Universe.* New York: Dutton, 1971.

———. 1910. "A Pluralistic Mystic." *Hibbert Journal* 8: 739–59.

———. 1912. *Essays in Radical Empiricism.* New York: Dutton, 1971.

Kohut, Heinz. 1971. *The Analysis of the Self.* New York: International Universities Press.

Küng, Hans. 1979. *Freud and the Problem of God.* New Haven: Yale University Press.

Levinson, H.S. 1981. *The Religious Investigations of William James.* Chapel Hill: University of North Carolina Press.

Linschoten, Hans. 1968. *On the Way towards a Phenomenological Psychology.* Pittsburgh: Duquesne University Press.

Meissner, William. 1984. *Psychoanalysis and Religious Experience.* New Haven: Yale University Press.

Niebuhr, Reinhold. 1941. *The Nature and Destiny of Man,* vol. 1. New York: Scribner's.

———. 1955. *The Self and the Dramas of History.* New York: Scribner's.

———. 1974. "Human Creativity and Self-Concern in Freud's Thoughts." In *Freud and the Twentieth Century,* ed. Benjamin Nelson, Gloucester, MA: Peter Smith.

Pellegrino, E., and Thomasma, D., 1981. *A Philosophical Basis for Medical Practice.* New York: Oxford University Press.

Ricoeur, Paul. 1966. *Freedom and Nature.* Evanston: Northwestern University Press.

———. 1970. *Freud and Philosophy.* New Haven: Yale University Press.

Tillich, Paul. 1951. *Systematic Theology,* vol. 1. Chicago: University of Chicago Press.

———. 1952. *The Courage to Be.* New Haven: Yale University Press.

————. 1959. *The Theology of Culture*. New York: Oxford University Press.
————. 1960. "The Impact of Pastoral Psychology on Theological Thought." *Pastoral Psychology* 11, 101 (Feb.): 17–23.
Whitehead, A. N. 1929. *The Function of Reason*. Princeton: Princeton University Press.

CHAPTER TWO

A ROMAN CATHOLIC PERSPECTIVE ON PSYCHIATRY AND RELIGION

Marie McCarthy, Ph.D.

The dialogue between religion and the healing arts and sciences is as old and as complex as cultures and religions. Throughout history both religion and the human sciences have responded to, reacted to, and shaped the cultures, customs, and philosophies of the worlds in which they exist. Our age is no exception. The dialogue between religion and the healing arts and sciences is vigorous and multifaceted. In the midst of this wide-ranging conversation, there is a growing concern on the part of both medical and religious professionals to understand more fully the relationship between psychiatry and religion and to articulate a public philosophy for psychiatry that might more adequately guide the practices and decisions of the psychiatric, ministerial, and legal professions in our society.

In order to articulate such a public philosophy for psychiatry it seems useful to examine how the various religious traditions have understood the relationship between religion and psychiatry and to explore the ways in which the normative visions of the human person that these traditions lift up can contribute to a public philosophy for psychiatry.

A public philosophy for psychiatry, it can be argued, should be rooted in a normative vision of the human person, a vision that can only be arrived at through an interdisciplinary dialogue in which the partners remain clear about their own proper enterprises and limits. It is not just that psychiatry and religion see things differently. In important respects they see different things.

Psychiatry, as a branch of medicine, is dedicated to diagnosing and treating disease whenever possible, using scientifically based knowledge, but always aims at comforting the sick and alleviating suffering. Unlike general medicine, psychiatry is a service profession dedicated to caring for the sick even in the absence of scientifically based knowledge of the sickness.[1]

Theology, as the discipline that reflects in an ordered fashion on religious experience and meaning, is a philosophical, metaphysical enterprise
concerned with ultimates, with value, meaning, and transcendence, and
with the search for something by which to live a life worthy of one's striving. At the same time it cannot be said that psychiatry is unconcerned
with issues of value, meaning, and transcendence, any more than it can be
said that religion and theology are unconcerned with health of mind.[2]

The common concern for the welfare of the human person and the
unity of that person forms the meeting ground for the dialogue between
psychiatry and religion. Our task here will be to explore the relationship
between psychiatry and religion from a Roman Catholic perspective in
order to lift up important aspects of a normative vision of the human
person which might be useful in articulating a public philosophy for psychiatry with special reference to its relation to religion.

A Historical Overview

The question of the relationship between health of mind and salvation of
soul, sanctity and sanity, psychological well-being and spiritual well-being,
has emerged repeatedly throughout the history of the Roman Catholic
Church. This discussion has been shaped by a fundamental set of questions concerning the nature of the human person. Questions concerning
the relationship between body and soul (or the material and nonmaterial
dimensions of the human person), between freedom and determinism,
and between nature and grace have been particularly significant in this
ongoing dialogue. Differing interpretations of the relationship between
these various aspects of the human being are present implicitly and explicitly throughout the history of Roman Catholicism and lead to widely
divergent understandings of the relationship between psychiatry and religion. This essay will review briefly the ways in which these issues have
been cast and then suggest a constructive interpretation based on the theology of Karl Rahner. This interpretation aims to provide useful frameworks for understanding the relationship between psychiatry and religion
and beginning to articulate a public philosophy for psychiatry.

In the early history of the Church, psychopathology was understood
as either a manifestation of demonology or as the presence of saintly mystical vision. Most often mental illness was considered a punishment for
sins; prayer, fasting, and even exorcism were considered the appropriate
forms of treatment for such affliction. During the Middle Ages and Renaissance, the demonological viewpoint held such sway that the mentally
diseased were often subject to bloody persecution; the burning of
"witches" was at times common practice (VanderVeldt and Odenwald
1952, 37–38). By the mid-eighteenth century, as Cartesian dualism be-

came the prevailing view in the Western world, the Church, incorporating the Cartesian split between mind and body, began to view mental disease as an illness of body rather than an affliction of the soul. By the turn of this century, the Church showed little concern with the question of the relationship between psychiatry and religion. Psychiatry was understood to deal with the sick mind, religion with the troubled soul, and the two enterprises were seen as quite distinct (Ford 1953, 58).

The Climate in Church and Society prior to the Second Vatican Council

By the middle of the 1940s a vigorous discussion was once again under way. Much of the discussion during this period preceding the Second Vatican Council was marked, on the one hand, by a theological positivism in which Catholic theology functioned as a closed system operating according to its own internal laws rather than engaging in genuine dialogue with the larger world (Rahner 1972, 71). On the other hand, much of psychiatric practice, and particularly psychoanalytic psychiatry, was locked into scientific positivism which, through the application of a reductive principle, saw all ritual and religion as merely expressive of certain psychodynamic factors and internal conflicts (Stern 1948, 31). The Church, which advocated "an unchangeable objective norm of morality" (VanderVeldt and Odenwald 1952, 19), found itself in tension with psychiatric and psychoanalytic practice, particularly as these professions expanded their interests and concerns, blurring the boundaries between the medical and nonmedical.

A fair number of Roman Catholic theologians and writers were locked into a theological positivism and a Cartesian dualism, which set a sharp boundary between body and soul, nature and grace, Church and world. They took a defensive and adversarial posture toward the burgeoning field of psychiatry. These writers were largely antithetic to all forms of psychiatric practice that were not dealing with strictly organic mental disease. They posited a fundamental incompatibility between Freudian psychology and Catholic truth (Conway 1954, 185), even asserting that it was a mortal sin for Catholics to employ psychoanalysis as a cure or to submit oneself to such a cure (George 1952, 12). The cultivation of this particular approach, with its emphasis on the separation of body and soul and the power of grace to overcome nature, gave rise to the mental hygiene movement in which the cultivation of virtue was seen as a prophylactic against mental disease, and a "sound spirituality [as] in many ways incompatible with a number of mental disorders" (Moore 1959, 147). In this view religious ideals were seen as preventing or curing some mental disorders and the reform of the moral and spiritual life was seen as a central ingredient in the therapeutic process (Moore 1959, ix–x).

Another type of response, quite different in kind and quality, was found in a smaller, but important, group of Catholic theologians and psychiatrists. It was rooted in the conviction that no fundamental contradiction or discrepancy should exist between religion and psychiatry, and that an exploration of the relation between religion and psychiatry would benefit both fields. The Church and world were not seen as absolutely split. Nature and grace were seen as integrally related to each other, and psychiatry was seen not as a threat but as a help to religion. These writers and thinkers, while deeply convinced of the truth of Catholicism, were equally convinced that there is no ultimate conflict between faith and reason and that a rightly interpreted theology and an authentic science could not be in contradiction (Dempsey 1956, x). These writers anticipated the changes in thought and interpretation of the Second Vatican Council. They likewise took an approach to the relation of religion and psychiatry that more accurately reflected the official position of the Church at this time.

The tone of the official response of the Church was cautious but friendly. It is captured in the address that Pope Pius XII gave to the Fifth International Congress of Psychotherapy and Clinical Psychology, in which he asserted that "theoretical and practical psychology, the one as much as the other, should bear in mind that they cannot lose sight of the truths established by reason and by faith, nor of the obligatory precepts of ethics" (Pius XII 1953, 428). He went on to articulate the fundamental attitude that is required of a Christian psychologist and psychotherapist:

> Psychotherapy and clinical psychology must always consider man 1) as a psychic unit and totality, 2) as a structured unit in itself, 3) as a social unit, and 4) as a transcendent unit, that is to say, as a unit tending towards God. (Pius XII 1953, 429)

When this view of the human person provided the orienting framework, Pius XII was supportive of the work of depth psychology in exploring the psychic aspects of religious phenomena. And while he suggested that prudence and reserve were called for on both sides of the dialogue, he concluded his remarks with the assurance that

> . . . the Church follows your research and your medical practice with her warm interest and her best wishes. You labor on a terrain that is very difficult. But your activity is capable of achieving precious results for medicine, for the knowledge of the soul in general, for the religious dispositions of man and for their development. (Pius XII 1953, 435)

One can discern in this address of Pius XII both the general tone of the Church's response and the range of the Church's concerns about psychiatric practice. It aimed to integrate the therapeutic advantages of psychiatric theory and practice with a Roman Catholic world view. This integration had to be made in such a way as to avoid undermining the authority of the Church in matters of faith and morals and to avoid the reduction of all religious experience, values, and morality to merely psychological dynamics (VanderVeldt and Odenwald 1952, 196). The goal of psychotherapy was seen as educating persons to become responsible, to face reality, not to use escape mechanisms, to act maturely rather than childishly, and to meet obligations and duties. At the same time responsibility included moral responsibility. Thus it was seen as acceptable to turn to the psychiatrist for problems such as an inability to make decisions. But when morals and values were involved, the Church and its teachings became determinative (VanderVeldt and Odenwald 1952, 26, 105).

The Response to Psychoanalysis

There was a marked difference between the intensity of the responses to psychiatry in general and to psychoanalysis in particular. This was due in large part to the prevailing dualistic world view in which a clear distinction was made between the organic and nonorganic dimensions of mental affliction. In general the Church had little difficulty with the medical side of psychiatric practice. Its concerns focused far more in the boundary-crossing areas involving attitudes, values, personal growth, and morality. Consequently, much sharper conflicts arose between religion and psychoanalysis (Ford 1953, 58–59).

Psychoanalysis itself was born and nurtured in an atmosphere of hostility to religion. Roman Catholicism responded in kind, issuing a blanket condemnation of Freud. Standard moral manuals asserted that "the system as a whole, in its pure Freudian form, must be rejected" (Ford and Kelly 1958). The philosophical, cultural, and religious views expressed in the Freudian system, coupled with Freud's reductive methodology, were mainly responsible for the strong opposition between Roman Catholicism and psychoanalysis. Some theologians solved this problem by distinguishing between the philosophical foundations of the Freudian system—with its religious and moral implications, psychological concepts, hypotheses, and theories—and the therapeutic value of its methods (VanderVeldt and Odenwald 1952, 142; see also Burns 1950, 121). Those portions of psychoanalytic psychotherapy that were of demonstrated benefit to suffering individuals, that were not logically derived from philosophical premises seen as erroneous, and that did not use means of treatment considered immoral were acceptable.

The Problem with Freud

Roman Catholic theologians raised four concerns about Freudian psycho-analytic theory and practice: Freud's views on (1) religion, (2) anthropology, (3) morality—in particular sexuality, and (4) freedom and determinism.

View of Religion

In the Freudian system, as Catholic theologians generally understood it, elements of belief and faith were treated as remnants of unanalyzed complexes; religion as infantile dependency and wish fulfillment; the religious attitude as basically feminine (that is, immature and infantile) and submissive; and religious practices as neurotic. This reduction of moral and supernatural values to extraneous and accidental determinants was unacceptable to Roman Catholic religious consciousness.[3] Thus, in his address to psychiatrists and psychologists, Pius XII asserted unequivocally:

> We know . . . that religions, the natural and supernatural knowledge of God and worship of Him, do not proceed from the unconscious or the subconscious, nor from an impulse of the affections, but from the clear and certain knowledge of God by means of His natural and positive revelation. (Pius XII 1953, 433)

Anthropology

Freud's views on human nature were as problematic as his views on religion for Roman Catholic theologians. For the Roman Catholic the human person is essentially a creature of desire who does and must seek after an absolute (Dempsey 1956, 33). That is, human nature has an inherent transcendent dimension. To the extent that Freud was a materialist, holding that there is only matter and not spirit in the universe, there is a cleavage between a Roman Catholic and a Freudian anthropology. Roman Catholic philosophy and theology insist on the spirituality of the soul (Conway 1954, 187). Thus, Roman Catholic writers pointed to Freud as a genius at exploring the instincts, feelings, and emotions that we share with the lower animals, but they insisted that he had left out essential dimensions of the human person. Thomas Verner Moore wrote that "the psychotherapy of the last decades had in general treated the patient largely on the animal level. It left out of consideration, therefore, moral and spiritual ideals and the free responsible action by which only they can be attained" (1959, 117). While the various unconscious determining factors of human personality that Freud brought to light were considered important, they were not seen as defining human nature.

In addition, Catholic philosophy insists that the human person must always be understood as a structured unity.[4] Body and soul are united as matter to substantial form in one living, psychological, psychosomatic composite. The psyche is not juxtaposed to the body, but is, rather, the form and act of the body. The person is a unity of rational and irrational factors, of conscious reason and instinctual and emotional forces (Dempsey 1956, 9–10).[5]

Morality and Sexuality

The area of the Freudian system that aroused the most vigorous response among Catholic theologians and the general Catholic public was the Freudian approach to morality, particularly sexuality.[6] Catholic theologians were concerned to uphold objective absolute principles that they understood to constitute divine law. Thus, while they acknowledged the existence of an irrational, even morbid guilt, they distinguished this from genuine guilt resulting from real offense. They were likewise concerned that therapeutic practice not offend against moral principles by encouraging behavior considered immoral on the grounds of its being necessary to achieve cure (Conway 1954, 187).

There was strong opposition to what was referred to as the "pansexualism" of the Freudian system. To some, the assumption in the Freudian system that sex constitutes the essential driving force in human nature marked a major cleavage between a Roman Catholic and Freudian view of the human person (VanderVeldt and Odenwald 1952, 144). While some noted that it is easier to charge Freud with pansexualism than to prove it, the majority of Catholic theologians and authors assumed the legitimacy of the charge (cf. Moore 1959, 187).

In addition to the concern with the central position given to sexual instinct in the Freudian system, there was major concern with the Freudian technique of free association about sexual matters. In the 1950s, the teaching of the Church was that the deliberate excitation of sexual feelings, fantasies, desires, and actions constituted grave sin (Ford 1953, 57, 64). It was thought that "the protracted consideration and discussion of sexual matters, not in the abstract but in their concrete setting, is bound to be a grave moral risk" (George 1952, 12). The general opinion was that, in matters of sexuality, emphasis should be on education and self-mastery. Inner release was not considered morally neutral, as one had to attend to which needs—the biological or spiritual—were to be released, and which self—the higher self with its lofty aspirations or the lower animal self—was to be released. The road to health had to be a moral road that included the whole self.[7]

While most Catholic writers of this period had grave difficulties with

Freud's understanding of sexual drives, a few discerned possibilities for rapprochement between the Freudian system and a Catholic world view. These writers pointed to the continuity between the Freudian understanding of libido and a Catholic understanding of love as the driving force in human nature. Thus, Maryse Choisy noted that Freud used the term *libido* in its etymological sense as referring to sense appetite or desire. It included not just sexual desire, but the whole range of human loves, from self-love, friendship, and love of children to love of humanity and devotion to concrete objects and abstract ideas. Eros was not to be understood as coinciding completely with sexuality (1951, 79–80). In addition Dempsey pointed to the continuity between the Freudian view of libido and a Thomistic understanding of human nature in which all the aggressive drives are seen as finally oriented toward love (1956, 74). These writers suggested that the Freudian theory of sexuality is useful and important in distinguishing between holiness and neuroticism, noting that a supernatural relation of love with God has to build on the foundation of our natural psychic structure. They pointed out that the choice of chastity should be rooted in love, not in neurotic flight from the risks of love.[8]

Freedom and Determinism

A further area of the Freudian system that presented major problems to Roman Catholic theologians was its understanding of freedom and determinism. A view of psychic mechanisms and unconscious motivations as absolutely determinative of human action is incompatible with a Roman Catholic anthropology.[9] The absolute determinism that many find in the Freudian system was seen as replacing the autonomy of the will with the heteronomy of instinctive dynamism (Pius XII 1953, 429). It was the absolute quality of determinism, the position that "certain factors *always* determine a person's action, even though he may labor under the illusion that he himself decides," that was objectionable (VanderVeldt and Odenwald 1952, 29). Dempsey points out that in the early years of depth psychology the discovery of unconscious motivating forces led to an overemphasis on the subterranean forces at work in human destiny. The inadequacy of reason, the feebleness of the conscious ego, and the rarity of full personal freedom were stressed (1956, 9), and the various determining factors were seen as necessitating rather than inclining (1956, 137).

    This concern with the nature and extent of the determinism present in the Freudian system was bound up with two central tenets of Roman Catholic anthropology and theology. These are the affirmations that grace builds on nature and that for an act to be human and therefore either virtuous or sinful it must be a free act. Neither virtue nor sin are seen as possible apart from free, responsible action. Thus, Louis Beinsert points out that just as "in the biological order a certain integrity of the nervous system is necessary for the full blooming of the conscience; also, in the order of salvation, a certain integrity of the psychic structure is necessary for the mystery's presence, the double mystery of sin and saving love" (Beinsert 1951, 41).[10] Since the full possession of one's intellectual processes is considered necessary to the exercise of free will, the actions of persons suffering from certain delusional or hysteric conditions are not considered imputable to them. In the Catholic position, "formal sin requires freedom of will, and the necessary condition of freedom is the use of reason" (VanderVeldt and Odenwald 1952, 27).

There were again some theologians and writers who found the Freudian theory of psychic mechanisms and Roman Catholic theology basically compatible. They saw the theory of psychic mechanisms as uncovering unconscious motivating factors and determinants of behavior which could, in the long run, leave one freer to choose and act in accord with higher values. Choisy points out that "authentic morality exists . . . only when man is completely free. As long as he is neurotic, he is not responsible. In this is not psychoanalysis in accord with theology which teaches us that it is necessary to be fully conscious in order to sin?"[11] (1951, 78). One should not see Freud's discovery of certain fundamental psychic structures as implying an absolute determinism. Acceptance of oneself means neither resignation nor giving of free rein to instinct. Rather, "liberty is born when determinisms are totally integrated. Freudian determinism is the liberty to create by starting out from mechanisms known and accepted" (Choisy 1951, 82). It is precisely through knowing oneself fully, knowing the motivations and drives at work in choices and actions, that one becomes free to choose the good.[12] Choisy summed up the importance of Freud's contribution to the expansion of human freedom:

> From the moment that he recognized a reality proper to the psychic life, from the moment when he discovered by his patient method that man can also free himself from his mechanisms, Freud emerged towards a psychology open on all sides, even toward heaven. (Choisy 1951, 76)

A Critique of the Roman Catholic Response to Psychiatry

The responses of pre–Vatican II Roman Catholicism to psychiatric and psychoanalytic theory and practice are problematic on several grounds. For one thing, many were reactionary and based on misinterpretations and misunderstandings of the Freudian system. But, more important, a number of the arguments advanced against psychiatry and psychoanalysis were inconsistent with fundamental doctrines in Catholic anthropology and theology. As has been noted, many of the positions were rooted in a dualism incompatible with a view of the human person as an integrated unity. From the Council of Trent up to the Second Vatican Council, the Church was locked into a body/soul schema for understanding human nature which actually undercut the fundamental unity of the person that it was trying to assert (Klinger 1975, 1618). The dichotomies between body and soul, nature and grace, and church and world which are evident in the conversation concerning religion and psychiatry preceding Vatican II contradict core theological affirmations about the goodness of creation, about grace building on nature, and about God's revelation and action within human history.

The views of the person and of suffering that separate bodily and spiritual reality deny the fundamental anthropology of Roman Catholicism, which understands the person as a centered whole. Persons get sick, not bodies or souls. The body without the soul is dead, not sick. The soul without the body is spirit, and spirits don't get sick (Dempsey 1956, 3). Approaches that try to deal with the bodily or spiritual dimensions of the human person as if these were clearly separable and distinct are inadequate.

Nature and Grace

Many of the positions that have been examined suggest a view of the human person in which nature and grace exist as two distinct layers carefully placed so as to interpenetrate each other as little as possible (Rahner 1975a, 176). It is this view of nature and grace as distinct realms that leads to an excessive reliance on religion, virtue, and sanctity to prevent and even cure mental affliction.[13] Those theologians who take seriously the affirmation that grace builds on nature are more faithful to the teachings of Roman Catholic theology and also better able to assess realistically the value of Freud's insights to growth and development of mature, responsible Christian persons. To take seriously the affirmation that grace builds on nature points to the necessity of attending to nature and the myriad ways it can be disabled. Charles Burns highlighted the difference in these two perspectives when he wrote:

> What I am after, in short, is a respect for the nature of man and a recognition of its shortcomings and its needs. To think that prayer and the sacraments, necessary and holy as of course they are, will put everything right no matter what the nature of the child or adult may be, no matter how warped the character or how desolate and depressed the state of mind; to think this is "supernaturalism," and again a case of "nothing but". . . . It is to think only in terms of body and spirit and not of their

meeting ground which is mind; it is, in other terms, to create an absolute antithesis between nature and grace. (1950, 124)

Freud's Views of Sexuality

The Church's reaction to Freud's theories of sexuality is subject to a similar critique. Many responses to Freud and his theory focused excessively, almost exclusively, on his theories of sexuality, missing entirely more serious and fundamental issues such as the impairment of freedom that accompanies much mental affliction. The extensive prohibitions surrounding sexual matters, whether explicit discussion or exploration of sexual fantasy, seem to deny the goodness of creation. There is likewise an implicit denial of the principle that grace builds on nature contained in the lack of appreciation for human sexuality.

Freedom and Determinism

The area of the Freudian system that has the greatest potential for undermining central principles in a Roman Catholic theological anthropology is the treatment of freedom and determinism. It is also the area where the Roman Catholic response, even prior to the Second Vatican Council, is most consistent with the basic philosophical and theological tenets of the tradition. While there were some who read the Freudian system as undercutting all real human freedom, others pointed to the essential relation between freedom and determinism in human action. They saw the uncovering and integration of psychic mechanisms within personality as the key to a genuine liberty. Thus Dempsey could write:

> ... a more genuine liberty ... is engendered when the deterministic mechanisms are known, accepted and integrated in the pattern of behavior. To know and accept the determining forces in personality does not signify to allow them free reign. To accept the instinctive side of our nature, to accept the unruliness of the erotic and aggressive instincts, to accept the shadow, means readily to see through it, to render it, as it were, transparent, and so to become independent of it. This knowledge and acceptance constitutes a vital step in the increase of the human power of freedom. (1956, 139; see also Choisy 1951, 82)

Methodological Issues

There are several methodological problems with the responses of Catholic theologians to psychiatric practice and psychoanalytic theory in the 1940s and 1950s. One is the tendency of the theologians, in their stand against the excessive reductionism of the Freudian system, to move too readily to the highest levels of explanation (Wallace 1983, 218).

In doing this the connection between the various levels of experience and explanation is lost. There is a confusing and blurring of the lines between religion and psychology, and in some instances a reduction in the direction of religious explanation. Thus we have writers like Moore asserting that holiness or sanctity prevents mental illness (1959).[14]

A further methodological problem in these responses is their theological positivism and epistemological exclusivism. These writings, which come out of a "siege" mentality in the Church, contain frequent references to Catholic truth and regularly assert positions as true without offering the philosophical and theological grounds on which the positions stand. This approach, which embodies a vision of the Church as over against the world, opposes the history and development of Roman Catholic theology. Historically, it has always been a theology that is explicitly philosophically grounded and in genuine dialogue with the culture and society in which it is located. A Roman Catholic perspective that is faithful to the tradition must incorporate these principles by engaging in public dialogue with the disciplines that describe and assess the human conditions in our times.

A Constructive Proposal

After the Second Vatican Council, there have continued to be a range of responses to the questions of the relationship between psychiatry and religion. These responses are again the result of varying interpretations of the relationship between body and soul, nature and grace, freedom and determinism. At the same time, the Council achieved several significant shifts in emphasis and interpretation which broaden and deepen the dialogue between religion and psychiatry and open the possibility for a genuine rapprochement between the two endeavors.

The theology of Karl Rahner is particularly useful to this ongoing dialogue, as it thoroughly incorporates the major shifts of the Council. Both his methodological principles and certain principles and insights from his philosophical and theological anthropology may prove useful in understanding the relationship between religion and psychiatry and advancing a public philosophy for psychiatry.

The work of Karl Rahner is not *the* Roman Catholic position on theological matters. Rahner himself was quick to point out that no one can speak in the name of a *single* Catholic theology (1972, 101). He recognized a pluralism both of theologies and of philosophies too great to be mastered and controlled. This recognition compelled him to struggle to articulate the philosophical and theological grounds for the positions which he took. As a result, Rahner forcefully and compellingly articulates a Catholic theological anthropology that is faithful to core affirmations within the tradition, that incorporates the vision of the Second Vatican Council, and that is sensitive and responsive to the findings of the human sciences.

Rahner moves beyond neo-Scholastic interpretations rooted in Cartesian dualism to what he calls transcendental Thomism. This takes him beyond the mind/body and Church/world split that informed much of Catholic theology prior to the Council. His theology is informed by a vision of continuity between psychic desires, the openness and longing of the human spirit, and the longing for God, and of continuity between our ordinary human loves and the love of God.[15] This underlying principle of continuity informs Rahner's understanding of the relation between Church and world and compels him to leave behind the theological positivism and epistemological exclusivism of neo-Scholasticism. Rahner articulates forcefully the necessity of this move when he writes, "A real theology must not . . . refuse to learn anew and must not think that it itself in its existing form does not bring with it clouded and one-sided elements, elements which originated in the unchristian spirit of earlier centuries. . ." (1969, 154).

Rahner combines a sensitivity to the historical conditionedness of all knowledge with the conviction that ". . . there can be no absolutely contradictory opposition between faith and knowledge" (1983, 17).[16] At the same time, he recognizes the historical existence of conflict between theology and the natural sciences and the need of theology to engage in critical dialogue with the natural sciences (1975b, 74–75).

Methodology

These basic principles form the underlying supports for Rahner's methodology, a methodology that requires critical reflection on and dialogue between personal experience, God's revealing word, and contemporary science, culture, and technology. The interdisciplinary dialogue called for in Rahner's methodology is characterized by a genuine mutuality between theology and the human sciences in which the considerations and calculations of theology and theology's pursuit of truth are recognized as being as subject to historical conditioning as any other human endeavor. Rahner insists that this conditioning must be made the subject of explicit reflection (1974, 74–77).[17]

A significant feature of this historical conditioning for Rahner is the philosophical and theological pluralism of our situation, a situation he refers to as "gnoseological concupiscence" (1974, 73); the fracturing of this original unity of the human person affects the dimension of human knowledge as much as it does will and freedom. Consequently we live within a situation of irreversible pluralism within the sciences, a pluralism within which theology must find its place (1983, 18). This means that the natural sciences, as autonomous and self-authenticating, have central relevance to theological understanding. "Their validity must be recognized even in the light of the very nature of the understanding of man produced by faith" (1983, 23).

Basic Principles of Rahner's System

Rahner's entire theological system grows out of a metaphysics grounded on the inner experience of the human person. He understands the Christian mysteries as intrinsically connected to the human experience of self and world (McCool 1975, xxiv-xxviii). His most basic ontological principle is the original unity of being and knowing, the belief that ". . . being and knowledge are related to each other because originally, in their ground, they are the same reality" (1975a, 7). Knowledge is fundamentally and originally self-possession, or a coming to oneself. But this absolute identity of being and knowing is present only in Being itself, the pure act of being. The being who inquires about being is, therefore, both being and nonbeing. It is being because it can ask the question about being. It is nonbeing because it has to ask the question.

Having argued for the prior unity of knower and known in Absolute Being as the condition for the possibility of their unity in the human person, Rahner turns to consider the nature of the human person as subject. He insists that we can arrive at a genuine philosophy and metaphysics only when, without undercutting objective reality as such, we attend to the subject that is always involved in every act of cognition (1974, 81). Rahner views the human person as spirit, as active self-transcendence, as being-present-to-itself, as a union of being and knowing able to listen to a possible revelation of God, "an historical, spatio-temporal being whose spiritual dynamism was consciously, although implicitly, directed toward Infinite Being" (McCool, xix). In Rahner's anthropology the human person is a being not only able, but compelled, to inquire about being. The human person, as such, is made to strive for wholeness, completeness, perfection.

Rahner explores those qualities peculiar to human knowing, pointing out that as a created, finite spirit, and as a discursive knower, the human person's knowledge must begin with sense knowledge. The human person attains self-consciousness only by going out from the self in order to return to the self, only by becoming conscious of something other than the self (1975a, 1; 1963, 269). Only by going out of oneself into the world can one enter into the depth of personhood where one stands before God

(1963, 273). Thus, "sense perception is to be understood merely as the condition for the possibility of spiritual knowledge" (1969, 167).[18]

The human person is thus by nature a "hearer of the word," able to receive and accept the love that God is, one who has a real potency for the love of God. The human person, according to Rahner, is created as the burning longing for God, and as such is "someone always addressed and claimed by this Love" (1961, 311). For Rahner, "love is the central and abiding existential" of the human persona as that person really is (1961, 312).

The Understanding of Body and Soul

Rahner's understanding of the relationship of body and soul is rooted in the fundamental Christian position which rejects "any ultimate, radical dualism of spirit and matter" (1969, 157). Matter and spirit form a unity in origin, history, and goal. In affirming the "innermost and ultimate unity and relationship of spirit and matter" (1969, 157), Rahner rejects the Cartesian dualism of much of Western thought as being inconsistent with a Christian anthropology. He points out that, since matter and spirit have their origin in the same ground, matter is not opposed to spirit. Matter, like created spirit, is fundamentally good. This understanding of matter and spirit is consistent with basic Christian dogma which views creation as good and rejects "any kind of dualism and gnosticism which see matter as something a-divine or anti-divine and anti-spiritual" (1969, 157).

Rahner builds his theological anthropology on an understanding of matter and spirit as interpenetrating and irreversibly related. In their unity "they constitute the one reality of the world" (1969, 162). One cannot exist without the other. The soul, the primary force of subjectivity and the vehicle by which human nature attains selfhood, is originally and perpetually related to matter (Klinger 1975, 1615–16).[19] For Rahner the human person is an embodied, historical spirit whose transcendence and fulfillment come in and through matter. For the human person corporeality is essential in attaining salvation and perfection (Alfaro 1975, 1036). Rahner points to the mystery of Incarnation as the ultimate statement of the unity of matter and spirit, writing:

> . . . the climax of salvation history is not the detachment from the world of man as a spirit in order to come to God, but the descending and irreversible entrance of God into the world, the coming of the divine Logos in the flesh, the taking on of the material so that it itself becomes a permanent reality of God in which God in his Logos expresses himself to us for ever. . . . Always and everywhere, man is regarded by Christianity, precisely in the history of his relationship to God in this the material constitution of his existence. (1969, 160–61)

Nature and Grace

Rahner presents an understanding of the relationship between nature and grace that is drawn from his theological anthropology; it contrasts sharply with the position that informed much of Catholic thinking and teaching in the nineteenth and early twentieth centuries. This position, which came out of the neo-Scholastic manuals, contained an extrinsicist approach to grace. It posited no intrinsic relation between self-understanding, human experience, and grace (McCool 1975, 173). The neo-Scholastic, manualist tradition presented a sharply circumscribed view of human nature, asserting that whatever human persons knew by themselves about themselves or in themselves belonged to their nature. This was in accord with the Council of Trent definition of human nature as "that which we know about ourselves without the world or revelation" (Rahner 1975a, 176). This understanding of human nature as mere nature led to a view of grace as a disturbance or an intrusion on the person (1961, 299).

Rahner opposed this manualist tradition in which nature and grace were conceived as two separate layers, in which grace could not be experienced, and in which coming to grace and coming to oneself did not coincide. In contrast Rahner advances the concept of the "supernatural existential" to explain the possibility of grace being received as gift, rather than as an intrusion on nature. He argues that God's gift of grace ontologically changes human nature and as a result nature is not precisely delimited from grace. Nature is never pure nature. "It is a nature which is continually being determined . . . by the supernatural grace of salvation offered to it" (1975a, 183–84). Nature, in the theological sense, is thus a "remainder concept." It is that which is left over if we subtract grace.[20] Rahner points to those realities in human experience that are signals of the openness and transcendence of the human spirit, of the capacity for grace. In arguing for the basic essence of human nature as open transcendence, as an already graced reality, he writes:

> The initial elements of such fulfillment are already present: the experience of infinite longings, of radical optimism, of unquenchable discontent, of the torment of the insufficiency of everything attainable, of the radical protest against death, the experience of being confronted with an absolute love precisely where it is lethally incomprehensible and seems to be silent and aloof, the experience of a radical guilt and of a still abiding hope, etc. These elements are in fact tributary to that divine force which impels the created spirit—by grace—to an absolute fulfillment. Hence in them grace is experienced *and* the natural being of man. (1975a, 184)

Rahner is concerned to preserve the unexacted nature of grace. Grace, to be grace, must be both freely given and freely received. Grace, as God's self-communication in love, requires "someone to whom it can address itself and someone to whom it is not owed" (1975a, 77). The human person must be so created as to be able freely to accept or reject God's self-communicating love, knowing that that love is not owed, but freely given as gift (1961, 310–11).

This understanding of the relationship between nature and grace requires that revelation always be given in terms the human person can receive. "In whatever way revelation may originally take place, it has to be transposed into the human word, if man is not to be taken by revelation out of his human way of existing" (1975a, 64). This means that the place of revelation and grace is within human history and struggle. Our development and growth as human persons in human communities is the place of the experience of grace. Nature and grace are experienced in the same place. Fulfillment in grace is necessarily fulfillment as a natural person (1975a, 75).

Freedom and Determinism

In his theology Rahner emphasizes both the historicity of the human subject and the role of freedom in the people's authentic grasp of themselves, their world, and the world's horizon. For Rahner, freedom is an essential, determinative element both for God's self-communication and for human reception of that revelation. "Freedom is first of all 'freedom of being'" (1969, 184). And this freedom of being refers both to Absolute Being and to created being. Rahner points out that "the finite has its ground in the free, luminous act of God" (1975a, 38). We proceed from God through an act of creative freedom and stand before God as responsible. Freedom, decision, responsibility, and knowledge are the essential determinants of the human person, the constitutive elements by which human existence is capable of attaining selfhood (1969, 184). Our responsibility toward God presupposes and requires freedom toward God. "It is decisive for the Christian doctrine of freedom that this freedom implies the possibility of a 'yes' or 'no' toward its own horizon and indeed it is only really constituted by this" (1969, 180).

The freedom of which Rahner speaks is not the freedom to choose individual acts or objects, but the freedom to choose oneself as a whole. "It is . . . the freedom of self-understanding, the possibility of saying yes or no to oneself, the possibility of deciding for or against oneself" (1969, 185). The freedom of self-choice and self-understanding constitute the subject nature of the human person. Our authenticity or inauthenticity

springs from our fundamental choice of ourselves. In all of our free decisions we choose and mold ourselves, we freely dispose of ourselves as a
whole (1975a, 43). We do not simply perform good or bad actions. We
become good or bad persons.[21]

Implications for a Model
for Relating Religion and Psychiatry

Rahner's theology, both in its methodology and its anthropology, is suggestive for relating religion and psychiatry. His understanding of the original unity of being and knowledge, joined with recognition of the
irreversible pluralism of our philosophies and theologies, points to the
nature of the relationship between theology and psychology that is
needed. The proper relationship between theology and the sciences is one
of interdependence and dialogue rooted in a genuine humility. No single
perspective or discipline can adequately articulate the human situation or
define human being and its possibilities.

Normative View of the Person

Rahner's normative view of the human person, with its affirmation of the
intrinsic relationship between both matter and spirit and nature and grace,
further grounds the necessity for interdisciplinary dialogue between theology and the social sciences. He offers an understanding of the human
person which moves beyond Cartesian dualism, viewing the person as an
essential unity of body-spirit. His understanding of the human person as
subject is coupled with the recognition of human persons as conditioned,
historical, and situated. As such the human person is always open for the
possibility of revelation, of God's self-communication in love. But because
of the nature of the human person this elevation can occur only in and
through the ordinary categories of human experience. The place of revelation is in the concrete, lived experience of the historical and conditioned
human subject.

Herein lies the relevance and necessity of the secular sciences and theology for each other. Through the human sciences we learn who the human person is in his or her concrete conditioned, historical existence. And
it is here that we can listen for a possible word of revelation. Through the
disciplines of philosophy, theology, and ethics we explore and understand
the realms of value and meaning in life. However, in insisting on the essential interrelatedness of spirit and matter, Rahner points to the impossibility of drawing a sharp line between the two. In his perspective one
cannot conceive of a spiritual disease that is not in the body, or of a bodily
disease which does not affect the spirit. Thus we cannot readily divide up

the care of persons, relegating the care of the body to the physician and the care of the soul to the priest.

Practical Implications

How, then, should these work together? Theology and psychiatry are two distinct disciplines with distinct areas of competence. In recognizing that it is not possible to mark off or delineate either a "purely religious" or a "distinctly nonreligious" sphere of human action, both religion and psychiatry must resist the temptation to reduce human dynamics and experience to either exclusively psychological or exclusively religious explanations. Religion must be concerned with psychological dynamics as these affect and qualify religious functioning. And psychology must be concerned with religious and moral issues as psychological factors insofar as they impact on psychological functioning (Burns 1950, 119).

Edwin Wallace suggests that psychoanalysis (and I would say psychology in general) can make several contributions to the understanding of religious phenomena. His view is one that Rahner could easily accept. These contributions include clarifying the relationship between religious beliefs and psychic economy, disclosing conflicts in which religion serves as a defense, and exploring the role that one's religion plays in overall adaptation (1983, 218–19). In other words, psychology in general and psychoanalysis in particular help us to uncover and understand the psychological meaning and dynamics of religious beliefs. Similarly, James Gill points to the advantages of approaching spirituality from the viewpoints of psychology and psychiatry, suggesting that

> They can say a great deal about the nature on which grace is acting. They can point out the human faculties and aptitudes that await education and development (for example, the imagination in relation to prayer, or motivation in connection with the will), and they can identify unhealthy attitudes and practices as well as unsuspected styles of self-deception. (1976, 28)

Development

In insisting on the essential historical nature of the human being, Rahner points to the developmental character of human knowledge and human personality, thereby highlighting the fact that all our knowledge is historically conditioned and in process of development. Our understanding of ourselves and our world is never complete (Rahner 1961, 301; 1969, 171). This awareness calls us to a greater humility and openness in the dialogue between the sciences.

At another level the recognition of the developmental character of all nature points once again to the usefulness of the psychological sciences to both theology and religion. For as the psychological sciences offer concrete descriptions of human developmental processes, they provide essential information for the articulating of an adequate theological anthropology and also the data necessary to assist the spiritual and moral development of persons. Our normal developmental experiences are the soil in which the spiritual life grows and matures (Gill 1976, 33).

Freedom and Determinism

Rahner posits a radical freedom at the core of human subjectivity. This is the freedom of self-choice, self-possession, and self-disposing. It is freedom as the capacity for wholeness (Rahner 1969, 203). The human person is called to be free and responsible, and it is fidelity to this subject based character of human existence that constitutes morality. However, Rahner could agree with Gregory Baum when he writes, "To the extent that we suffer from neurotic or psychotic disturbances we are unable to exercise our freedom" (Baum 1982, 55). Thus, the therapeutic disciplines enhance the capacity for freedom and self-determination. As Wallace points out, the proper objective of therapy according to Freud is to increase the freedom to choose (1983, 234). Maryse Choisy powerfully articulates the support that psychoanalysis can provide to human freedom and spiritual growth:

> We may say then of psychoanalysis what Bacon wrote formerly of science. A little psychoanalysis separates us from God; a great deal of psychoanalysis brings us closer to Him.
> We know—and Freud himself admitted it—that the unconscious contains the best as well as the worst. The psychoanalyst who is in daily contact with the unconscious can help man win the battle between his instincts and his inspirations. He can make him free again to receive the best. But it is then up to the liberated man to know what he will do with his liberty. . . . The tasks of the confessor and the investigator of the unconscious are complementary. Their rapprochement will give the spiritual man a power such as he has never before known. (1951, 90)

The Place of Values

In interrelating religion and psychiatry, the role of values becomes a central issue.[22] We need to ask whether mental health is possible without sound moral principles and ideals. If the therapeutic process enhances the capacity for choice, how is one to know what to choose? Once we have regained our health, what are we to do with our lives? The mutually informing character of theology and psychology is particularly important to a consideration of value in human life. The realm of value is inevitably and essentially present within therapy, and must be attended to. It is evident in the goals of the therapeutic process and the vision of human fulfillment that these goals advance. Dempsey, in describing the ideal personality of psychoanalysis, highlights the coherence between psychoanalytic and Christian values. He writes:

> The ideal personality of psychoanalysis is the individual in whom predominate reason and love, in whom the influence of the unconscious superego coheres benevolently with the rational insights and judgments of conscience, and the ego-ideal in turn corresponds to the real potentialities and talents of the individual and is capable of satisfying them. Truth then and goodness become the normative forces in personality, and reason nature's guide. (1956, 105)

Both therapy and religion seek to enhance capacities for choice, for adaptation, and for transformation. Both are concerned, not only with actuality, but also with possibility, with self-choice and self-creation. And both have an essential contribution to make to the understanding and the continuing development and transformation of the human being-in-the-world. A Roman Catholic theological perspective such as Rahner's has much to offer to the dialogue between religion and psychiatry. With its understanding of existence as graced and the human person as genuinely free, it offers symbols of hope and transcendence and points to the real possibility that we can change. We can choose to make a difference.

Notes

1. This definition of psychiatry was offered by Dr. Patrick Staunton, a psychiatrist who was a member of the group that reflected on these issues for three years.

2. Drane (1984, 83) points out that attempts within the psychiatric community to change the way mental afflictions are described quickly become philosophical debates about the nature of the human person.

3. The issue here is reductionism. Peter Dempsey (1956, 37) points out that a number of the arguments Freud raises for rejecting religion would also lead Catholic theologians to reject religion or to find it inadequate. Thus, a Catholic theologian would not find it sufficient to believe because our ancestors believed, nor to believe because of the antiquity of the proofs, nor to believe because it is forbidden to raise questions concerning the authenticity of doctrine.

4. Pius XII spoke of the centrality of this concept of the person when he said: "Man is an ordered unit and whole, a microcosm, a sort of state whose character, determined by the end of the whole, subordinates to this end the activity of the parts according to the true order of their value and function. This charter is, in the

final analysis, of an ontological and metaphysical origin, not a psychological and personal one" (1953, 430).

5. It is helpful to note that, while the Church was always taught that the human person is a structured unity, the pervasive Cartesian dualism in the nineteenth- and early twentieth-century Western world profoundly affected the understanding, interpretation, and application of this basic assumption.

6. A typical response to these areas of the Freudian system can be seen in Moore's statement that "the principles of right conduct are dictates of reason. Man even independently of any revelation is bound to obey them by the natural law. Unfortunately, there are psychiatrists who look upon morality as nothing more than the customs of the time and in dealing with patients who have a moral conflict by ridding them of their concepts of morality" (1959, 118–19).

7. This concern about the means being moral was expressed clearly by VanderVeldt and Odenwald when they wrote: "Even if it be granted for the sake of argument that the free satisfaction of immoral impulses might help the patient to regain his mental balance, yet sound ethics forbid him to buy his health at that price" (1952, 163).

8. Choisy argues for the usefulness of Freud's discoveries in living an authentic Christian life, writing: "Too often the Christian choice is made on the basis of a negative virtue, on a fear of risk, on a flight from love, while on the contrary it ought to be the choice of the best out of an ardor, an elan, an overflow of life. Behavior in love is the mobilization of sexuality for the adoration of value. Sexuality ought to be healthy in order not to vitiate adoration itself. Our religious life, like our sexual or social life, can serve as a vehicle or means of expression of an infantile or morbid affectivity" (1951, 81).

9. Note that, while this misrepresents Freud, it represents the popular understanding of Freud among Catholics of the time.

10. Dempsey makes a similar point when he writes: "Morality is possible only where an active human reason is functioning and men can place fully human acts" (1956, 103). A bit later he refers to the distinction Thomas Aquinas makes between acts of man and human acts. According to Thomas, human acts must proceed from a fully deliberate will. All other acts performed by a person may be "acts of man," but they are not human acts (1956, 131–32).

11. It is interesting to note that much of the controversy surrounding lobotomies in Catholic circles centered around the issue of free will. While some saw lobotomies as interfering with free will, others argued that free will was even more impaired in the psychotic state. Similar issues were raised with regard to electroshock and drug therapies, though lobotomy, because it was irreversible, was considered more serious. (VanderVeldt and Odenwald 1952, 67)

12. The effort to free oneself from hidden motivations and drives is particularly important to a Catholic viewpoint on morality. For neurotic psychic structures and processes limit one's freedom and one's vision. They can restrict and cloud the proper functioning of conscience. The proper formation of conscience is centrally important as, in Catholic teaching, one is obliged to follow one's conscience even if it is erroneously formed or is in disagreement with the public teaching of the Church. This principle is articulated by VanderVeldt and Odenwald

when they write: "A man must obey the directions of his conscience, regardless of whether it be true or false, because conscience is the only means that an individual possesses for becoming aware of the objective orders of the Lawgiver" (1952, 24–25).

13. Thomas Verner Moore offers numerous examples of this kind of thinking. He writes: "Heroic virtue means that grace is dominant in the soul and nature has retired into the background" (1959, 190). "A non-Catholic psychiatrist should know that a devout Catholic gets his main help in the difficulties that confront him from . . . the sacramental life of the Church" (1959, 51). "Sound spirituality is in many ways incompatible with a number of mental disorders" (1959, 147). "If a paranoid patient could be led in the early stages of his disorder to give up his dreams of the great things that are going to come to him and forget all about himself in the service of God and man, not letting his left hand know what his right hand does, his condition would not progress to dementia" (1959, 111).

14. Moore titles the second part of his book, *Heroic Sanctity and Insanity,* "Mental Disorders and Sanctity at Its Therapeutic Level" (1959, 100).

15. This view of continuity expresses the Catholic model of *caritas.* It is an understanding of the relationship between the human and divine that has been at the heart of the tradition since the time of Augustine (see David Tracy 1979). Yet, not all contemporary Roman Catholic theologians take this position. Henri DeLubac, for instance, distinguishes sharply between psychic desire and the longing for God, suggesting a radical discontinuity between the two (1984, 27, 223).

16. He elaborates further on this position: ". . . fundamentally and in the light of historical experiences, in such cases of conflict between theology and natural science, theology is equally and frequently compelled to reexamine itself, to understand itself better, to give way to natural science. Even in a case like this the revision of theology may certainly consist in a return to a better understanding of its own principles. But this in no way alters the fact that this return to its own principles is in practice caused and necessitated by the conclusions of the natural sciences. In practice, therefore, there is an open relationship between natural science and theology: possible situations of conflict, even though they can be solved in principle, are not *a priori* avoidable" (1983, 20).

17. Rahner does state that "we are assuming that every science is *per definitionem* a particular branch of human knowledge, but that this does not apply to divine revelation and theology, at least so long as these do not betray their own true nature, and . . . that this fundamental difference must have a decisive influence upon the relationship between theology and the sciences" (1975, 95). However, this need not be construed as affording a privileged place to theology in the dialogue, as Rahner carefully and repeatedly points out the ways in which in concrete, historical reality, theological positions are as conditioned as any other positions. While divine revelation may not be one branch of human knowledge among others, our experience and interpretation of that revelation surely are.

18. Rahner sums up his understanding of human spiritual dynamism when he writes: "Man is spirit, i.e., he lives while reaching unceasingly for the absolute, in openness towards God. And this openness towards God is not something which may happen or not happen to him once in a while, as he pleases. It is the condition

of the possibility of that which man is and has to be and always also is in his most humdrum daily life. Only that makes him into a man: that he is always already on the way to God, whether or not he knows it expressly, whether or not he wills it. His is forever the infinite openness of the finite for God" (1975, 20).

19. An interesting implication of Rahner's thought emerges at this point, for this material origin of the soul and its consequent perpetual relatedness implies the possibility of transcendence for all reality. Klinger points out that "the soul's 'material' origin brings with it its perpetual (dependence) relatedness. Since then matter appears in the soul as a relation, the substantial nature of the soul's transcendence reveals the equally substantial transcendence of all reality—as a natural process" (1975, 1616).

20. Rahner points out the impossibility of even pursuing the question of nature and grace without the help of revelation which lets us know that in us which is of grace.

21. Rahner does recognize the different degrees of freedom and responsibility present in concrete human beings in concrete historical circumstances. He says of this, "the sovereignty of the subject in his free decision about opening itself actively towards the motives trying to move him is determined by causes pre-existing the free decision. The number of thus offered possibilities for freedom is always finite, can be very limited and thus can so hem in freedom materially without destroying it formally that it becomes almost or even absolutely nil, since in a concrete case there may no longer be a plurality of motives among which one could choose" (1969, 207). Real freedom, according to Rahner, is "not the possibility of infinite revision, but the capacity to do something uniquely final, something which is finally valid precisely because it is done in freedom" (1969, 186).

22. Edwin Wallace, in speaking of the conflict between Freudian psychology and religion, insists *"it is the place of attitude or value rather than that of fact, upon which this battle must be fought out"* (1983, 219).

References

Alfaro, Juan. 1975. "Nature and Grace." In *Encyclopedia of Theology: The Concise Sacramentum Mundi,* ed. Karl Rahner, 1033–38. New York: Seabury Press.

Baum, Gregory. 1982. "Theology Questions Psychiatry: An Address." *Ecumenist* 20 (May–June): 55–59.

Beinsert, Louis. 1951. "Does Sanctification Depend on Psychic Structure?" *Cross Currents* 1 (Winter): 39–43.

Burns, Charles. 1950. "Psychology and Catholics." *Blackfriars* 31 (March): 118–24.

Choisy, Maryse. 1951. "Psychoanalysis and Catholicism." *Cross Currents* 1 (Spring): 75–90.

Conway, William. 1954. "Analytical Psychology and Catholic Teaching." *Irish Theological Quarterly* 21 (April): 185–88.

De Lubac, Henri. 1984. *A Brief Catechism on Nature and Grace,* trans. Brother Richard Arnandez, F.S.C. San Francisco: Ignatius Press.

Dempsey, Peter. 1956. *Freud, Psychoanalysis, Catholicism.* Chicago: Regnery.

Drane, James. 1984. "Philosophy of Psychiatry: A Defense of the Medical Model for Mental Afflictions." *Cross Currents* 34 (Spring): 83–105.

Ford, John C., S. J. 1953. "May Catholics Be Psychoanalyzed?" *Linacre Quarterly* 20 (August): 57–66.

Ford, John C., S. J., and Gerald Kelly, S. J. 1958. *Contemporary Moral Theology* Vol. I. Westminster, MD: Newman Press.

George, Gordon, S. J. 1953. "The Pope on Psychoanalysis." *America* 88 (October 4): 88.

Gill, James J., S. J. 1976. "Psychiatry, Psychology and Spirituality Today." *Chicago Studies* 15 (Spring): 27–37.

Klinger, Elmer. 1975. "Soul." *Encyclopedia of Theology: The Concise Sacramentum Mundi*, ed. Karl Rahner, 1615–18. New York: Seabury Press.

Loftus, John Allan. 1981. "The Integration of Psychology and Religion: An Uneasy Alliance." *National Guide of Catholic Psychiatrists Bulletin* 27: 88–103.

McCool, Gerald A., ed. 1975. *A Rahner Reader.* New York: Seabury Press.

Michaels, Peter. 1946. "Sanctity Is Sanity." *Catholic Digest* (10 August): 41–46.

Moore, Thomas Verner. 1924. *Dynamic Psychology.* 2nd ed., revised. Chicago: Lippincott.

———. 1959. *Heroic Sanctity and Insanity.* New York: Grune and Stratton.

Papenfus, S. C. 1976. "Christianity and Psychiatry." *Irish Theological Quarterly* 43 (3): 211–16.

Pope Pius XII. 1953. "Psychotherapy and Religion." An address to the Fifth International Congress of Psychotherapy and Clinical Psychology, April 13, 1953. *Catholic Mind* 51 (July): 428–35.

Rahner, Karl. 1961. *Theological Investigations,* Vol. 1, trans. Cornelius Ernst, O. P. New York: Seabury Press.

———. 1963. *Theological Investigations,* Vol. 2, trans. Karl H. Kruger. New York: Seabury Press.

———. 1969. *Theological Investigations,* Vol. 6, trans. Karl H. and Boniface Kruger. New York: Seabury Press.

———. 1972. *Theological Investigations,* Vol. 9, trans. Graham Harrison. New York: Seabury Press.

———. 1973. *Theological Investigations,* Vol. 10, trans. David Bourke. New York: Seabury Press.

———. 1974. *Theological Investigations,* Vol. 11, trans. David Bourke. New York: Seabury Press.

———. 1975a. *A Rahner Reader,* ed. Gerald McCool. New York: Seabury Press.

———. 1975b. *Theological Investigations,* Vol. 13, trans. David Bourke. New York: Seabury Press.

———. 1979. *Theological Investigations,* Vol. 16, trans. David Marland. New York: Seabury Press.

———. 1983. *Theological Investigations,* Vol. 19, trans. Edward Quinn. New York: Crossroad Publishers.

Stern, Karl. 1948. "Religion and Psychiatry." *Commonweal* 49 (October 22): 30–33.

Tracy, David. 1979. "The Catholic Model of Caritas: Self-Transcendence and

Transformation." *The Family in Crisis or in Transition,* Concilium Vol. 121. New York: Seabury Press, pp. 100–111.

VanderVeldt, James and Robert Odenwald. 1952. *Psychiatry and Catholicism.* New York: McGraw-Hill.

Wallace, Edwin R. IV. 1983. "Reflection on the Relationship between Psychoanalysis and Christianity." *Pastoral Psychology* 31, 4 (Summer): 215–43.

CHAPTER THREE

THE JEWISH RESPONSE TO PSYCHIATRY: CONTRIBUTIONS TO A PUBLIC PHILOSOPHY FOR PSYCHIATRY

Steven Kepnes, Ph.D.

Although many religious Jews have expressed opinions about psycho-analysis and psychiatry, there has not been systematic reflection about psy-chological theory and practice until very recently. Protestant theologians have easily outstripped the Jews in attending to the philosophical presup-positions and implications of modern psychiatry. In seeking Jewish con-tributions to a public philosophy for psychiatry, however, it is important to point out that theology—systematic philosophical reflection upon fun-damental beliefs—has not received a great amount of attention in Juda-ism, where central religious concern has been focused on law and practice over and above belief. To the extent that one has theology in Judaism, it is found in story and its interpretation, in what is called *aggadah* and *mid-rash*. Because Judaism has not developed an elaborate philosophical the-ology, few of its thinkers have reflected on philosophical connections between Judaism and psychiatry.

In addressing the issue of the Jewish response to psychiatry, we are also faced with the issue of the plurality of forms of modern Jewish expres-sion. If by Judaism we mean the more liberal Reform and Conservative movements, we find a generally very positive response to modern psychia-try. If, on the other hand, we define Judaism by the various movements in Orthodoxy, the response is more mixed. In addition, the issue of the Jew-ish response to psychiatry is complicated by the facts that the founder of modern psychiatry, Sigmund Freud, was a self-proclaimed "godless Jew" and that Jews are grossly overrepresented in all fields of modern psychol-ogy and psychiatry. Freud's own ambivalence toward his heritage, his si-multaneous appreciation for its power and his desire to replace it with his own modern moral science of psychoanalysis (Rieff 1979), has colored the response of all Jews to their fellow Jew's creation of psychoanalysis and psychoanalytically oriented psychiatry.

Until very recently the only serious resource for a public philosophy for psychiatry could be found in the work of Martin Buber and his particular brand of Jewish existentialism. Buber's reformulation of Jewish theology in terms of the interpersonal I-Thou relationship provides a model for interhuman relationships and a philosophical anthropology that has had a significant impact on contemporary psychiatry (Abramovitch and Kepnes [forthcoming]) and remains a major resource for those interested in a philosophy for psychiatry. Since Buber, a second highly interesting but little-known figure, Mordechai Rotenberg of the Hebrew University of Jerusalem, has begun to question implicit assumptions about mental illness and its psychoanalytic treatment. Rotenberg's work is particularly interesting because it uses the *aggadic* and *midrashic* theological principles that are intrinsic to Judaism to develop an alternative philosophical understanding of the strategies and aims of psychoanalysis. Both Buber and Rotenberg criticize the individualism of psychoanalysis and call into question its ability to replace the moralizing functions of Judaism. In their ethical critiques, Buber and Rotenberg are joined by a number of Orthodox Jewish thinkers who have castigated psychoanalysis and modern psychiatry for undercutting traditional Jewish values such as family loyalty and social responsibility. These figures have struggled to articulate the positive ethical, social, and psychological import of concepts long under psychoanalytic attack, such as guilt and shame (Klein 1979; Amsel 1982).

In this paper I shall begin with Freud and then move to an in-depth analysis of the works of Martin Buber and Mordechai Rotenberg; these two, I believe, will provide the most constructive Jewish resources for a philosophy for psychiatry.

Freud and Judaism

In the preface to the Hebrew translation of *Totem and Taboo,* Freud very clearly reveals his ambivalence toward Judaism.[1]

> No reader of [the Hebrew translation of] this book will find it easy to put himself in the emotional position of an author who is ignorant of the language of holy writ, who is completely estranged from the religion of his fathers—as well as from every other religion—and who cannot take a share in nationalistic ideals, but who has yet never repudiated his people, who feels that he is in his essential nature a Jew, and who has no desire to alter that nature. (Freud [1939] 1950, ix)

Here, Freud tells us that he is "completely estranged from the religion of his fathers"—and that he is "in his essential nature a Jew." Freud's estrangement from religion in general and from the religion of his fathers in particular can be explained in a number of different ways. In his central text on religion, *The Future of an Illusion* ([1927] 1961), Freud makes it clear that he locates religion's major cultural purpose in its ability to make people moral. Through fear of religious authority, humans are forced to give up antisocial wishes; through religious ritual, individuals dramatically express and cathartically release their incestuous and murderous impulses; through religious symbols, individuals receive substitute satisfactions that compensate them for the privations caused by civilized life. Yet Freud argues that religion has no true future because it is an illusion based on childhood wishes and childish, primitive psychological mechanisms. Most of religion's claims about the fundamental reality of religion, God, cannot be empirically verified, and therefore its foundation is sure to crumble with the onslaught of the modern scientific world view. To fill the moral and cultural vacuum caused by the demise of religion, Freud offers psychoanalysis as the branch of science that will assume religion's moralizing functions. Through psychoanalytic knowledge, man can replace the crude, primitive and often unsuccessful moralizing mechanisms of religion "by the results of the operation of the intellect" (Freud [1927] 1961, 14).

Freud's analysis in *The Future of an Illusion* obviously leaves as little room for Judaism as it does for any other religion. Freud makes it obvious that psychoanalysis was, in part, fashioned with the idea of replacing all religions in modern culture. When Freud specifically speaks about Judaism as a cultural edifice, he presents it in less positive terms than he presents Christianity. In his last book, *Moses and Monotheism* (1939), Freud analyzes Judaism as a religion of unresolved oedipal conflict based upon the conjectured parricide of Moses by the Israelites in the desert. Freud basically accepted a Hegelian and Christian view of Judaism by asserting that Judaism, a "father"-based religion, was supplanted by the more highly developed "son" religion of Christianity (Freud 1939a, 111).

On the less theoretical and more personal level, Freud harbored animosity toward Judaism as an impediment to his professional advancement. Freud was well aware that his Judaism not only blocked an appointment for him to a university but also, as he put it, "had a share in provoking the antipathy . . . to psychoanalysis" (Freud 1925, 222).

On the positive side—and perhaps the reason why Freud never renounced his Judaism—he felt that it gave him certain qualities indispensable for his success. In a letter to the liberal Jewish B'nai Brith organization, of which Freud was a member, he stated:

> It was only to my Jewish nature that I owed the two qualities that have become indispensable to me throughout my difficult life. Because I was

a Jew I found myself free of many prejudices which restrict others in the use of the intellect; as a Jew I was prepared to be in the opposition and to renounce agreement with the "compact majority." (Freud 1926, 274)

Freud seemed to believe that in distancing him from the inner circle of Viennese high culture, his Jewishness gave him a sense of independence that propelled him toward the formulation of his unique, new discipline of psychoanalysis. Dennis Klein suggests that "the Jewish consciousness of Freud and his colleagues strengthened their confident independence, provided a basis for mutual encouragement, propelled the resolve for ambitious work, and gave substance to the conviction that they were fulfilling a revolutionary mission" (Klein 1981, xi).

The facts that Freud and his immediate circle were Jewish and that they were ambivalent about their Judaism have affected the attitude of modern believing Jews toward psychoanalysis and toward psychiatry. Their reactions, to use a Freudian term, are "overdetermined." On the one hand there are those who, wanting to claim Freud as one of their own, go out of their way to praise psychoanalysis and psychiatry, overlooking some of its negative statements about religion and about Judaism. On the other hand there are those who, precisely because Freud was a Jew who did not adhere to the tenets of traditional Judaism, express virulent hate for one of their own whom they see as an apostate. By and large, those religious Jews who applaud Freud and psychiatry accept such tenets of modern culture as personal autonomy, the primacy of reason, democratic process, and equality, which Freud championed in *The Future of an Illusion*. They share many of Freud's views about traditional religion and differ from him only in their belief that Judaism has a future if it can be refashioned in accordance with the major premises of enlightenment culture (Franzblau 1956, Steinbach 1956). In this refashioning, psychoanalysis itself, as a tool of self-knowledge and critique of pathological, illusory, and idolatrous elements in religion, is a welcomed aid.

Buber and Rotenberg: Jewish Contributions to a Public Philosophy for Psychiatry

Most of the sustained Jewish responses to psychoanalysis and psychiatry have failed to address themselves to overarching philosophical issues and concentrated on extending Freud's own writings on Judaism or drawing rough parallels between psychoanalysis, psychiatry, and Judaism. For example, Richard Rubenstein, in his *The Religious Imagination* (1968), extends Freud's analysis of Judaism by pointing out that oral-phase conflicts over an enveloping archaic mother image are more prevalent in rabbinic literature than castration fears and oedipal-patricidal wishes. Mortimer

Ostow draws parallels between Judaism and psychoanalysis, arguing that they both share a passion for truth at all costs and a notion that through special knowledge of the truth one can find salvation (Ostow 1982, 3–5). Reuven Bulka draws parallels between talmudic thinking and Victor Frankl's logotherapy (Bulka and Spero 1982, 298ff.). And a variety of rabbinic authorities and psychiatrists have written on the psychotherapeutic aspects of various Jewish observances, including mourning rituals, the sabbath, and the High Holidays (Bulka and Spero 1982, 298ff; Spero 1981).[2] These studies, as interesting and helpful as they may be in relating Judaism and psychiatry, do not address themselves to overarching and foundational philosophical issues. For this we will need to look first to Martin Buber and then to Mordechai Rotenberg.

Martin Buber

In his well-known book *I and Thou* (1923) Buber attempted to reformulate and re-present traditional Jewish conceptions of human social relationships in the terms of modern existentialism.[3] He used the terms *I* and *Thou* to speak about an ethical mode of human relating which maximizes communication and care. When I treat my friend, my wife, a colleague at work, even a stranger whom I casually meet, as a unique and whole person, a person whom I am interested only to meet and not to use for my own personal aggrandizement and gain, I am offered not only the opportunity to enter into this other person's special "world," but also, I am offered an opportunity to "hallow" this earthly life. Soon after the publication of *I and Thou* in Germany, psychiatrists recognized that Buber's philosophy of I-Thou, shorn of its more explicit religious references, could provide a model for the type of human relationships that therapists hope their patients will be able to have as a result of therapy. Beyond this, some conjectured that if one could have an I-Thou meeting with a patient in psychotherapy, the results would be curative.

Buber had a lifelong interest in mental illness and psychiatry, and in 1957 he was encouraged by Lesley Farber and Maurice Friedman to come to the United States to give the William Alanson White lectures at the Washington School of Psychiatry. In this series of lectures, titled "What Can Philosophical Anthropology Contribute to Psychiatry?" Buber attempted to elaborate his views on the nature of persons with a special eye towards psychotherapeutic applications. Buber's objective was not to provide psychotherapeutic technique or diagnosis, but rather, to provide an overarching view of the nature of man that could give psychiatry what Farber came to call "some steady conception of the fully human" (Farber 1967, 579).

Buber developed an "ontology of the interhuman" which highlighted the human capacity for "I-Thou" relationships as that essential trait which makes humans human. In fully articulating the different dimensions of the interhuman, Buber has provided psychiatry with images and concepts to address the issue of the goal of therapy. If we can conceive therapeutic "cure" as in some way helping people to reach their human potential, how should we conceive of this potential? What is the "realized person?" Buber's focus on I-Thou relationships and on the area between persons suggests that self-realization necessarily entails relationships to others and activity in and for society. Buber's philosophical anthropology runs counter to a primary philosophical presupposition of modern psychiatry, which conceives of the individual as separate from others and from society and tends to concentrate on individual fulfillment to the exclusion of communal fulfillment. The cliches of modern individualism—"express yourself," "find yourself," "do it your way"—are implicit in and have been fostered by modern psychiatry. In Buber's view, psychological individualism has not only led to a deterioration of social life but has also led to a deterioration of the individual's ability to find self-fulfillment. For self-fulfillment is intricately tied to the fulfillment of others and of society.

Distance and Relation

Buber began to articulate his particular notion of the fully human in his first William Alanson White lecture, "Distance and Relation" ([1950] 1965). He argued that it is the two-fold capacity for "distance" and "relation" that separates humans from all other earthly creatures. Distance "provides the human situation" and relation "provides man's becoming in that situation" ([1950] 1965, 64). Human beings, unlike animals, can distance themselves from their natural habitat. Lacking the "hard-wired" instincts of animals, they have freedom to alter their behavior and their world. What is crucially important for Buber is that their ability to distance themselves from their world allows humans to see it separate from their own needs, to see it as it is in and for itself. Man is the "creature (*Wesen*) through whose being (*Sein*) 'what is' (*das Seiende*) becomes detached from him and recognized for itself" ([1950] 1965, 61). Taking distance from the world, the human being and only the human being is able to see the world in its wholeness and in its unity.

The German title for Buber's lecture is *"Urdistanz und Beziehung"* ("primal distance and relation"). Buber spoke of a primal distance not only because the ability to take distance from the environment establishes the difference between man and beast, but also because distance is required before relation can occur. Distance is the "presupposition" for relation. Without distance there can be no relation. "One cannot stand in relation to something that is not perceived as contrasted and existing for itself"

([1950] 1965, 62). Distance allows other human beings to be seen as "separate" and "independent." But though distance is the presupposition of relation, it is not the "source" of relation. For distance is "universalizing" and objectifying, and relation is "personal" and particularizing. Distance provides the primal conditions for the possibility of relationship; but it is relation that allows for human growth and realization. "Relation provides man's becoming" ([1950] 1965, 64).

In Buber's view, it is only by entering into relation with another human being that a person becomes a person. Entering into relation is a complex activity that properly moves to deeper and deeper levels of intimacy. What one does when one first enters into relationship is to "confirm" the other person "in [his or her] personal qualities and capacities" ([1950] 1965, 67). Confirmation says yes to the special, unique qualities of another being. Confirmation affirms the present reality and future possibilities inherent in a person. I confirm "what he is, even what he can become" ([1950] 1965, 68). Buber speaks of confirmation as a "need" of man. Being separate, distanced, from the environment and from the security of set instinctual behavior patterns, human beings need to be confirmed in their unique ways of being.

> The human person needs confirmation because man as man needs it. An animal does not need to be confirmed, for it is what it is unquestionably. It is different with man: Sent forth from the natural domain of species into the hazard of the solitary category, surrounded by the air of a chaos which came into being with him, secretly and bashfully he watches for a Yes which allows him to be and which can come to him only from one human person to another. ([1950] 1965, 71)

Buber explained further how one person says yes to another with his concept of realization or "making present" *(Vergegenwärtigung)*. Making present rests on the capacity that Buber calls "imagining the real" *(Realphantasie)*. Here I imagine the reality of the other person.

> I imagine to myself what another man is at this very moment wishing, feeling, perceiving, thinking, and not as a detached content but in his very reality, that is, as a living process in this man. ([1950] 1965, 70)

In his second Alanson White lecture, Buber emphasized the active quality of imagining the real. He referred to it as a "bold swinging— demanding the most intensive stirring of one's being—into the life of the other" (Buber 1954, 81).

In sum, distance and relation are two terms used to map out Buber's philosophical anthropology, his answer to the question, What is the human being? Human beings are distanced from nature; this distance allows them to be unique, to find their own way. Yet they can only find this way, they can only become themselves, through relation to other human beings. It is the other that bestows upon me the gift of myself. As Buber puts it, "It is from one man to another that the heavenly bread of self-being is passed" ([1950] 1965, 71).

The primacy of relationship in Buber's philosophical anthropology, if taken seriously by psychiatry, draws attention away from concern with psychological mechanisms, coping techniques, and drugs toward the patient's capacities for human relationships. In therapy, the focus becomes the relationship between therapist and patient. The relationship referred to here is not the transference relationship, it is a meeting of selves that cuts through the masks of transference and countertransference and brings the therapist and patient face to face as the persons they simply are. If self-being is passed from one person to the other, then, Buber's anthropology suggests, it is the therapeutic relationship that helps the patient to grow and develop. One German psychiatrist, Hans Trueb, after studying Buber, came to speak of the entire process of psychotherapy as a matter of "healing through meeting" (1952). A genuine human meeting in therapy is a moment of reality, a sacred contact with something that is real and true, a foundation on which the patient builds the ability to truly meet others outside of therapy.

Although Buber intended to provide an overarching image of the human for psychiatry, psychiatrists have been quick to also see direct practical implications of Buber's concepts of "distance and relation," "confirmation," and "imagining the real."

"Too close" and "too distant," this dynamic of distance and relation is crucial to psychotherapy. As intimacy is something that many patients fear, the good therapist is sensitive to modulating the extent to which he or she gets close to his or her patient.[4] Buber's notion of "confirmation" provides a helpful way of talking about many forms of supportive therapy that aim to provide an affirming "holding environment" for the patient. And the concept of "imagining the real" articulates dimensions of what many therapists have referred to as "empathy" (see Katz 1975; 1985).

Dialogue and Monologue

In his second Alanson White lecture, "Elements of the Interhuman," ([1954] 1965), Buber speaks of the "dialogical" as the unfolding of the sphere of the "interhuman." Dialogue, for Buber, means communication between persons. It means conversation and speech. But the term does not only have a linguistic reference for Buber. Buber uses the term *dialogue* as a metaphor for mutuality, for "vital reciprocity" (Buber [1954] 1965, 84) between persons. It is a term that refers to a special kind of communication—communication that builds and tells of selves, conversation that addresses existential truths. The opposite of dialogue is *Gerede,* what the English translation refers to as "speechifying" and what I would somewhat loosely translate as "monologue." *Gerede,* as Buber uses the term, is speech used to communicate one's views without regard to the reality of the listener. Here a true relationship between persons is hindered by the desire of one person to impose his views, his self, his reality on another. Unlike the distance-relation polarity, which properly works dialectically, each assisting the other, monologue and dialogue are true opposites which defeat one another.

Buber's notion of dialogue further articulates elements of good psychotherapy. Since Freud's first patient, Anna O., labeled psychoanalysis the "talking cure," therapists have been aware of the importance of speech and language to psychotherapy. Buber's philosophy suggests that the quality of the dialogue in psychotherapy is correlated directly with the quality of therapy. Psychotherapy may be seen as a workshop in dialogue. Its goal is to bring about honest, mutually confirming speech between therapist and patient. Maurice Friedman has used Buber's work on dialogue to speak of the "healing dialogue in psychotherapy" (Friedman 1985). "Healing," in Friedman's sense, means that from the strength of the dialogue that occurs in therapy the patient is empowered to move from monologue to dialogue in his or her relations outside of therapy.

Buber also explicates his polarity of dialogue and monologue by introducing another related polarity, that of "being" and "seeming." For dialogue to occur, being must predominate over seeming. Being and seeming represent attitudes taken to life in the interhuman realm. In being, one "proceeds from what one really is," and in seeming, one acts "from what one wishes to seem" to others (Buber [1954] 1965, 76). Buber, intoning central themes of existentialism, asserts that yielding to seeming is "man's essential cowardice" and resisting seeming and asserting being "is his essential courage" ([1954] 1965, 78). Buber, however, differs from many existentialists in that for him, the "courage to be" (Tillich 1952) is not primarily a matter of a self-transcendent assertion of the will in the face of anxiety, but a courage to be vulnerable in the realm of dialogue. It involves "granting to the man to whom he communicates himself a share in his being" (Buber [1954] 1965, 77).

In psychotherapy, the patient often does not have the courage to be vulnerable and to speak from his or her "being." The therapist directs much attention to getting the patient to speak from true feelings and true thoughts, from the level of "being" and not from thoughts or feeling he or she wants to have or thinks the therapist wants him or her to have (the level of "seeming"). Often, arriving at one's "being" and speaking from it is fraught with fear, pain, and overwhelming emotion. Thus, bringing the patient to this level of "being" requires a great deal of trust—trust based upon the strength of the relationship between the patient and therapist.

A final issue that Buber discusses in his second lecture is the effect on dialogue of inequality in human relations. Dialogue requires each partner to regard the other as unique and whole. When a relationship has inherent inequalities—for example, in relations between old and young, ill and well—Buber argues that the stronger partner must imagine the future or "possible" wholeness of the weaker partner "even if his wholeness, unity, and uniqueness are only partly developed" ([1954] 1965, 80).

Buber addresses two types of strategies to affect the weaker partner in situations of inequality which correspond to the monological and the dialogical. He refers to them as "propaganda" and "education." The propagandist tries to "impose himself, his opinion and his attitude" ([1954] 1965, 82) on the other, often without any regard for who the other person is and what he or she thinks. The individual qualities of the other person "are of importance only in so far as [the propagandist] can exploit them to win the other" ([1954] 1965, 83).

The educator, on the other hand, tries to elicit from the other, from the nascent possibilities of the other, the view he or she believes is right. The educator

> wishes to find and to further in the soul of the other the disposition toward what he has recognized in himself as right. Because it is right it must also be alive in the microcosm of the other, as one possibility. The other need only be opened out in this potentiality of his. ([1954] 1965, 82)

Although some of Buber's writings[5] have suggested that the unequal relationship that obtains between the therapist and patient does not allow for an I-Thou relationship and for "dialogue" to occur, Buber's statements on the educator suggest that dialogue can indeed occur in therapy despite the inequality that necessarily exists. Recently the classical psychoanalytic model of the all-knowing, all-powerful, healthy doctor and the ignorant, weak, and sick patient has been challenged. Psychiatrists know that they are not omnipotent and that fostering an image of themselves as omnipotent can support the patient's own counterproductive fantasies about an all-powerful doctor who will magically "cure" them. Particularly with borderline and narcissistic cases and with character disorders, it is important that the therapist be known to the patient as a human being complete with frailties and inadequacies. A person with a weak sense of self needs not a blank screen to project herself on but a real person who will provide a model for her and who will respond to her naturally and genuinely. Therapy, properly, is not an equal relationship. The patient seeks help from a therapist who has special training and experience. Therapy must concentrate more on the patient than the therapist. Yet in the move away from the hierarchical doctor-patient relationship, Buber's more mutual educator-student relationship and his thoroughly equal I-Thou relationship provide important alternative models.

Guilt and Guilt-Feelings

In his third lecture, "Guilt and Guilt-Feelings" ([1957a] 1965), Buber moves away from concern with the existential quality of the therapeutic relationship and addresses issues of human responsibility and ethics outside the narrow confines of therapy. He argues for the positive ethical dimension of guilt (cf. Tillich 1952, 52–53). The guilty person is the person aware of his or her responsibility to others and to the world. Guilt is part of the glue of interpersonal relations. It can motivate persons to repair an injury to another and rebuild a human relationship. Buber recognized that there is pathological guilt, there are excessive "guilt-feelings", which paralyze and destroy both the individual and relationships. Yet there is also an existential guilt, a guilt that, if attended to, leads the patient out into the larger world to repair broken strands of relationship and rebuild a responsible social life. Because the self is never whole alone but only when related to others, psychological healing means interpersonal healing. As Buber puts it, the self "is never sick alone, but [there is] always a between-ness also, a situation between it and another existing being" (Buber [1951] 1974, 97). The therapist who fervently tries to alleviate all guilt may remove an essential psychological mechanism for the interpersonal healing that is a required concomitant to personal healing.

In his lecture Buber gave an example of a woman called Melanie, who, out of sport and not love, broke up the engagement of a friend and married her friend's fiance. Her friend then attempted suicide. Soon after, Melanie's new husband divorced her, and Melanie then became ill, plagued by guilt. Through psychiatric treatment Melanie was relieved of her guilt, but she never again married and never treated men as more than "objects to be seen through and directed by her" ([1951] 1974, 129).

Buber argued that the therapist successfully treated the guilt feelings but in so doing prevented Melanie from facing the original wrong she had done to her friend. She was therefore prevented, not only from reconciliation with her friend and from further relations with men, but also from becoming a truly better human being.

> With the silencing of the guilt-feeling there disappeared from Melanie the possibility of reconciliation through a newly won genuine relationship to her environment in which her best qualities could at the same time unfold. ([1951] 1974, 129)

For Buber, the totality of the individual's relationships to others gives him or her a "share in the human order of being." Doing harm to one of these relationships injures this human order of being ([1951] 1974, 132). This injury leads to existential guilt, and assuaging the guilt and restoring the order can only be accomplished by the person who caused the injury. It is not the job of the therapist to thrust the patient out into the world to make reconciliation with the injured party. At the very best, the therapist can prepare the patient to "glimpse his personal way" to reconciliation ([1951] 1974, 133). But a restorative action with the injured person and with the world lies at the horizon of truly dealing with any act that causes existential guilt. The therapist who is unaware of the ontological dimension of a patient's guilt and fails to perceive its import will not only fail the patient but also fail the wider human order.

For Buber, the person exists in a web of human relationships: in a family, in a community, as part of a people, and in the human world, in what Buber calls a "manifold We" ([1936] 1965, 80). Buber's interpersonal view of the person and his concept of interpersonal responsibility has made him an important figure in the growing field of family therapy. Ivan Boszormenyi-Nagy, one the founding theorists of family therapy, has developed a form of such therapy based on notions of dialogue, intergenerational responsibility, and familial trust inspired by Buber's writings (Boszormenyi-Nagy 1987). In addition Buber's concepts have been used in marriage therapy (Fishbane [forthcoming]) and group therapy (Kron and Yungman 1987) and in addressing tensions between social groups (Gordon 1983; Katz and Kahanov [forthcoming]).

Martin Buber's ontology of the interhuman, as we have it in the three William Alanson White lectures now available in Buber's *The Knowledge of Man* (1965), should serve to remind the psychiatrist of what is sometimes forgotten. Psychiatry is directed to people first. Though metapsychology, psychodevelopmental theory, diagnostics, and therapeutic techniques are important, they can never fully comprehend the whole human person sitting opposite the therapist. This whole person comes, not alone, but with an elaborate network of relations to other persons and to the world; and it is ultimately these relationships that must be repaired if the patient is to be helped.

Mordechai Rotenberg

In his most recent book, *Re-biographing and Deviance* (1987),[6] Rotenberg focuses on the recent turn to narrative in psychoanalysis and gives this turn a particular rabbinic twist through which he engages in a thoroughgoing critique of underlying assumptions of psychoanalysis and attempts to forge a new model for the psychotherapeutic process. Rotenberg argues that psychoanalysts like Roy Schafer (1980; 1983), who have used structural linguistics and the work of the French psychoanalyst Jacques Lacan to argue that psychoanalysis is a matter of helping the analysand to form a coherent life-narrative, have resurrected the most archaic element of Freudian orthodoxy: the oedipal conflict. Thus, the literary turn in psychoanalysis has exhumed the original Freudian myth, the myth of Oedipus and his oedipal guilt, elevated this story again to the status of paradigm, and sent its analysts out into the fields to convert patients and force their life stories to conform to the oedipal plot.

Rotenberg, it must be emphasized, does not dispute the validity of the literary turn in psychoanalysis; in fact, he applauds it. That human beings conceive their lives as a story, which provides temporal pattern and coherence—a sense of a past (narrative beginning), a present (narrative middle), and a future (narrative end)—is not disputed by Rotenberg. He affirms that mental illness can often bring with it a disjointed, confused, or fragmented life narrative and an inability to forge a coherent story. He believes that therapy can be seen as a process of story construction or "rebiographing."

What Rotenberg questions is the oedipal presupposition, the oedipal "meta-code" (Rotenberg 1987, 25) or "root-narrative" that has been resurrected by contemporary narrative psychoanalysis and brought out to rule the process of retelling one's life story to the exclusion of all other models. In addition, he questions certain patterns of self-development, forms of human relating and attitudes toward family and tradition that the oedipal narrative establishes as normative. Rotenberg explores biblical stories and rabbinic *midrash* (interpretation) of these stories to find alternative "root-narratives" and patterns for retelling life narratives that are less restrictive to the individual and that function to preserve familial cohesion and relation to tradition.

In first developing his argument, Rotenberg points out that the primacy of oedipal conflict is expressed apodictically by Freud in the last line of *Totem and Taboo* ([1939b] 1950): "in the beginning was the deed," the primal parricide by the sons against their father. In Freud's foundational text, *The Interpretation of Dreams,* he states, "It is the fate of all of us . . . to direct our first sexual impulse towards our mother and our first hatred and our first murderous wish against our father" (1900, 262). Psychoanalysis then becomes, in Rotenberg's terms, "a confession and 'cleansing-admission' process of unfolding one's past unavoidable parricide: original sin" (Rotenberg 1987, 80). People do not necessarily have oedipal conflicts but "acquire" them through analysis.

I propose that this analytic relearning to tell one's life story in terms of "infantile modes of sexual-aggressive actions" which may enhance, at least initially, one's self-destructive and self-blaming guilt, is, in fact, acquired through what is known as therapeutic "insight." (1987, 41)

Rotenberg argues that psychoanalysis "chains" its patient to a retrospective guilt-producing self-search that enhances self-depreciatory impulses and discourages optimistic, future-directed orientations. Psychoanalysis presents oedipal hate as an "original sin" which determines the patient's identity and from which he or she is never free. In addition, the oedipal root-narrative suggests that personal development and autonomy are won only at the price of the symbolic killing of the father (1987, 80). Rotenberg argues that the oedipal model for self-development has also been adopted by much of Western society and culture, so that social and cultural "development is contingent on the *elimination* of the 'no more fitting' old ruling class or Oedipal father" (1987, 93). Rotenberg is pointing to the fact that the modern West has been built upon the repudiation of the past, of tradition, and of our forefathers—a repudiation codified and taught by psychoanalysis.

As an alternative to the oedipal master plot and its peculiar prescriptions for psychotherapy, individual development, familial relationships, and attitudes towards tradition, Rotenberg looks to biblical stories and their rabbinic interpretations. First he concentrates on attitudes toward human faults or sins. Here he finds that the personal faults of central biblical figures—Jacob, Saul, David, Reuven—are not dwelled upon by the rabbis but corrected and reinterpreted to present the figures in the best possible light. The figures are given a "rehabilitative biographic rereading" that neutralizes their sin.

> For example, Jacob's "holy cheating" of his father Isaac when stating, "I am Esau thy first born" (Gen 27:1) is reread by separating between the words "I am" and "Esau (is) thy first born." The words "I am" are then transferred to the "I am the Lord your God" appearing in the ten commandments which Jacob presumably had in mind when he said "I am" to reaffirm his loyalty to God. (See Midrash Rabba 65:18). Similarly, Rachel's stealing of her father Laban's images (Gen 31:32) is reinterpreted by asserting that she took the images "for the sake of Heaven" in order to prevent her father from idol worshipping (Midrash Rabba, 71:5). And finally, with Joseph, we have the reconsideration of a seemingly detrimental callous act as an eventual useful event for humanity. What first appeared as the "sinful" selling of Joseph is reinterpreted by Joseph himself, when he assures his brothers (Gen 50:20) retroactively: "Ye thought evil against me: but God meant it unto good . . . to save many people alive" (Gen 50:20). (1987, 53)

Rotenberg finds within the Talmud an extension of rabbinic midrash toward a form of midrashic psychotherapy. The Talmud asserts that the person who commits a sinful act for which he is guilty must, as Buber suggested, seek restitution, or in more traditional terms "repentance" (1987, 45). But after serious repentance has occurred, the individual should not be chained to his or her sinful act, as Rotenberg claims as is done by psychoanalysis, but given a "new leaf" chance and allowed to reinterpret the sinful past.

> The Talmud seeks to institutionalize a social-cultural norm by which re-penters will not merely be given a "from now on" a "new leaf" chance, but be granted full "biographic rehabilitation" by being permitted to correct, reinterpret and assign new meaning to their past failing history. (1987, 52)

Narrative psychotherapy, in Rotenberg's rabbinic interpretation, be-comes not a matter of establishing a definitive "history" of the patient's past based on the oedipal theme. Personal story should not be a static monument to a person's past, a "closed book" (1987, 64) or a "case his-tory" that locks a person into a one character, one role, one clinical diag-nosis. Rather, personal story should be a "hermeneutic" and not a "hermetic" creation, a tale open for reinterpretation and retelling. Rab-binic midrash suggests that we should be able to "rebiographize" our lives using a variety of story models. Rotenberg argues *against* what he calls the dogmatic "fundamentalistic" quality of orthodox psychoanalysis, which is based on one oedipal meta-code, and *for* a "multiple hermeneutic code."

> Psychotherapy need not enforce new fundamentalistic techniques for re-framing and reinterpreting but should help troubled people who are cap-tured by any fundamentalistic belief system to accept a multiple hermeneutic code that will enable them to free themselves from any fun-damental internalized code. They will then be able to freely choose their own personality suited life story interpretation. (1987, 4)

Rotenberg stresses the need for a future and not past orientation to psychotherapy, but he argues that the past must not be cut off from the future. Instead, the past should be reinterpreted in terms of future goals to give the person a sense of temporal continuity.

> A future-oriented self-renewal is only possible through a reinterpretive temporal dialogue that reestablishes cognitive consistency between one's failing and sinful past and one's aspiring future. (1987, 74)

Rotenberg's "biographic rehabilitation," in structure, has affinities with certain psychoanalytic theorists and Jungian analysts of which he does not seem to be aware (see Cohler 1982; Hillman 1975; cf. Kepnes 1982; 1985). Given that many psychoanalysts have moved away from an oedipal-stage focus and have recognized the importance of other psycho-sexual and psychosocial conflicts, Rotenberg might be beating a dead horse in focusing his attack on the oedipus conflict. Yet there are some surprisingly reactionary aspects of certain literary critical and narrative therapeutic reapplications of Freud which Rotenberg has put his finger on. And his attention to rabbinic methods of rehabilitating biblical figures breaks new ground for the dialogue between Judaism and psychiatry.

If Rotenberg's characterization of narrative psychoanalysis may be a little overdrawn, he is certainly on the mark when he suggests that the oedipal pattern of renouncing the father to establish individual autonomy and cultural advancement is dominant in the modern West. It has become a given that children need to do something different from their parents and are expected to surpass them in learning, success, and status. If we look at the cultural giants of the modern West—Freud, Marx, Nietzsche—each has repudiated the past and developed a philosophy of repudiation to build a dream for the future. If we take religion as a symbol of tradition and a symbol of the past, each figure has developed a program of renun-ciation of religion to build his vision of the future. Lest the reader fail to notice, two of the three modern figures mentioned, perhaps the two most powerful, are Jews. Freud, through psychology, could be argued to rule the modern culture of the West, and Marx, through Communism, the East. Rotenberg suggests that these Jews have adopted a Pauline-Hegelian logic in which progress occurs through an *aufheben*—in positive terms, an "integrating elevation," or in more negative terms, a renunciation of for-mer thesis by antithesis. In terms of the history of religions in the West, this means, for Paul and Hegel, the "integrating elevation" or renunciation of Judaism by Christianity. In terms of personal development this means, for Freud, the oedipal renunciation of the father by the son, and in terms of social and economic advancement this means, for Marx, the socialistic renunciation of capitalism by the proletariat.

In the face of this Hegelian renunciatory model for progress and for attitudes toward the past, Rotenberg explores resources in the oldest liv-ing religious tradition, in Judaism, for establishing continuity from past to present to future and articulating a vision of the future without neces-sarily negating the past. In biblical stories and midrashim, Rotenberg finds "a systematic effort to establish the possibility of dialogic progress and intergenerational continuity" (Rotenberg 1987, 104). Rotenberg uses the Buberian term "dialogic progress" in contrast to Hegelian "dialectic prog-ress," and by the former term he means a "dynamic coexistence" of thesis and antithesis, past and present, and a notion of advancement that does not require repudiation of the past.

"Dialogic progress" would generally refer to the possibility of growth in which an "I" may emulate and even surpass the "Thou" with whom he or she interacts and through whom he or she develops, without having to destroy him or her. (1987, 95)

The biblical story that symbolizes dialogical progress is the paradigmatic tale central to all Judaism, the Akedah, or binding of Isaac. Here the hateful destructive impulses that exist between father and son, symbolized (in reverse to Oedipus) by the father's attempt to kill Isaac, are restrained, at the last moment, to allow for coexistence and continuity. Rotenberg argues that the Akedah offers an alternative paradigm, a

dialogic paradigm that idealizes Isaac's "parricidal" faith in a last-minute avoidance of Abraham's "filicidal" pressure to facilitate continuity of the son ruling *after* the father. (1987, 105)

The Akedah offers a model for growth that suggests that the son need not renounce his father and the past to establish his autonomy and move into the future, but can move forward "without having to destroy his cultural heritage" (1987, 99). Rotenberg does not deny that there are tensions between father and son, between past and present, between tradition and modernity. But his focus is on solutions to these tensions that lead to coexistence and continuity instead of a focus on the conflict and *aufheben* models of negation which, in his view, serve to perpetuate conflict and tension. The motto that killing begets killing is apt here. There is something entirely nihilistic about our modern myths of supersession of the old by the new. The new, of course, never remains new, and it too must be negated to make way for the future. In this *aufheben* model for progress, every son subconsciously knows that he too will be negated by his son. In killing my father to be me, I know that my son will kill me to be him; the cycle is unending. Is it not strange then that Freud, in the latter part of his life, came to formulate the death principle? Indeed, there is something deeply life-threatening about our modern oedipal myths. Rotenberg asks a rhetorical question whose answer is obvious: "Is [not] growing and branching impossible if the tree's roots are dead?" (1987, 93). If the past is destroyed, there can be no real future.

Despite the modern Jewish masters of suspicion, Freud and Marx, Judaism holds out alternative myths of life and interpretive methods that foster continuity between past, present, and future. This is Rotenberg's central argument, an argument that this author finds particularly compelling. One could easily argue that the forces that threaten continuity from one generation and one epoch to the next are at least as great as those that work to keep them in dialogue. In the cultural and personal struggle to remain vibrant and set off into the future, there is a tendency to want to cut ties to the past. Yet this move, as Rotenberg tries to show, has deadly consequences.[8]

In his concern for forging a dialogue between the past and future, between children and their parents, between Judaism and psychiatry, Rotenberg joins Buber in his attempt to map out the paths through which relationships are repaired in the face of the conflicts and tensions that threaten to destroy them. Since Freud, there have been tensions between philosophy and religion on the one hand and psychiatry on the other. The truly constructive contribution of both Buber and Rotenberg to psychiatry may be in pointing to resources to forge continuity between the great Western religious and philosophical traditions and the modern disciplines of psychiatry. As a result, the life-preserving and life-enhancing aims of psychiatry may be advanced.

Notes

1. For a collection of articles on Freud's Judaism, see Ostow (1982). For an overview of the growing literature, see Miller (1981).

2. The work of Moshe Halevi Spero (1980, 1981) certainly represents a serious attempt to provide psychiatry with a Jewish philosophic grounding. Where Rotenberg uses primarily rabbinic midrash and aggadic materials to provide a Jewish philosophy for psychiatry, Spero uses halakhic or legal materials to formulate what he calls a "metapsychology" (1980, ch. 2) for psychiatry. Spero begins from the orthodox view that "Halakhah precedes reality in the form of an *a priori* structure. This *a priori* structure . . . includes the givens of human psychology" (1980, p. 19). Spero then shows how halakhic notions of free will and determinism and prescriptions for mourning, repentance, and confession can provide psychiatry with halakhic justification and Jewish religious depth. I do not review Spero's work extensively in this paper because it is directed toward the strictly observant Jewish community and to problems unique to it. Spero's work, I am afraid, will not have a great amount of relevance to non-Orthodox Jews, Christians, and secular psychiatry. Still, Spero's extensive knowledge of rabbinic and talmudic literature and his equally vast knowledge of psychology and psychotherapeutic theory make his work very interesting, and he is without doubt the leading figure in relating Halakhic Judaism to psychiatry.

3. This section on Martin Buber was written in consultation with Henry Abramovitch, Ph.D., of the Sackler School of Medicine, Tel Aviv University, Israel.

4. Leston Havens (1986) who explicitly states his indebtedness to Buber has developed a variety of techniques to vary the degrees of distance and relationship in therapy.

5. In Buber's dialogue with Carl Rogers (1957), Buber asserted, in opposition to Rogers, that the therapeutic relationship could not be a form of I-Thou

relationship (1957b, 170ff). Yet, in a recent letter (Dec. 15, 1986), Rogers informed me that after their formal dialogue Buber explained that when he said dialogue could not occur in therapy he was speaking of therapy with the most severe schizophrenic cases. With less severe cases, he believed, a form of I-Thou relationship could take place.

6. In his earlier book, *Dialogue with Deviance,* Mordechai Rotenberg begins with Buber and moves back through Hasidism (eighteenth-century Jewish pietism) to develop a Jewish "egalitarian 'I-Thou' model for interpersonal relations." Arguing against Western Protestant and psychological models for the self, which suggest that the self "constructs" itself autonomously, Rotenberg presents a Hasidic model, which suggests that the self "contracts" with others to build itself. For Hasidism "development depends not on an ego-centered *construction* of the self but on one's inter- and intra-personal self-*contraction* and opening up to let the natural and social world infiltrate and imbue one's being" (xv). Rotenberg takes a social view of many mental illnesses, arguing that the mentally ill are often people who are different or deviant. Our modern Western society, with narrow views of normalcy, views many deviants as mentally ill. Less structured societies such as the Hasidic embrace all members of their community and make a place for members who are "different." Rotenberg, who teaches at the Hebrew University School of Social Work, favors community-based treatment centers and community integration for those labeled mentally ill.

7. Rotenberg quotes Schafer on his form of "narrative psychoanalysis." When "the analyst retells these [the analysand's] stories . . . certain features are accentuated while others are placed in parenthesis" (Schafer 1980, p. 35). "The analysand . . . may be an unreliable narrator, highlighting the persecutory actions of others and minimizing the analysand's seduction of the persecutor. . . . The analyst slowly and patiently develops an emphasis on infantile or archaic modes of sexual and aggressive action (1980, p. 39).

8. Lest Judaism be presented as the sole Western tradition with resources to counter the forces that separate present and future from the past, the simple fact that the Hebrew scriptures were preserved as the "Old Testament" in the face of supersession by the New Testament attests to wisdom and resources for strategies to preserve continuity within Christianity.

References

Abramovitch, H. and S. Kepnes, eds. Forthcoming. *Toward a Psychology of Healing Through Meeting: Buber and Psychotherapy.*

Amsel, Abraham. 1982. *Judaism and Psychology.* New York: Philipp Feldheim.

Boszormenyi-Nagy, Ivan. 1987. *Collected Papers.* New York: Brunner/Mazel.

Buber, Martin. 1923. *I and Thou.* New York: Scribner's, 1958.

———. 1936. "The Question to the Single One." In *Between Man and Man,* trans. R. G. Smith. New York: Harper and Row, 1965.

———. 1950. "Distance and Relation." In *The Knowledge of Man,* ed. and trans. M. Friedman and R. G. Smith. New York: Harper and Row, 1965.

————. 1951. "Introduction to H. Trueb 'Healing Through Meeting.'" In *Pointing The Way*. New York: Schocken, 1974.

————. 1954. "Elements of the Interhuman." In *The Knowledge of Man,* ed. and trans. M. Friedman and R. G. Smith. New York: Harper and Row, 1965.

————. 1957. "Guilt and Guilt Feelings." In *The Knowledge of Man,* ed. and trans. M. Friedman and R. G. Smith. New York: Harper and Row, 1965.

Buber, Martin, and Carl Rogers. 1957. "Dialogue Between Martin Buber and Carl Rogers." In *The Knowledge of Man,* ed. and trans. M. Friedman and R. G. Smith. New York: Harper and Row, 1965.

Bulka, Reuven and Moshe H. Spero, eds. 1982. *A Psychology and Judaism Reader.* Springfield, IL: Charles Thomas.

Cohler, Bertram. 1982. "Personal Narrative and Life Course." In *Life Span Development and Behavior,* ed. P. Baltes and O. Brim, Jr. New York: Academic Press.

Farber, Leslie. 1967. "Martin Buber and Psychotherapy." In *The Philosophy of Martin Buber,* ed. M. Friedman and P. Schilpp. LaSalle, IL: Open Court.

Fishbane, Mona DeKoven. Forthcoming. "Buber and Couple Therapy: An Integrative Systematic Approach." In *Toward a Psychology of Healing Through Meeting: Buber and Psychotherapy,* ed. Abramovitch and Kepnes.

Franzblau, A. N. 1956. "Psychiatry and Religion." *Judaism and Psychiatry,* ed. S. Noveck. New York: United Synagogue.

Friedman, Maurice. 1985. *The Healing Dialogue in Psychotherapy.* New York: Aronson.

Freud, Sigmund. 1900. *The Interpretation of Dreams.* Standard Edition, Vol. 4. London: Hogarth.

————. 1925. "The Resistances to Psychoanalysis." Standard Edition, Vol. 19. London: Hogarth.

————. 1926. "Address to B'nai Brith." Standard Edition, vol. 20. London: Hogarth.

————. 1927. *The Future of an Illusion.* New York: Norton, 1961.

————. 1939a. *Moses and Monotheism.* New York: Vintage, 1955.

————. 1939b. *Totem and Taboo.* Jerusalem: Kirjeith Zefer. (New York: Norton, 1950)

Gordon, Haim. 1983. "Trust: A Method Developed in Buberian Learning Groups." *Israel Social Science Research* 1, 1: 65–78.

Havens, Lesley. 1986. *Making Contact.* Cambridge: Harvard University Press.

Hillman, James. 1975. "The Fiction of Case History: A Round." *Religion as Story,* ed. James Wiggins. New York: Harper.

Katz, Israel and Maya Kahanov. Forthcoming. "Dilemmas in Leading Group Meetings Between Jews and Arabs in Israel." In *Toward a Psychology of Healing Through Meeting: Buber and Psychotherapy,* ed. H. Abramovitch and S. Kepnes.

Katz, Robert. 1975. "Martin Buber and Psychotherapy." *Hebrew Union College Annual* 46: 412–31.

————. 1985. *Pastoral Care and the Jewish Tradition.* Philadelphia: Fortress Press.

Kepnes, Steven. 1982. "Telling and Retelling: The Use of Narrative in Psychoanalysis and Religion." *The Challenge of Psychology to Faith,* ed. S. Kepnes and D. Tracy, Concilium Vol. 156. New York: Seabury.

———. 1985. "Freud and Judaism: The Path to Rapprochement." *Listening: The Journal of Religion and Culture* 20 (Fall): 230–43.

Klein, Dennis. 1981. *Jewish Origins of the Psychoanalytic Movement.* New York: Praeger.

Klein, Joel. 1979. *Psychology Encounters Judaism.* New York: Philosophical Library.

Kron, Tamar and Rafi Yungman. 1987. "The Dynamics of Intimacy in Group Therapy." *International Journal of Group Psychotherapy* 3,7: 52.

Miller, Justin. 1981. "Interpretations of Freud's Jewishness, 1924–1974." *Journal of the History of the Behavioral Sciences* 17: 357–74.

Ostow, Mortimer. 1982. *Judaism and Psychoanalysis.* New York: KTAV.

Rieff, Philip. 1979. *Freud: The Mind of the Moralist.* Chicago: University of Chicago Press.

Rotenberg, Mordechai. 1983. *Dialogue with Deviance.* Philadelphia: ISHI.

———. 1987. *Re-biographing and Deviance.* New York: Praeger.

Rubenstein, Richard. 1968. *The Religious Imagination.* New York: Bobbs-Merrill.

Schafer, Roy. 1980. "Narration in the Psychoanalytic Dialogue." *Critical Inquiry* 7: 29–53.

———. 1983. *The Analytic Attitude.* New York: Basic Books.

Spero, Moshe Nalevi. 1980. *Judaism and Psychology: Halakhic Perspectives.* New York: KTAV.

———. 1981. "Remembering and Historical Awareness: Part II. Psychological Aspects of a Halakhic State of Mind." *Tradition* 19, 1: 59–75.

Steinbach, A. A. 1956. "Can Psychiatry and Religion Meet?" *Judaism and Psychiatry,* ed. S. Noveck. New York: United Synagogue.

Tillich, Paul. 1952. *The Courage to Be.* New Haven: Yale University Press.

Trueb, Hans. 1952. Heilung aus der Begegnung, ed. E. Michel and A. Sborowitz. Stuttgart: Ernst Klett Verlag.

CHAPTER FOUR

ENEMIES OR FELLOW TRAVELLERS?

RELIGION AND PSYCHIATRY

IN THE NINETEENTH CENTURY

James P. Wind, Ph.D.

In 1896, the founding president of Cornell University, Andrew Dickson White, published his *History of the Warfare of Science with Theology in Christendom*. The book's title proposed what became a dominant metaphor for the complex relationship that had emerged between science and religion in modernity. For the scientist seeking emancipation from religious fetters and for the religionist threatened by the troubling new discoveries of nineteenth-century giants like Darwin and Freud, warfare seemed to be the most apt way of describing relations.

That metaphor, although subject to serious reconsideration by some in our "postmodern" context, has continued to appeal to many who think about the relationship—especially the early modern one—between religion and psychiatry. The clashes between modern psychoanalytic perspectives and traditional religious ones have often seemed like warfare, whether declared or not.

But such a confrontational view tells only part of the story. There were—as this essay will demonstrate—other patterns of relating. What is more, whether religionists and psychiatrists were clashing, coexisting, cooperating, or simply ignoring each other, they were also sharing a common odyssey that subtly transformed their theories and practices. As Alexis de Tocqueville noticed during his famous visit to the United States in the 1830s, Americans were shaping a new individual-centered culture that was altering almost every aspect of life. As recent observers like Robert Bellah and his colleagues have noted, this powerful tradition of individualism, although unnoticed by most, was reshaping American life along public and private lines (Tocqueville 1969; Bellah et al. 1985). This reshaping was a larger and determinative context for both religion and psychiatry. While leaders in each realm of thought attempted to provide public interpretations and systems of meaning for the culture, they were participating in a cultural transformation that ultimately made their theories and practices private affairs. This essay seeks to temper the reigning "warfare" portrait of religion and psychiatry's relations at the same time that it helps account for a contemporary situation in which representatives of both religion and psychiatry are searching for public philosophies that will overcome the estrangement between them.

For those who appreciate an occasional bit of tidiness in the midst of all the contradictory trends, data, forces, and factors in history, 1844 is an appropriate year at which to begin an inquiry into this relationship. This was the year when William Miller and his followers watched October 22 come and go with no hint of Christ's return—in spite of all of their hopes and predictions. Their ardent premillennialism, dashed on the rocks of this "great disappointment," was but one form of the popular religious fervor that "burned over" the northeastern United States and swept along its constantly moving frontier. The Millerites, soon to become Adventists, had the unsought distinction of frequently serving as "Exhibit A" when the subject of religious insanity arose in the middle third of the nineteenth century. Their relations with the forerunners of American psychiatry often resembled warfare (Numbers and Numbers 1986).

By way of contrast, the constituting meeting of the Association of Medical Superintendents of American Institutions for the Insane, held in Philadelphia six days before the Millerites' "great disappointment," seems almost bland. Yet this small and almost completely forgotten meeting of the association's "original thirteen" members represented a nodal point for American psychiatry. These physicians had created the United States' first *national* medical society (it preceded the American Medical Association by two years). And they had given birth to the organization that eventually became one of the most important forces in the field of mental health care—in 1921 the AMSAII changed its name to the American Psychiatric Association (McGovern 1985).

When viewed together, the new religious enthusiasms fostered by American revivalism and the new model of caring for the insane championed by the asylum superintendents epitomize two fundamental dynamics that shaped the relationship between religion and psychiatry during the remainder of the nineteenth century.

On the one hand, religion in America flourished and proliferated during this period. The great waves of immigrants that spilled across the land during the century—especially its second half—bore a wide variety of religious traditions which challenged the Anglo-Saxon Protestant hegemony of colonial Presbyterians, Congregationalists, and Anglicans. But even if one were momentarily to ignore the newcomers, America's religious efflorescence still impresses. Already in colonial days there was a sizable diversity of religious belief and practice. When itinerant preachers like George Whitefield made their north-to-south journeys they had to pass through communities settled by Puritans, Quakers, German Reformed, Lutherans, Anglicans, Deists; not infrequently they encountered a Roman Catholic or Jew.

The transformations of religion during the First and Second Great Awakenings (1737–43 and 1796–1802) guaranteed that religious pluralism would become an ever more potent reality in the new land. These two great outpourings of revivalism launched new denominations and divided old ones. They revealed a peculiar American penchant for intense religious experience, and set a style that put a premium on personal opinion, conversion, and spiritual searching. For those disenchanted old-stock Americans who found both mainline and revived religion too confining, the spacious national landscape provided ample room for experimenting with new religious beliefs and practices. Throughout the nineteenth century, groups as diverse as Shakers, Raapites, Transcendentalists, Mormons, and Millerites took advantage of their religious and geographical freedom to shape a colorful panoply of new options for those who hungered for religious meaning and experience. When taken as a whole, America in the nineteenth century was a place of religious intensity and conflict, of spiritual creativity and competition.

On the other hand, far outnumbered by the religious questors were those represented by the asylum superintendents. Some, both within and beyond the motley pale of the nation's denominations, sought to organize the care of mentally troubled people in more systematic and humane ways than those afforded by the poorhouses and jails of colonial America. These people, typified by those whom Constance M. McGovern calls "masters of madness," were not all enemies of religion, although they often harbored deep suspicions of its more extreme forms. But a stronger motive was an incipient professionalism. They wanted to single out a specific problem, "insanity," and then create specialized institutions, therapies, and experts to address it. Their efforts to specialize in one zone of life preceded the more visible reorganization of American society along professional lines which occurred later in the nineteenth century, when graduate education and professional associations became dominant features on the national horizon. As an advance platoon for the "culture of professionalism," these first physicians embodied a style and set of concerns that increasingly became the norm (Bledstein 1976). While outnumbered, they, like the religionists, were bearers of an ethos that would set some of the terms for the relationship between religion and psychiatry.

When these superintendents, or psychiatrists as they would one day be called, began to classify certain Millerites as religiously insane, two powerful impulses collided. The needs for religious people to express their beliefs and advocate them according to their own wisdom and convictions intersected with a nascent profession's attempt to define a problem and treat it.

Such a collision suggests several things. First, religion and psychiatry did not need Sigmund Freud's theories to create their conflict. On the contrary, the theories about religion and the psychoanalytic model of therapy invented by Freud and developed by his followers were latecomers on a scene where a wide variety of relationships already existed between various religious groups and those who sought to care for the mentally ill. Further, Freud's theory triumphed largely because of its congruence with a situation created by the American religious efflorescence on the one hand and the culture of professionalism on the other.

A second factor is foreshadowed in this prior interrelationship between religious America and incipient professional psychiatry. Unwittingly, religiously plural Americans and self-consciously professional asylum superintendents were becoming coconspirators in the relegation of personal belief and mental therapy to the private sphere. Even as they clashed, they were adding to America's mounting confusion about matters of meaning and well-being. The collision of the Millerites and the superintendents occurred at an early stage of a culturewide process whereby matters of personal belief and perception moved from the public to the private sides of life. Once upon a time in America—as the Salem witchcraft and Anne Hutchinson episodes of the seventeenth century remind us—personal belief, perception, and mental health were public matters. But as the nation came of age, as its religious dissensus became more pronounced, and as its professionalization of life proceeded, matters like these increasingly became the problems for the therapist's office, the clergyperson's study, or the individual's private domain. As religion proliferated and psychiatry professionalized, the possibility of public interaction, cooperation—and eventually even sustained conflict—seemed to disappear.

Nineteenth-Century Options

Pastoral Care

Where did people with mental and spiritual problems turn for help during the nineteenth century? At the beginning of the century most people with mental and spiritual maladies depended upon their own resources, or those of families and local communities. No specialized institutions existed. In his recent book *The Invention of the Modern Hospital,* Morris J. Vogel found only two other general hospitals in the United States at the time of the founding of Boston's first general hospital in 1821. Half a century later, a survey by the United States Bureau of Education counted 120 such institutions, a far cry from the more than 6,000 in existence in the 1920s (Vogel 1980, 1). Throughout most of the century little help for mental illness could be found in even the most advanced of these institutions. As for the modern mental health professions themselves, the *Oxford English Dictionary* reminds us that the word *psychiatry* did not make its first appearance in the English language until 1846. The first instance of identifying someone as a psychiatrist occurred in 1890. On the other hand, psychology, psychiatry's older sibling, had been part of English parlance from 1693, and psychologists had been part of this linguistic world since 1727.

These institutional and linguistic clues indicate that when a given individual became too difficult for a family or community to absorb into its daily way of life, the best that could be offered during the seventeenth and eighteenth centuries was a cell in a jail or a place in the community's poorhouse—if it had one. In his *Madness and Civilization*, Michel Foucault described the variety of options employed in European contexts—options that served as paradigms for those who migrated to the New World. In Renaissance times there had been ships of fools and wandering groups of mad vagabonds. Towns hired soldiers to keep these people out and to round up those who somehow slipped in. According to Foucault, a pivotal moment in Western history occurred when the Hôpital Général was established in Paris by the royal edict of April 27, 1656. With the establishment of this institution, the era of The Great Confinement of the mad—often indigent, ignorant, and powerless—began. A year later, on May 13, the "archers of the Hôpital," as the militia came to be known, were commissioned to hunt down the marginal and institutionalize them. Within four years between five and six thousand French men and women were confined, not to be treated, but to be isolated (Foucault 1965). This era of confinement—never replicated in the United States, although it was echoed in the small poorhouses and jails of its villages and cities—lasted until 1794, when Philippe Pinel began his reforming work at Bicêtre by unchaining patients—many of whom had been restrained for thirty to forty years. Pinel's alternative understanding of mental illness and treatment became a precursor of the approach employed by the asylum superintendents in the United States.

Prior to the development of the asylum model, the only American institution that had any kind of developed theory or therapy for responding to people with this sort of need was the local church or synagogue. There an explanatory system and even a plan of cure might be found.

Most of the evidence for how churches and synagogues responded to the needs of people with mental problems is lost to modern probers. Occasionally, a diary or pastoral handbook provides a glimpse into America's earliest way of dealing with problems of mind and spirit. E. Brooks Holifield, in *A History of Pastoral Care in America* (1983), has explored a good deal of the extant literature, especially within mainline Protestantism. There, for example, readers will encounter the pastoral technique of Ichabod Spencer, whose book *Pastor's Sketches* (published in 1850) sold more than six thousand copies in a nation served by twenty-seven thousand clergy. Spencer, himself a victim of a series of nervous breakdowns that disrupted his ministry at a prominent Presbyterian church in Brooklyn, was an expert in the "answering method" of pastoral counsel, which had been the norm for almost two centuries. Spencer's manner of dealing with a depressed middle-age parishioner illustrates one of the main responses given to the problem of mental anguish in his era. He called upon a woman one day because he was concerned about her "taciturn manner." She responded that her day was "gone by" because the "Holy Spirit has left me." Spencer set out to "remove her error" by asking a series of questions. How long had she felt that way? Eighteen years. Had she prayed? No. Why? "Prayer from me would not be heard." "Madam," the pastor replied, "you are in error. . . . And I can convince you of it." He asked to come again; his conversation partner resisted at first but finally gave in to her persistent pastor. For five or six weeks he visited her at regular intervals, working until he got the answer he wanted. When she responded "I can be saved! I can be saved!" he knew his mission was accomplished.

Spencer's pastoral goal was consistent with the main thrust of the Christian tradition. Of primary concern to him and to his pastoral colleagues was salvation, the deliverance of people held captive by forces of evil that lurked within and beyond them. The Puritan heritage, which stands behind Spencer's technique, placed a premium on personal appropriation of the deliverance won by Jesus of Nazareth. To feel his job was done, to expect that a depressed patient would be decidedly better off once she made her own what his tradition offered, to rely on the words of spiritual conversation alone as therapeutic means, were all part of the Protestant assumptive world in antebellum America.

But as Holifield persuasively suggests, beneath the surface of pastoral consistency, a tremendous transformation was taking place. The subtitle of his history, *From Salvation to Self-Realization,* identifies the process. For a variety of internal and external reasons, pastoral care was moving away from the assumptions and goals of the Spencers. For one thing, America was reorganizing itself around the modern processes of industrialization, urbanization, and specialization. Life was becoming segmented as homes became separated from work places, churches became sanctuaries for escaping from the problems besetting society, and social classes began to draw more distinct boundaries between each other.

As this "chopping up" of life proceeded, new ideas about the self began to emerge. Spencer and most of his mainline Protestant colleagues were good Baconians: they employed a prevailing "faculty psychology" that divided human mental actions into those of the understanding, the will, and the affections. As Baconians, they developed dexterity at classifying mental activity and employed a variety of typologies that could accommodate the temperament, dispositions, beliefs, behavior, and experience of their people. They observed, categorized, and generalized.

This manner of thinking about the self, usually called "mental philosophy" and usually done by clergy, prevailed until the post–Civil War era, when a new pastoral theology appeared. It turned away from the static categories of faculty psychology and employed new dynamic and natural metaphors. The new pastoral theologians began to speak of powers, forces, and energies that impelled humans. As people surrounded by powerful and often unprecedented social forces, they began to develop a portrait of the self that was much more congruent with the flux, dynamism, and complexity of their context. This was the era of "manly" ministers and virile portraits of Jesus—selves capable of mastering the changes occasioned by modernity. They advanced a "muscular Christianity" that championed a Jesus whom the age's most flamboyant evangelist, Billy Sunday, called "the greatest scrapper that ever lived" (Holifield 1983, 164–72).

During the years when the United States refashioned itself following its fratricidal Civil War, Americans responded to their uprooting, innovations, and loss of old ways of life by first cultivating and then mastering the self. These were years when lyceums, lectureships, museums, libraries, colleges, debating clubs and other institutions offering ready-made culture appeared all over the land. The churches followed the trend and often played key shaping roles in providing opportunities for self-culture and self-mastery. They invented a new kind of space, the "church parlor," to host the variety of meetings for purposes of self-expression and self-development. In these and many other ways, Americans continued down the individualistic road that Tocqueville had described earlier in the century.

In the midst of these cultural and metaphorical changes, many practitioners of pastoral care quietly (and perhaps unknowingly) shifted their goal from salvation to self-realization. Holifield cites one W. T. McElveen, pastor of First Congregational Church in Evanston, Illinois, who near the turn into the twentieth century embodied many of the aspects of the new, more natural style of pastoral care. On one occasion an alcoholic stranger approached Pastor McElveen for help. Although their one conversation did include moments of prayer, McElveen "won" his battle against this alcoholic's dependence by being a manly friend. McElveen in essence challenged his visitor to a wager: "You here, MacDonald. . . . You can't keep your promises." The alcoholic accepted the challenge and in so doing set out on a journey that led (the pastor claimed) to the personal mastery of alcohol (Holifield 1983, 181–83). Cases like these indicate that by this time theological reticence had become part of clerical technique. In essence, a de facto schism between care for mental health needs on the one hand and the religious beliefs of a congregation on the other was already visible within pastoral practice—long before the advent of Freud!

Moral Treatment

For those who chose not to make use of pastoral care, or for those whose needs exceeded the resources of the clergy, there were other options. Chief among these was the moral treatment offered by asylum superintendents. When the "original thirteen" superintendents held their organizational meeting in 1844, there were twenty-five asylums in the United States (McGovern 1985: 3). The oldest was the Friends' Asylum for the Insane, founded by Quakers in 1817 and located near Philadelphia. It was modeled after William Tuke's York Retreat, a British farm established by and for Quakers in 1792. Tuke's *Description of the Retreat,* published in 1813, served as their blueprint.

Prior to the establishment of Friends' Asylum, there had been a few glimpses of medical approaches to the problem of insanity. Occasionally doctors would take insane patients into their own homes for care. Under the impulses of an optimism fostered by the Enlightenment, a number of physicians began to attempt to find somatic cures for some of the problems of the insane. Thus they bled, purged, blistered and provided opium for their patients. Some, like Dr. Perley Marsh of New Hampshire, attempted a cold "water cure." By keeping the individual immersed to the point of unconsciousness, Marsh hoped that the "stupefaction of the life forces" would break the "chain of unhappy circumstances" in his patients' lives (McGovern 1985, 38). Others like Dr. Benjamin Rush of Philadelphia theorized that insanity came from a chronic inflammation of the brain's blood vessels brought on by emotional disturbances which in turn were occasioned by too much religious or political activity. Rush advocated employing patients and providing them with recreational activity as ways to provide a stable environment that would lead to recovery.

The "moral treatment" model received its most significant early articulation in the practice and writing of Philippe Pinel (mentioned above). This enlightened physician did not break with the idea of confinement, although he significantly remolded it. His goal was to provide a carefully designed total environment that could counter the effects of a previously unmanageable one. The treatment model that evolved from Pinel's early attempts is well summarized by McGovern (1985, 10):

Moral treatment was relatively simple. The sick person had to be hospitalized in order to remove him or her from an environment that doctors believed had been both the precipitating and a contributing cause of insanity. In the hospital the doctors' individual attention, firm but kind treatment, and reluctance to use physical or mechanical restraint gained the confidence of the patient. Doctors then put into effect a program that interjected stability into the patient's life by its very regularity. Each asylum had a daily schedule of rising, eating, exercising, and socializing that varied only according to summer or winter hours.

Next the doctors had to break up the "wrong association of ideas" of the patients and help them to form "correct habits of thinking as well as acting." They did this by planning a series of activities including manual labor, religious activities, and recreational and intellectual pursuits.

The total therapy regimen of these asylums was worlds removed from earlier methods of care. Building upon Pinel's foundation, the superintendents kept their patients busy with manual labor, lectures, libraries, picnics, carriage rides, harbor excursions, and evening Scripture readings.

The chief problem these physicians had was the image of success they cultivated and projected. McGovern documents how they manipulated statistics in order to be able to present high cure rates to the public. Depending upon state legislatures for revenue and intent upon serving a middle-class clientele, the superintendents quickly found themselves fighting and losing a rear-guard battle with a public that wanted them to expand their institutions beyond the optimum population of 250. By the end of the century the typical asylum population had doubled, making the type of care intended an impossibility. According to McGovern, the superintendents succeeded in carving out their own professional niche. The irony in their victory was that by the end of the century they had lost the possibility of achieving their moral treatment goal and ended up presiding over a new set of custodial institutions that housed the increasing population of social outcasts who could not adjust to modern America.

Before turning from the moral treatment advocates, it is important to note their stance towards religion. While they mentioned religiously insane patients in their annual reports, and while several of the superintendents expressed grave concerns about certain types of religious expression (such as that represented by the Millerites), most of the medical superintendents welcomed religion into their programs of cure. Moreover, several of the leaders of the asylum movement drew upon religious impulses for their vision. Thomas Kirkbride, the author of the Kirkbride plan that served as model for many asylums built in the 1850s and 1860s, for example, drew upon Quaker roots. Without doubt the dominant figure in the "original thirteen," Samuel Woodward, was "regarded with much doubt by the federal and orthodox Calvinists." There were "whisperings" about his infidelity. Yet Unitarians welcomed the fact that he "accepted the prevailing faith in the perfectibility of man" and supported his work. Dorothea Dix, an official Unitarian, was so affected by her experience teaching a Sunday school class at the East Cambridge (Massachusetts) jail where the mentally ill were indiscriminately mixed with criminals that she set forth on a crusade to build asylums. Her work resulted in the establishment of St. Elizabeth's Hospital, at that time the only institution for the mentally ill sponsored by the federal government (McGovern 1985, 64–66, 79, 107–8; Lavan and Williams, 1986, 364).

The examples of Kirkbride, Woodward, and Dix, along with the official place for religion in the treatment plans of the superintendents, suggest that for much of the nineteenth century, certain kinds of religion were quite able to peacefully coexist with certain kinds of mental treatment. Such coexistence would continue to be the case until the 1920s, when a fundamentalist virus would infect both religion and psychiatry and overwhelm the accommodation achieved by the superintendents.

Mind Cure

There was still another major option for those seeking mental health during the nineteenth century. Clergy like Ichabod Spencer and physicians like Samuel Woodward were not the only ones offering therapy to Americans. The medical superintendents kept their eye on the Thomsonians, who challenged established medical models with their herbal prescriptions. In addition there were phrenologists, mesmerists, and a variety of popular healers, each offering a cure for whatever problem people presented. All of these alternative curers made America's religious and medical leaders very nervous. But none of them triggered as large a reaction as that occasioned by the mind cure movement.

When Phineas Parkhurst Quimby heard French lecturer Charles Poyen expound upon hypnotism in Maine in 1827, a tradition of American mind cure began. Although Quimby would eventually abandon the technique of hypnosis, his 1838 experience of self-cure on the basis of mental suggestion set him on a course of mental healing that drew many followers. One of them, the Reverend Warren Felt Evans, left behind Methodism and Swedenborgianism to follow Quimby. In 1869 he published the first book of the new religious movement, *The Mental Cure*. Evans, soon to be surpassed by Mary Baker Eddy, sought to demonstrate how the "divine influx" of God's spirit healed.

In 1862 Mary Baker Eddy sought out Quimby for cure. Then forty-one years old, Eddy had suffered from "colds, fevers, chronic dyspepsia, lung and liver ailments, backache, nervousness, gastric attack and depression." In addition she had sampled many of the self-help remedies and sectarian cures of her era. As had happened on several other occasions, Eddy experienced "an immediate but temporary cure." She kept returning to Quimby and continued to find temporary relief. However, she discovered that, as she attempted to practice Quimby's therapy with others, she "vicariously acquired" her patients' symptoms. In 1866, less than a month after Quimby's death, Eddy slipped on the ice and was seriously injured. This time no one was able to cure her. Instead she found help by herself, reading the biblical accounts of Jesus' miracles. Her core discovery: "There is but one creation, which is wholly spiritual." With that "healing Truth" came spontaneous recovery. By 1875 she had developed her insight into a textbook, *Science and Health*. In 1879, the Church of Christ, Scientist, was formed with Mrs. Eddy as pastor. A new religion had been institutionalized and an alternative therapy had been proclaimed. By 1882 Eddy was serving as Professor of Obstetrics, Metaphysics, and Christian Science at her own Massachusetts Metaphysical College. Soon her practitioners were practicing on their own. By 1890 she had 8,724 members of her new denomination. Sixteen years later that number had grown to include 55,000.

While there were other variants of mind cure than Eddy's most visible version, the important point here is to note that it presented a distinct alternative to the somatic and social approaches to illness advocated by mainstream American medicine. Yet it seized upon the fascination with science that typified the age. It also capitalized on the discontent of the medically and religiously disenfranchised—women outnumbered men in the Christian Science movement five to one in the 1890s (Schoepflin 1986). And it forged an explicit and simple linkage between faith and therapy, an accomplishment that its followers did not find equalled in any other religious or medical group. Mind cure would never be a majority movement in the nineteenth century. Yet it claimed to offer a union where others increasingly found only schism. At the same time it served as foil for new scientific, psychotherapeutic, and religious approaches to mental illness.

Medicalization

For some in the nineteenth century, religious solutions or accommodations of any sort seemed beside the point. The late nineteenth century seemed to be presenting a new environment that was hazardous to American mental health. The new discoveries made by neurologists and other scientists seemed to render traditional approaches obsolete. There were compelling new scientific explanations for many of life's mysteries. In such cases, religion was not so much an enemy to be vanquished as a distraction to be ignored. There were simply better ways to look at things.

One example of the attempt to redescribe modern mental illness in medical terms was George M. Beard's campaign, beginning in 1869, on behalf of the disease category neurasthenia. Dr. Beard hoped to give those who experienced profound physical and mental exhaustion the same status as those who suffered from smallpox or cholera. This peculiarly—and for several decades quite fashionable—American disease was believed to be a product of the onslaughts of modernity. Beard singled out the telegraph, steam power, and other features of urban life as causes for the enervating illness. Stresses of a new way of life left Beard's patients in a condition that many likened to an overloaded electrical circuit or an overdrawn bank account. Neurasthenia's essential feature was a pronounced loss of energy.

The disease manifested itself in amazingly diverse ways. Barbara Sicherman catalogues its characteristic symptoms: "sick headache, noises in the ear, atonic voice, deficient mental control, bad dreams, insomnia, nervous dyspepsia, heaviness of the loin and limb, flushing and fidgetiness, palpitations, vague pains and flying neuralgia, spinal irritation, uterine irritability, impotence, hopelessness, and such morbid fears as claustrophobia and dread of contamination." She has also observed that the category was so broad and imprecise that a later scholar in Beard's field came to call neurasthenia "the newest garbage can of medicine."

By 1920 the many conditions and symptoms that Beard had lumped together in his neurasthenia diagnosis had become so unwieldy that few made use of the term. Many of the physical symptoms and mental conditions that had gathered under this nosological umbrella had become discrete diseases in their own right, with very specific symptoms and etiologies. What had once been the "disease of choice" soon became passé.

Of interest here is that Beard serves as an exemplar of the newer form of professionalism that was reshaping American life in the late nineteenth century. Like the asylum superintendents of the preceding generation, Beard singled out a specific problem and offered an expertise about it. But Beard's type of professional response was a challenge to the older model of the superintendents. Neurasthenia became the new alternative to older disease categories like insanity, hypochondria, and hysteria—the prevailing categories of the superintendents. It didn't carry the stigma associated with "insanity," nor did it require institutionalization in an asylum for cure. Regarded as a treatable early warning of potentially more serious mental illness, the disease could be dealt with at home or at one of the nation's new "nerve retreats." Clothed in the garb of medical disease, neurasthenics could fit into the new scientific ethos rather than experience marginalization. And the new generation of specialists who treated these patients in their clinics and private offices had in their new disease a powerful weapon for breaking the by then creaking monopoly of the asylum superintendents.

A minister's son who chose medicine over ministry for his profession, Beard had first-hand experience with the "lack of vitality" that afflicted his patients and many of the leading figures of his age—people like William James and Jane Addams. In his attempt to find physical, environmental, and disease explanations for his own experience and that of many others, Beard stands as exemplar of the nascent but soon to become powerful trend to medicalize mental illness. His own alternative may have had only episodic significance. But his quest to find a medical explanation and cure for mental illness, as well as his quiet professional turn away from religion, represents another of the century's powerful options (Sicherman 1979).

The Emmanuel Movement

In *Ministry After Freud* Allison Stokes proposes the thesis that a significant "religion and health movement" emerged in the twentieth century. The movement's leaders attempted to forge an accommodation between the new psychology of modernity and the Christian tradition. This movement, unnoticed by historians of both medicine and religion, was located within the liberal stream of mainline Protestantism and played a significant role in reshaping pastoral care in America. Stokes's chapters on the roles of Anton Boisen, the founder of clinical pastoral education, and theologian Paul Tillich reach beyond the time frame of this essay. However, her attention to the origins of the religion and health movement provide one more glimpse of the pre-Freudian relationships possible between religion and psychiatry.

In 1904 the Reverend Doctor Elwood Worcester accepted the call to Emmanuel Church, the largest Episcopal congregation in Boston. After completing college and seminary training in the United States, Worcester had gone to the University of Leipzig to earn a Ph.D., which he received in 1889. At Leipzig he had studied psychology under Gustav Fechner and Wilhelm Wundt and developed the conviction that scientific methods could be applied to "the immaterial and spiritual" as well as to physical and material realities. When he arrived at his new post in Boston, Emmanuel was at the forefront of the burgeoning social gospel movement, which was responding to the very social forces that had sent people flocking to neurasthenia experts like Beard. Emmanuel had chosen to respond to these new urban problems with a complex set of institutional ministries: clubs, classes, camps, a gymnasium, hospital programs, and a settlement house in one of Boston's less privileged neighborhoods. Sympathetic to the goals of the social gospel, Worcester nonetheless found the movement incomplete.

> It can change the environment, but as yet it seems to have no means of changing the heart. It can help men in the bulk, but it has no direct access

to the depth of the individual conscience. We therefore venture to believe that the social movement will soon by supplemented by a psychical movement which speaks in the name of Christ to the soul. (Stokes 1985, 22)

There can be little doubt that Worcester's Boston neighbors, the Christian Scientists, were an important additional concern as he fashioned his new ministry. Rejecting Mrs. Eddy's type of practical science, he sought to fashion a scientific approach to people's inner turmoil that made a practical difference while remaining congruent with mainline American religion. Here there was to be no need for an either/or decision between science and a religious tradition. Nor was it necessary to invent a new religion as Mrs. Eddy had. Instead, the psychology of Leipzig and evangelical liberalism would merge their resources.

Together with another clergyman, Dr. Samuel McComb, Worcester fashioned a team of medical and religious professionals into what Stokes (1985, 25) describes as "the first American venture between clergy and doctors in the cure of souls." The appeal of Worcester's new approach was immediate. The day after announcing in his November 1906 lecture that he, McComb, and two physicians would be available for counsel, 198 people appeared. Focusing on functional nervous disorders (just as Beard had), the Emmanuel team conducted health classes and private consultations. By 1909 they had five thousand applications for therapy and counted six hundred people in the opening session of one of their classes. Before the Emmanuel movement peaked in 1911, McComb and Worcester had become popular on the lecture circuit, and their program had been written about in magazines like *Good Housekeeping* and *Ladies' Home Journal*.

Eventually the physicians who were instrumental in launching this unique joint venture—James Jackson Putnam, Richard C. Cabot, Isador Coriat—would become nervous about clergy's encroachment upon medical territory, a sign that professionalism continued to shape the relationship between religion and psychiatry as much as new ideas or therapies. But before leaving the short-lived movement, it is instructive to let one of them describe the therapy offered. Cabot, a faculty member at Harvard Medical School and one of the early shapers of clinical pastoral education, defined the psychotherapy they offered as "the attempt to help the sick through mental, moral, and spiritual methods." This form of therapy was "scientific, rational mind cure," something physicians were nervous about because the Christian Scientists and faith healers were already claiming the field for themselves. Granting that there was some truth even amidst the "antics and extravagances of Mrs. Eddy," Cabot believed psychotherapy addressed the whole personality of a human—mind, soul, intellect, moral life. Minister, doctor, and social worker all had roles to play in this type of treatment. Various professions, and various therapeutic sects (osteopaths, Christian Scientists, and hospital physicians, for example) "ought to get together" in this all-encompassing version of therapy (Stokes 1985, 25).

The Emmanuel Movement soon faded from view, an indication of the difficulty of achieving accommodation between the new medicine and traditional religion. Stokes's counterclaim, that this first effort at accommodation was seminal for a movement that grew and came to prominence in the 1940s, suggests that we not dismiss it too quickly. It stands as an early example of an American attempt to blend and reconcile, a reminder that separation of religion from psychiatry was not the only option on the American landscape.

Sigmund Freud's New Total View

The shadow cast by Sigmund Freud over modernity is so sizable that it threatens to obscure almost every other part of the religion-psychiatry story. While the "Freudianity" hypothesized by novelist Peter DeVries may be the overstatement of a gifted satirist (DeVries 1973), Freud's vision of the inner workings of human consciousness and unconsciousness have become virtual commonplaces for moderns. Few except for the specialists know about the asylum superintendents, the Ichabod Spencers, the George Beards, or the Elwood Worcesters. At the same time, so taken for granted is Freud that we are tempted to accept shorthand versions of his story. Because so much has been written about him, it is difficult to imagine that anyone can say anything new about him. We assume that our conventional knowledge is adequate.

One fresh reading of Freud that offers an added dimension to the overview offered in this essay is that provided by Edwin C. Wallace. In essence, Wallace claimed that Freud made a number of mistakes that have been enormously important for subsequent relations between religion and psychiatry. First, he too facilely transferred psychoanalytic insights "from office to culture." On the basis of his own self-discoveries and those gained from hours of therapeutic conversation with patients (many of whom were pronouncedly pathological and thereby extreme rather than representative cases), Freud made important discoveries about the unconscious dimensions of individual psyches. Those discoveries Wallace and others affirm as of tremendous value for our modern self-understanding.

But Freud's "direct" transfer of those discoveries to culture was both unscientific and misleading. This fundamental mistake depended in turn upon other mistakes that he shared with many of the Viennese materialists of his day. Like them, Freud too readily embraced "the cornerstone doctrines of cultural evolutionism—psychic unity, the comparative method, the notion that cultures everywhere develop along a fixed and unilinear evolutionary scheme, psychic Lamarckism and the biogenetic law, the idea that contemporary 'primitive' cultures may be equated with those of pre-historic men, and the doctrine of survivals" (Wallace 1984, 133).

Rather than take up each of those assumptive "mistakes" individually, it is important to grasp the overall force of Wallace's criticism. Following Philip Rieff, Wallace contended that Freud did much more than design a therapy for troubled individuals. Instead, he constructed a total view that had to contend with other total views, especially religious ones. Or, as Rieff described it, Freud proposed a *Weltanschauung* that was "the last great formulation of nineteenth century secularism complete with substitute doctrine and cult" (Wallace 1983, 222–23).

Those interested in detailed discussion of the fine points of Freud's alternative doctrine should consult Wallace. But here it is instructive to note that the same individual who equated religion with psychopathology, labeling it at turns "neurotic relics," "mass delusion," and "blissful hallucinatory confusion," constructed an alternative to it that had remarkably similar features. Wallace pointed to similarities between the method of psychoanalysis and the exegetical techniques of the Judaism of Freud's home world. Freud himself suggested that the analyst was really a "secular pastoral worker (*Seelsorger*)." Speculating on the basis of such statements, Wallace asked if "at least to some degree, albeit largely unconsciously, Freud saw himself laboring in the service of a new priesthood and a new temple?"

As an answer to his own question Wallace proposed a thesis that cannot help but create controversy. It also sheds light on the main concern of this essay. "My thesis is that because psychoanalysis for Freud (largely unconsciously) partook of the character of a 'positive community' with its own therapeutic and reintegrative symbolism, he had to oppose it to all the more traditional 'positive communities' and commitment therapies—foremost among which was religion" (1984, 150). Here again Wallace follows Rieff, who suggests that Freud's therapy emerged at the very moment when the positive communities that had traditionally provided meaning and mechanisms for responding to mental illness were breaking down. Most particularly the religious communities that had provided frameworks within which such phenomena could be placed were failing to fulfill that longstanding task. "From the ashes" of that collapse Freud built a new positive community which Wallace suggests may have been an ersatz form of the Jewish community that was breaking down in Vienna (1983, 238–39). That community began in the group that gathered for the "Psychological Wednesday Evenings," which became the Vienna Psychoanalytic Society in 1908. Regarding that group "of mostly Jewish

young men" Wallace states: "I maintain that there is not a considerable
difference between the organization Freud founded for himself and more
traditional therapeutic communities" (1984, 150).

Freud did not set foot in America until 1909, and while a few scholars
knew of his work prior to his arrival, the kind of conflict between religion
and psychiatry which he precipitated was *not* the dominant mode of relation for most of the nineteenth century. But even though Freud is really
more a part of the twentieth century American story than the nineteenth,
it is important to note the quest for a new total view and new positive
community that he represents. That quest was part of the American experience before Freud arrived. The nation's positive communities were
being overwhelmed by modernity. That nineteenth-century experience
helps account for the ready reception accorded to Freud's therapy in the
next part of the American story. In essence Freud's turn to the neurotic
individual's own deepest experience provided an alternative source of
meaning and authority for those whose positive communities were failing
them. Such a move from publicness to privateness was quite congruent
with the major dynamisms of the American experience.

The Need for a Public Philosophy

The varying approaches to mental illness described here—asylums, pastoral care, new medical diagnoses, new religious movements, new forms
of psychotherapy (whether Freud's or Emmanuel's)—demonstrate the
cultural confusion about mental illness which proliferated during the nineteenth and early twentieth centuries. Within these options were a variety
of understandings of the source and cause of mental illness and its treatment. Some, like the asylum superintendents, found the source in environmental configurations. Others, the early neurologists, looked to somatic
explanations. Still others, like the Christian Scientists, opted for spiritual
rather than materialistic theories. And still others—chief among them
Freud—posited new psychological and psychodynamic realities. A few—
represented by the early Emmanuelists—attempted to find mediating approaches that could bring together elements from various approaches into
a more comprehensive understanding of the self and its workings. But all
(largely without self-awareness) made it more difficult to articulate a common language or understanding that could bridge the deep gaps between
the materialists and the spiritualists, the accommodationists and the pur-
ists, the competing sects within medical or religious professions. Yet the
professions continued their drive toward social dominance, and the public
became, for better and worse, an amalgam of private consumers.

Perhaps no turn-of-the-century individual felt this need for a public
philosophy as acutely as William James, a figure whose name can stand as

an eponym for the modern search for mental health. An M.D. who preferred philosophy to medical practice, a victim of an almost total nervous collapse occasioned by insoluble theological and philosophical problems, the author of both a basic textbook on psychology and the classic *Varieties of Religious Experience,* James attempted to construct a new philosophy that could bridge the gaps between empiricism and absolutism ([1892] 1958; [1902] 1962). Calling his approach first pragmatism, then radical empiricism, James attempted to "build out" a philosophy from the basic fact of personal consciousness. By carefully studying the ways human consciousness worked, James was able to propose a via media between the physician's medical facts and the philosopher's or theologian's concerns about the "more" ([1892] 1958, 387–91). In James's capacious and incomplete universe there was room for research into the physiological workings of synapses, the religious experience of once-born and twice-born individuals, and even the unorthodox reports of psychical experience.

For our purposes, James's goal is more significant than the specifics of his proposal. Attempting to forge a basic understanding that could allow religion and psychiatry, science and philosophy, faith and reason to share common ground, James was one of the early pioneers in modern America's search for a public philosophy that allows private worlds to become more accessible, or public, for each other.

Equally important is James's fate. While the many competing approaches to mental health built their new schools, faded out of existence, or transformed themselves, few of their adherents followed James's public path. An irony of American history is that the public philosophy advocated by James has remained the private perspective of a stream of theologians and philosophers, while the private-minded religionists and psychiatrists have attracted much larger followings. The result has been a legacy of misunderstandings, of partial relations, of counterproductive hostility and competition. James's particular approach has not proved to be a solution to our national style of professionalism, privatization, and occasional hostility between religion and psychiatry. However, his quest for a public discourse and understanding of the great mystery that is human consciousness in all of its manifestations still stands before us as an overarching challenge.

References

Bellah, Robert N., Richard Madsen, William M. Sullivan, Ann Swidler, and Steven M. Tipton. 1985. *Habits of the Heart: Individualism and Commitment in American Life.* Berkeley: University of California Press.

Bledstein, Burton J. 1976. *The Culture of Professionalism: The Middle Class and the Development of Higher Education in America.* New York: Norton.

Cabot, Richard C. 1908. "The American Type of Psychotherapy." In *Psychother-apy: A Course of Reading in Sound Psychology, Sound Medicine, and Sound Religion,* vol. 1, ed. W. B. Parker, 5–13. New York: Centre Publishing Co.

DeVries, Peter. 1973. *Forever Parting.* New York: Penguin Books.

Foucault, Michel. 1965. *Madness and Civilization: A History of Insanity in the Age of Reason.* New York: Random House.

Holifield, E. Brooks. 1983. *A History of Pastoral Care in America: From Salvation to Self-Realization.* Nashville, TN: Abingdon Press.

James, William. [1902] 1962. *Psychology: Briefer Course.* New York: Collier.

———. [1892] 1958. *The Varieties of Religious Experience.* New York: New American Library.

Lavan, Spencer and George Huntson Williams. 1986. "The Unitarian and Universalist Traditions." In *Caring and Curing: Health and Medicine in the Western Religious Traditions,* ed. Ronald L. Numbers and Darrel W. Amundsen. New York: Macmillan.

McGovern, Constance M. 1985. *Masters of Madness: Social Origins of the American Psychiatric Profession.* Hanover, NH: University Press of New England.

Numbers, Ronald L. and Janet S. Numbers. 1986. "Religious Insanity: History of a Diagnosis." *Second Opinion* 3: 56–77.

Schoepflin, Rennie B. 1986. "The Christian Science Tradition," In *Caring and Curing,* ed. Numbers and Amundsen, 424–31. New York: Macmillan.

Sicherman, Barbara. 1979. "The Uses of a Diagnosis: Doctors, Patients, and Neurasthenia." In *Nourishing the Humanistic in Medicine,* ed. William R. Rogers and David Barnard, 217–44. Pittsburgh: University of Pittsburgh Press.

Stokes, Allison. 1985. *Ministry after Freud.* New York: Pilgrim Press.

Tocqueville, Alexis de. 1969. *Democracy in America,* trans. George Lawrence, ed. J. P. Mayer. Garden City, NY: Doubleday.

Vogel, Morris J. 1980. *The Invention of the Modern Hospital: Boston, 1870–1930.* Chicago: University of Chicago Press.

Wallace, Edwin R. 1983. "Reflections on the Relationship Between Psychoanalysis and Christianity." *Pastoral Psychology* 31, 4 (Summer): 222–23.

Wallace, Edwin R., IV. 1984. "Freud and Religion: A History and Reappraisal." In *Psychoanalytic Study of Society,* vol. 10, ed. W. Muensterberger, L. B. Boyer, and S. Grolnick. Hillsdale, NJ: Analytic Press.

White, Andrew Dickson. 1896. *History of the Warfare of Science with Theology in Christendom.* (Reprint). New York: Free Press, 1965.

CHAPTER FIVE

AMERICAN SOUL-DOCTORING AT THE TURN OF THE CENTURY: TOWARD A PSYCHIATRY OF THE SPIRITUAL

Thomas Jobe, M.D.

The three decades between 1890 and 1920 witnessed a curious transformation in the development of medical psychology in both Europe and North America. An essentially European tradition of individualistically oriented, strongly secular, organicist medical psychology had grown up around the new profession of psychiatry since its inception in the mid nineteenth century (Hoeldtke 1967). This tradition had fought a battle with established religion and with popular forms of spiritualism that left it free to speculate about the causes of insanity without the trappings of a theologically tinged physiology. Yet, between 1890 and 1920, this medical psychology began to exchange its physiologically grounded associationistic psychology for speculation about the unconscious, subconscious, and subliminal mind. It was during this period that competing versions of the unconscious were advanced; some of them entertained questions about the ontology of the soul or of the spiritual. Some writers used older concepts such as "unconscious cerebration" but abandoned their hostility to theological ideas and incorporated notions of the spirit interacting with the unconscious mind. Henri Ellenberger has provided a solid analysis of the dependency of the dynamic psychologies developed by Pierre Janet, Theodore Flournoy, and Carl Gustav Jung upon the fascination with the occult that these authors had at the beginnings of their respective careers (Ellenberger 1970). Anton Muller has given us an excellent study of the inclusion of occult ideas into the systems of medical psychology of Charles Richet, Schrenk-Notzing, Enrico Morselli, and Cesare Lombroso (Muller 1967). J. P. Williams has exposed the points of connection between British medical psychology and the explosive field of psychical research between 1880 and 1900 (Williams 1985). Nathan Hale, Jr., has provided comparable documentation of American medical psychologists' interest in the spiritual at the turn of the century. He has argued that "American religious therapy," as William James referred to it, helped provide the content for the reception and early popularity of psychoanalysis in America (Hale 1971). Finally, Robert Powell has carried Hale's thesis further by examining the works of Edwin D. Starbuck, George B. Culten, James Hyslop, and others to show that the American scene was richly textured by theories that permitted subliminal contact with the spirit world—contact that could be used to explain a great range of psychopathology previously attributed to pathophysiological phenomena (Powell 1979).

This essay will retrace and largely confirm these previous researches into turn-of-the-century psychiatry of the spiritual. However, I will argue by way of addition to the Hale-Powell thesis that this tradition did not completely disappear but went underground and continued to assert itself in secularized versions, most notably in the unorthodox views of Trigant Burrow. The American founder of group psychotherapy and originator of phyloanalysis, Burrow has been largely ignored by both psychoanalysts and American psychiatrists, who have not been able to assimilate his complex and unorthodox ideas about society and human nature. Burrow went against the mainstream of American psychiatric thought by proposing a radical notion of human communality and the concept of the neurosis of normalcy. Despite the fact that Burrow repudiated religion early in his career and attempted to be rigorously scientific in his work, I will argue that his view of humanity is strongly influenced by his religious background and by the open dialogue between religion and psychiatry that characterized this era. My argument, however, will be largely to show the remarkable analogy between his ideas and the spiritual anthropology of Saint Augustine. To prepare for my argument concerning the Augustinian influences upon Burrow, I will discuss the ideas of the Canadian psychiatrist Richard Maurice Bucke (1837–1900). In his concise biography of Bucke, S. E. D. Shortt argues that the concept of the unconscious provided late-Victorian alienists the only alternative to a rigidly deterministic hereditarian view of insanity (Shortt 1986). Looking back from the present, the concept of the unconscious carries with it either the Victorian idea of counter-will or the Freudian notion of rigid determinism. What is missing is the "liminal" view that Shortt and Powell have uncovered in the works of Bucke, Hyslop, Myers, and others. This view of a plastic substance that may interact with spirits or molecules is further secularized in Burrow's concept of phylum as the embodiment of consciousness.

The emergence of psychiatry as a medical specialty in the 1840s and 1850s in Europe and America coincided with the gradual abandonment of, and development of hostility toward, therapies that relied upon persuasion, suggestion, and other psychological interventions. Thus, mesmerism, phrenology, phenomesmerism, neurypnology, and later hypnosis, and even moral therapy were all attacked, abandoned, or retained only as ways to demonstrate psychopathology, not as viable therapies. The reason for this attack, I believe, was to distinguish clearly the new medical specialty from traditional, largely religious, approaches to the psyche, specifically from the cure of souls and faith healing, and to create the strongest scientific image for the new specialty as akin to medicine in general. This combination of factors led to the so-called somatic style of theory and therapeusis that dominated the last quarter of the nineteenth century. This somatic style required a strong allegiance to physiological principles for the explanations of insanity and a preoccupation with speculations concerning brain function.

Key to the establishment of secular psychiatry's priority over religious views of psychopathology was the attack on mid-nineteenth-century spiritualism. The advocates of the physical manifestations of the spirit world and the practitioners of the arts of parapsychology proved a great embarrassment to established religion. Spiritualism was viewed alternatively as a species of religious enthusiasm, heresy, superstition, charlatanry, or heterodox sectarianism by Protestants and Catholics alike. The new medical psychologists or psychiatrists found a perfect platform for discrediting spiritualism in their new physiological theories of the origin of hallucinations and delusions. The psychiatrists themselves were almost entirely devout churchmen and opponents of philosophic materialism, and so they found themselves in the unusual position of advancing both their new science and their personal faith by attacking spiritualism.

Typical of the style of the "medical materialists'" later attack of the 1870s is a work by William W. Ireland, M.D., entitled *The Blot upon the Brain: Studies in History and Psychology,* published in 1885. In this work, Ireland, a prominent asylum superintendent in Scotland and close associate of Dr. Clauston of the Royal Asylum at Morningside, and Dr. Grierson of the Roxburgh District Asylum ranks the hallucinations of Mohammed and Luther with those of Caligula, Heliogabalus, Ivan the Terrible, Paul of Russia, and Francis Xavier, not to mention the delusions that characterized the "hereditary neurosis" of the Royal Family of Spain. Ireland seemed to consider Luther's preoccupation with the devil as particularly injurious to the development of an enlightened view of mental illness. Thus he quotes Luther's *Table Talk* extensively as evidence of the reformer's delusive and hallucinatory encounters with the devil and how these encounters impaired Luther's understanding of science. Thus, "idiots, the lame, the blind, the dumb are men in whom devils have established themselves; and all the physicians who heal those infirmities as though they proceeded from natural causes, are ignorant blockheads who know nothing about the power of the demon" (Ireland 1885, 52). Luther's *Table Talk* continued to excite pathographical attention, even among those who abandoned the somatic style, as is evidenced by the psychoanalytic treatment connecting Luther's demonic scatology to the anality of infantile sexuality. In fact, Norman O. Brown, in his work, *Life against Death: The Psychoanalytic Meaning of History,* published in 1959, goes so far as to state that "The Devil is a middle term connecting Protestantism and anality" (Brown 1959, 230).

Because of the popularity of Ireland's work, in 1889 he published a sequel entitled *Through the Ivory Gate: Studies in Psychology and History.* This work provided a detailed account of the life and writings of Emmanuel Swedenborg (1688–1771), the founder of Swedenborgianism, a religion with a scientistic framework, not dissimilar to the views of Gustav Fechner's psychophysics of the mid-nineteenth century. Ireland concluded that one should "look in Swedenborg's case for the symptoms of the mania of grandeur and of the mania of persecution. Here, we must bear in mind how much he transferred his thoughts and interests to a world of his own fancy and how much he had withdrawn from them the ways of ordinary men. In his claim to direct intercourse with the Divine Being, we find the loftiest delusion of grandeur, and in his complaints of "being infested for whole days by wicked spirits," we recognize the delusions of persecution (Ireland 1885, 129). But even Ireland noted the contradiction between his diagnosis and Swedenborg's actual behavior. To handle this problem, a physiological concept resolved the matter in a way characteristic of the somatic style. "It is surprising that through such strange experiences, Swedenborg should have preserved so much serenity of disposition and displayed in many things so much sagacity of thought. This would imply that the higher centers of the brain were less affected than the lower, which is the rule in what is called delusional insanity" (Ireland 1889, 129).

A variant of the pathographical tradition in which a religious phenomenon is reduced to a case of delusional insanity is the mass delusion or mass hysteria concept applied to those who followed a religious leader. A case in point can be found in William A. Hammond's work, *Spiritualism and Allied Causes and Conditions of Nervous Derangement,* published in 1876. In this work, Hammond attributes John Wesley's extraordinary success to his capacity to hypnotize or otherwise manipulate groups of women inclined to hysteria. In describing the effect of Wesley's preaching, Hammond concludes that

> hysteria from any other cause is marked by exactly such phenomena—the emotional disturbance, the falling, the loss of consciousness, the spasms, convulsions, coma—are all so many symptoms which physicians see every day arise from very different factors than the 'spirit of God.'.
>
> But the relations of hysteria to religion have never been more distinctly shown than in the fact that women under its influence have been able to gather numerous followers and actually to originate new religious faiths of such preposterous tenets and practices as to inevitably lead to

the conclusion that the adherents are either fools or knaves. (Hammond 1876, 239)

Michael Clark, in his article "The Rejection of Psychological Approaches to Mental Disorders in Late 19th Century British Psychiatry," articulated the essence of the problem when he concluded that psychiatrists of the somatic style perceived psychological techniques as essentially immoral:

> Since mental disorder was conceived psycho-physiologically as a lapse from a dualistic or parallelist norm of physical and mental health, and psychologically as a state of dangerous moral irresponsibility, not only were psychopathological phenomena regarded as by definition inaccessible to rational scientific explanation, but also treatment was envisaged exclusively in terms of the restoration of this norm of health and with it, the patient's capacity for exercising individual responsibility. The medical treatment of mental disorder was to consist almost solely in the relief of intercurrent physical disorders and the "moral" treatment in the repression of selfish instincts and emotions and the cultivation of more "altruistic" or "social" sentiments—that is, in the enhancement of the voluntary power of responsible self-determination; the discouragement of introversion and self-absorption; and the encouragement of a less subjective, more extroverted attitude toward external reality." (Clark 1981, 301)

This attitude, which shunned introversion to focus on the clear light of day, was consonant with the muscular Christianity and ministerial manliness of the late-nineteenth-century pastoral theology. How then did this attack on spiritualism and psychological approaches to therapy turn into its opposite, namely, the development of a psychiatry of the spirit? In the first place, none of the "medical materialists" ever substantially altered their views on spiritualism. Rather, those who were developing toward a nonreductionistic orientation from the start were given encouragement by the change in intellectual climate. As one of the new spiritual psychiatrists, R. Osgood Mason, Fellow of the New York Academy of Medicine, expressed it in his book, *Telepathy and the Subliminal Self* (1987):

> And first, in August, 1874, twenty-two years ago, at the moment when the materialistic school was at the height of its influence, both the scientific and religious world were brought to a momentary standstill—like a ship under full headway suddenly struck by a tidal wave—when one of the most eminent scientific men of his time [Tyndall], standing in his place as president of the foremost scientific association in the world, spoke as follows: "Abandoning all disguise, true confession which I feel bound to make before you is that I prolong the vision backward across the boundary of experimental evidence and discover . . . the promise and

potency of every form of life." On that day the taproot of materialism was wounded, and materialism itself has been an invalid of increasing languor and desuetude ever since. (Mason 1897, 313)

Mason then proceeded to praise the writing of Swedenborg as an extraordinary example "of the wonderful work of the subliminal self" (Mason 1897, 322). Other influences that must have encouraged those inclined to develop and publish their views on the spiritual from a medical-psychological point of view were the philosophic idealism of William James's *Varieties of Religious Experience* (1902) and his interest in the paranormal; the establishment of the London Society for Psychical Research; the publication of *Human Personality* (1903) by Frederic W. H. Myers, the theoretician of the subliminal self, and the publication of J. Milne Bromwell's *Hypnotism* (1903), which brought into vogue the use of a spiritual diagnosis of symptoms thought to be purely psychopathological.

Another factor that contributed to this transformation was the rise in respectability of spiritualism through its institutionalization as the new science of psychic research (Hyslop 1919). Critical methodologies for such studies were developed. Thus, James H. Hyslop established his American Institute for Scientific Research with two sections, the American Society for Psychical Research and the Abnormal Psychology Section, which would devote itself to "functional melancholia and vicarious or sympathetic mental aberrations; neurasthenia and psychasthenia; hysteria and hystero-epilepsy; obsessions, fixed ideas or monomanias; phobias; delusions; alcoholism; and all functional troubles that may ultimately be made to yield to the various forms of suggestions" (Hyslop 1907). The popularity of spiritualism or psychical research—or the paranormal, as it was beginning to be called—was evident in the popularity of works like Frank Podmore's *Is Communication with the Spirit World an Established Fact?* (1903), and his *Mesmerism and Christian Science, Modern Spiritualism* (1902), and *The Newer Spiritualism* (1910). These works anticipated Sir Arthur Conan Doyle's *History of Spiritualism* (1926).

William James would complain to the Swiss psychologist Theodore Flournoy that Freud had "condemned the American religious therapy (which has such extensive results) as very 'dangerous because so unscientific.' Bah!" (Hale 1971, 229). In the vanguard of this "American religious therapy" milieu was the Emmanuel movement. The founder of the movement, Reverend Elwood Worcester of the Emmanuel Church in Boston, critiqued the strenuous life of muscular Christians and sounded the alarm of a coming epidemic of neurasthenia. As E. Brooks Holifield pointed out, the Emmanuel movement was "the first serious effort to transform the cure of souls in light of the new psychology and theology." Beginning in

1905, it spread from Boston to the "Congregational clergy in Baltimore, Presbyterian in Cleveland, Unitarian in Portland, Baptist in Chicago, and Universalist in Brookline, Massachusetts" (Holifield 1983, 201). Holifield divides the relationship between the cure of souls and the new psychology and psychiatry into three phases: a pre–World War I phase, when psychotherapy was helped and promoted by Protestant pastoral theology; a post–World War I phase, when academic, military, and industrial psychology established themselves and began to dominate pastoral theology with concepts of adjustment; and finally, a post–World War II phase in which clinical psychiatry added its established strengths to new psychologies of self-realization, thus dominating pastoral psychology and theology with new metaphors of self-realization.

While it has been acknowledged that the Emmanuel movement strongly promoted the development of psychotherapy and the acceptance of psychoanalysis in the United States, little attention has been devoted to the actual doctrines, especially to the ideas of Isador Coriat, an early psychoanalyst at Worcester State Hospital, who coauthored the bible of the Emmanuel movement, *Religion and Medicine* (1909). Worcester, McComb, and Coriat explained their concern with functional nervous disorders as follows:

> An attack of typhoid fever may spring from no moral cause and it may have no perceptible influence upon character, but neurasthenia, hysteria, psychasthenia, hypochondria, alcoholism, etc. are affections of the personality. They spring from moral causes and they produce moral effects. In this domain the beneficent action of drugs and medicines is extremely limited, and the personality of the physician is everything. (Worcester, McComb, and Coriat 1908, 5)

While it is impossible to separate the views of Coriat from those of Worcester and McComb, it is probable that several of the points relating to the person of the physician belong to him. For example,

> Dr. Weir Mitchell, who is the teacher of us all, has proved the great value of rest, isolation, and abundant nourishment in a brilliant series of cures extending over a long term of years. But, on the other hand, Dr. Mitchell's patients owe even more to their contact with his remarkable personality, as is proved by the fact that his rest cure, valuable as it is in itself, in other hands, fails to produce the astonishing results that are associated with his name. (Worcester, McComb, and Coriat 1908, 50)

The message clearly given to the medical profession is that the active agent in all "so-called moral recoveries is faith." This faith must be instilled in the patient by the physician. Dr. A. T. Schofield is cited to the effect that "when the eye of the patient meets the eye of the physician, the cure begins if it is likely to take place" (Worcester, McComb, and Coriat 1908, 51). Besides Schofield, the authors rely heavily upon Myers, Bramwell, and Sidis. The authors predict a revolution in medicine and psychiatry in which "the next great development of medicine will be along psychical lines" (Worcester, McComb, and Coriat 1908, 52). Furthermore, the authors attack Charcot and Janet and, by implication, Freud for seeing the unconscious as exclusively pathological. They praise, on the other hand, those authors like Liebault, Bernheim, Forel, Bramwell, Moll, and Lloyd for developing notions of the unconscious or subconscious that have positive powers and spiritual properties. They conclude that authors like Charcot and Janet had very few patient contacts compared to the thousands of patients treated, for example, by the Nancy school. This larger induction of the facts, the authors believed, led to the proper discovery of linkage between the phenomenon of faith and the unconscious.

The linkage between faith, the spiritual or spirit, and the unconscious was reasonably developed in the writings of Alfred T. Schofield, M.D. While Schofield borrowed heavily from Myers, he developed his own system for connecting consciousness, the subconscious, and spirit in a continuum. Schofield critiqued unidimensional concepts of the subconscious in which conscious life is graded into the level of matter of the nervous system. He argued that the life of the spirit, or the soul, is also largely subconscious and has to be made conscious by effort—i.e., meditation, prayer—just as traumatic memories come to light only by diligent effort:

> Indeed, as these invisible rays extend indefinitely on both sides of the visible spectrum (in the radiation spectrum), so we may say that the mind includes not only the visible or conscious part, and what we have termed the subconscious, that lies below or at the (infra)red end, but the supra-conscious mind that lies beyond at the other end—all those regions of higher soul and spirit life, of which we are only at times vaguely conscious, but which always exist, and link us on to eternal verities, on the one side as surely as the subconscious mind links us to the body on the other. (Schofield 1901, 94)

Schofield argued that, just as thoughts best surface out of the subconscious when the activity of the conscious mind is momentarily paralyzed, so spiritual influences are best developed when the conscious mind is inactive.

> The Spirit of God is said to dwell in believers, and yet, as we have seen, His presence is not the subject of direct consciousness. We would include, therefore, in the supra-conscious, all such spiritual ideas, together with conscience—the voice of God—which is surely a half-conscious

faculty. Moreover, the supra-conscious, like the sub-conscious, is, as we have said, best apprehended when the conscious mind is not active. Visions, meditations, prayers and even dreams have been undoubtedly occasions of spiritual revelations. . . . (Schofield 1901, 95)

Dreams should be scrutinized for their encoding of spiritual messages as well as, and in conjunction with, their instinctive or subconscious ones. For Schofield, the *unconscious* encompassed both the supraconscious and its linkage with God and the subconscious and its linkage with the body.

> The truth apparently is that the mind as a whole is in an unconscious state, but that its middle registers, excluding the highest spiritual and lowest physical manifestations, are fitfully illuminated in varying degree by consciousness; and that it is to this illuminated part of the dial that the word "mind," which rightly appertains to the whole, has been limited. (Schofield 1901, 95)

A more serious plunge into the psychiatry of the spirit than the work of Coriat and Schofield is to be found in the work of the Canadian psychiatrist Richard Maurice Bucke (1837–1902), who spent most of his professional career as medical superintendent of the Asylum for the Insane at London, Ontario. Bucke's major work, *Cosmic Consciousness* (1901), was a great success and went through numerous printings during the 1920s. Bucke died a year after its publication and so did not live to enjoy its reputation, but he did receive a letter from William James who gave him encouragement with these words:

> I believe that you have brought this kind of consciousness "home" to the attention of students of human nature in a way so definite and unescapable that it will be impossible henceforward to overlook it or ignore it. . . . But my total reaction on your book, my dear Sir, is that it is an addition to psychology of first rate importance, and that you are a benefactor to us all. (Bucke 1901, Preface)

Bucke's notion of the cosmic consciousness developed in relation to his study of the sympathetic nervous system. The first theoretical discussion that linked the function of the sympathetic nervous system to higher levels of consciousness can be found in the second of Bucke's articles for the *American Journal of Insanity*, published in 1877. In that article, Bucke argued that all mental contents can be divided into four moral states or affections—faith, love, fear, and hate—and into an infinite number of conceptions and perceptions. Each experience is a complex combination of moral states and cognitive states. To Bucke, faith was synonymous with trust, confidence, and courage, but clearly different from belief, which involved complex cognitive components. According to Bucke,

The faith which substitutes the higher belief for the lower is the most valuable of all our possessions. It is through this association that belief came to be considered so important; since man having a certain grade of faith associated with a certain belief easily fell into the error that the belief was the cause of the faith—was necessary to it—was even the faith itself, though a greater error than this, and in some senses a more injurious one to humanity, could scarcely be imagined. (Bucke 1878, 233)

By an extensive statistical study, Bucke tried to quantify the amount of faith different persons possessed. From his physiological study he concluded that the sympathetic nervous system was the seat of the moral affections and that the brain contained the cognitive and appetitive functions. He also concluded that a healthy sympathetic nervous system accounted more than any other organ for longevity. Therefore there must be a correlation between moral excellence and longevity. Bucke found just such a correlation, particularly when he used the Jewish faith as the criterion of moral excellence. Though nominally Christian, Bucke argued that

No one, I fancy, will dispute, if he is capable of understanding what he is talking about, that the race which produced the law-givers, psalmists, prophets and finally, Jesus, himself, was and is the race which possessed and possesses the supreme moral nature of this planet. (Bucke 1878, 248)

Since the demographic studies of the times, cited by Bucke, clearly gave the Jews a lifespan six to eight years longer than that of non-Jewish Europeans, Bucke felt he had further confirmation of his hypothesis.

Bucke extended his study of the epidemiology of old age and discovered that longevity is not only a property of Jews but also of great men, married people, and women. He took this as further confirmation for his hypothesis that moral excellence is correlated with longevity. First, women live longer than men generally because they have greater endowments of love and faith. This is clearly shown, Bucke argued, in their "power of endurance and . . . greater patience under suffering and ill-usage" (Bucke 1878, 250). Married persons live longer than nonmarried persons because marriage indicates, according to Bucke, a higher capacity for love. Finally, great men live longer on the average, not because the time required to attain their achievements preselects them, but because they have the largeness of spirit implied by greater faith in their creative potential. Thus Bucke concludes: "The fact is that the only thing that can be shown, as far as I can see, to be common to Jews, great men, married people, and women—as against non-Jews, ordinary men, unmarried people, and men—is a higher moral nature" (Bucke 1878, 252).

These epidemiologic and physiologic studies provided the background for Bucke's theory of consciousness. His observation of mental disorder led him to the view that psychosis occurred more frequently in rapidly evolving organisms, and that man's rapid evolution led to an incidence of insanity seemingly greater than in any other animal. Furthermore, higher levels of consciousness were subject to more profound regressions. The most recently acquired faculty from an evolutionary standpoint would be the most sensitive to dysfunction and breakdown. It is for this reason that man's self-consciousness, while almost infinitely above the animal level of simple consciousness, is subject to marked degradation.

Bucke argued that self-consciousness was the uniquely human faculty and that it evolved only a few hundred thousand years ago. It is characterized by an awareness of personal identity and an intersubjective understanding of other persons. It is constituted by the moral affections, particularly love, hate, and fear. Faith, on the other hand, has continued to evolve, and the human race is experiencing instances of an evolutionarily further advanced stage termed cosmic consciousness. This kind of consciousness is radically different from self-consciousness, and it bursts through as a kind of illumination or mystical experience in those capable of it, usually in the early thirties when such persons are at the peak of their careers.

Cosmic consciousness can only be studied empirically, according to Bucke, by direct experience of it or by the study of those who have experienced it. Eventually, Bucke envisioned, the whole human race will evolve to a point where cosmic consciousness will be as commonplace as self-consciousness is now. Here is Bucke's vision of a world inhabited by a race of humanity, each and every member of which is endowed with cosmic consciousness.

> In contact with the flux of cosmic consciousness, all religions known and named today will be melted down. The human soul will be revolutionized. Religion will absolutely dominate the race. . . . The evidence of immortality will live in every heart, as sight in every eye. Doubt of God and of eternal life will be as impossible as is now doubt of [personal] existence; the evidence of each will be the same. Religion will govern every minute of every day of all life. . . . Each soul will feel and know itself to be immortal, will feel and know that the entire universe with all its good and with all its beauty is for it and belongs to it forever. The world peopled by men possessing cosmic consciousness will be as far removed from the world of to-day as this is from the world as it was before the advent of self-consciousness. (Bucke 1901, 5)

The fourth part of Bucke's work, *Cosmic Consciousness,* analyzes the experiences of persons who he felt had certain evidences of this highest form of awareness—in whom a sense of unity of all things, called the cosmic sense, was definitely present. They include Plotinus, Mohammed, Jacob Boehme, Jesus the Christ, Gautama the Buddha, William Blake, Walt Whitman, and Swedenborg. Interestingly, many of these had received extensive analysis for pathography at the hands of the "medical materialists" just twenty years earlier. Like James's *Varieties of Religious Experience*, Bucke's book also describes the experiences of approximately thirty unknown persons who experienced cosmic consciousness.

What happened to the psychiatry of the spirit after 1920? It apparently disappeared from the writings of psychiatrists. They turned to evolutionary theory and organismic biology to supply the underpinnings of psychiatric theory. This can be seen not only in the influence of Adolph Meyer (1866–1950), whose concept of "ergasia" provided a biological framework for schizophrenia, but in the efforts of psychoanalysts to establish a biological metapsychology more palatable than Freud's thanatos concept or death instinct. This biologizing was further fueled by the apparent success of insulin coma treatment, psychosurgery, and electroconvulsive shock therapy in the 1930s. Curiously, one psychiatrist of the 1920s–1940s, who was also very determined to establish the biological basis of psychopathology, represents at a deeper level the culmination of a psychiatry of the spirit but as an underground influence. This was the inventor of group therapy in American psychiatry, Trigant N. Burrow (1875–1950). Burrow remains an enigma in the history of American psychiatry because he rejected almost every basic assumption of his contemporaries. He found himself ostracized by his fellow psychoanalysts despite his early contributions to that field, and was rejected by men as influential as Adolph Meyer.

Yet Burrow founded an institute, The Lifwynn Foundation, to carry on his work and published several large volumes detailing his discoveries. On the surface it would appear to be the height of folly to assert that Burrow, who frequently debunked religion and who tried always to find empirical verification for his theories, could be an explorer of religious consciousness disguised by secular scientific language. In fact, despite the rejection of his ideas by the psychiatric community, Burrow was consistently admired for his scientific rigor, his caution, and his objectivity. The closest thing to a religion practiced by Burrow was indeed an apotheosis of science. But his ideas about human nature and the "social neurosis" are deeply informed by religious ideas, and I will argue that his entire system, though putatively pure biology, is actually a kind of biological model of the Augustinian theology to which he was exposed by his strongly Catholic upbringing. Despite his break with his mother's religion, Burrow remained devoted to the woman until her death. His letters to his mother, Anastasia Devereux Burrow, indicate that she was a true intellectual partner who shared in the development of Burrow's ideas, even after Burrow rejected the dogmas of the Roman Catholic Church soon after his graduation from Fordham University (Galt 1958).

Organized religion was, for Burrow, an accentuated version of the neurosis of normalcy, which he took upon himself to expose in every detail. This extensive quote gives an example of his mature ideas about religion:

> An overwhelming number of people build up entire systems of prejudice and pattern their lives in accordance with these systems. Indeed, to a far greater extent than we realize, people fashion their "God" out of the material of their own systematized prejudices. In their interrelational dissociation, they design their deity out of an arbitrary image of the parent and they like nothing better than to pin this fanciful label upon other people. I recall a patient—an unusually sensitive, intelligent woman—for whom the image she has fashioned of me had up to now proved an entirely adequate parent-surrogate. There was, however, just one reservation. But, "knowing me," she could not doubt that I would satisfy her affect-longing on this point, too. Only, as yet, she was not quite fully assured. Finally, she decided to settle the matter. "Dr. Burrow," she said, "there's one question I must ask you. Do you believe in God?" I replied wholeheartedly that I did not believe in anything else. Her face lighted with seraphic satisfaction for she wanted nothing to interfere with her liking for me. But on my adding that I could not guarantee that I believed in her God or in the personal God of anyone else, her face fell perceptibly. But I went on. I said that the concept of "God" is too generally fabricated out of the wishful yearnings of man's self-interested affects. I explained that the God of wishful hearsay and tradition is at variance with the principle of action and reaction, of cause and effect existing throughout the world of objective experience. I said that religion does not consist of an all-powerful parent; that what is needed in this disordered world is living in and by the principle of unity that abides alone in the prevailing order and consistency of the surrounding universe. (Burrow 1953, 161)

Burrow believed only in God, but his God was an objective unity between the outside physical universe and the communal life of mankind. For Burrow, the biological species essence of mankind constituted the essence of human nature. The individual's identity and willfulness, the affects that drive the self-seeking of the ego, are illusive and dangerous and the source of all discontents. The "I persona," the rightness of the individual, and the partitive affects that feed this system are the product of the *parencephalon* or the "neural areas whose function controls the partitive of paratonic pattern of tension" associated with conflict, strife, greed, and psychopathology. On the other hand, the phylic or species behavior of interrelational adaptation and unity are the product of the *orthencephalon,* "the functional areas of the cerebrum that regulate the organism's ortho-tonic pattern of tension as a whole" (Burrow 1953, 367). Similarly the *nomen* denotes the concrete consistency of mankind's organismic response to environmental phenomena, while the *numen* represents the "affecto-symbolic deflection superimposed upon man's primary feeling-reactions" that is conditioned by the self-aggrandizing, divisive "I persona" (Burrow 1953, 529). Burrow summarized his critique of the numenal in this state-ment:

> In the division within man's whole brain, there is division within his whole organism, within the whole motivation and behavior of man. It is because of this division in man that he seeks to find compensation in the fanciful unity of imaginal Gods rather than in the actuality of his own unitary organism and its continuity with the environment. Nor are those nations which in their autopathic strivings have set aside their Gods in favor of their own autopathic political State in any different pass. Their State is but another God. In his love of his imaginal Gods, man destroys himself, but he still continues to cherish and depend upon his Gods. We may not forget that Nazism is also a religion, that the massacre of St. Bartholomew was a religious ceremonial, that the crucifixion of Jesus was also the performance of a religious rite. Did they not rend their garments and cry: 'He hath spoken blasphemy'? Though through war after war, man pleads with his Gods for deliverance from Strife and bloodshed (and not infrequently both contestants plead with identical Gods), the Strife and the Gods and the pleading continue hand-in-hand without arousing in man any suspicion that all are of one texture, that the Strife, the Gods, and the pleading are of one piece with a conflict that is not outside man but within him. This is inevitable as long as man remains unaware that in apotheosing his many symbolic recourses to unity, he wholly misses the internal sense of the strength and solidarity of his own integrity as a phylum. (Burrow 1953, 333)

Burrow established his new science of phylobiology and phyloanalysis to explore the scientific basis of the species solidarity and how it becomes perverted by partitive affecto-symbolic processes. He traced the origin of this perversion to humanity's inability to tolerate the accentuated degree of self-awareness triggered by evolutionary advances in the development of consciousness. "To see ourselves as others see us" is the goal of this evolutionary advance, which brings persons into a higher level and inten-sity of group awareness and potential solidarity. But rather than realize this higher transcendent species awareness, in which each sees himself or herself *as* the collectivity sees them, mankind has caved into self-deception and misrepresentation of the self to be *more* than the collectivity sees. The "I persona" has emerged as a "king's-new-clothes" phenomenon. People are not strong enough to allow others to see them for what they are, so they conspire among themselves to create false selves or egos that provide the fundamental etiology of the neuroses. The normal self or "I persona" becomes the nidus of the social neurosis. The true God is the species collectivity in its organismic knowing of the individual. To turn away from this organismic species knowing is to turn away from God into sin or partitive affecto-symbolic processes. The creation of the "I persona" means a separation from the species essence and an intolerable and unbearable feeling of separateness and isolation. The creation of the false gods of traditional culture constitutes a desperate attempt to reestablish the organismic species unity, but now in a false, purely symbolic form, lacking the concrete feelings of solidarity. To quote Burrow's formulation of the organismic fall of mankind:

> The phyloorganism of men was split up into the knowing elements or social images constitutive of the "I persona" of each individual, as of each group, and the earth was accused in the symbolic division man had wrought. . . . In the intolerable dichotomy and conflict of his self-awareness—in his unbearable separateness as a person—man felt naked and alone and he sought to hide himself. He had forfeited his organismic security as a total entity in relation to the environment, and from now on man was repressed, secretive, divided, introverted; he was guilty and full of fear. In short, man was neurotic. Fanciful images had begun to replace factual reality. In his psychoneurosis, in his biologically insupportable isolation, man was driven to project the image of a larger Presence than his own. He was driven to compensate for the loss of his organism's bionomic integrity as a total functioning unit by conjuring the presence of a stronger, wiser Persona who, as an all-powerful parent, would henceforth counsel and protect him. . . . in his phylic plight, in his loss of a sense of species articulation, it is quite understandable that man should have employed this social numen to compensate for the absence of his organism's primary unity of motivation and behavior." (Burrow 1953, 297).

Burrow went a step further in his attempt to reveal the true God.

> I realize that whoever presumes to write objectively of Deity treads upon ticklish ground. . . . And so, while the theocratic affect-pretensions of the "I" persona undoubtedly merit thoughtful examination of the scientist, to attempt to bring to book these anomalous factors in man's adaptation is to appear to desecrate the age-old sanctuaries of our most sacred institutions. . . . However inept his digressions of fantasy, at heart man has been profoundly conscious of those cosmic motivations that underlie and integrate the processes of the phenomenal world. To some of us this universal order and harmony is all we know, all that we care to know

as God. And to the phylobiologist these unitary principles abide no less within the internal universe of man's own organism. (Burrow 1953, 298)

In the end, Burrow's God was never accepted by his psychiatric colleagues, who seemed to suspect all along that he was more concerned with pursuing his biotheology than his studies of psychopathology.

Despite the criticism he received from many sources, Burrow had a very extensive correspondence. He never doubted that his experiments would bear out the truth of his claims regarding the organismic unity of human consciousness. Each step along the road of this thought was shadowed by some empirical demonstrations, and it is to these that we now must turn. Before entering medicine, Burrow earned a Ph.D. in psychology at Johns Hopkins University under George Stratton. The subject of his dissertation provided him the empirical foundations of his later work. He studied visual attention and learned the techniques necessary to master eye tracking (Burrow 1909).

The advance in the technology of eye-movement tracking provided Burrow with greater and greater precision in his attempt to discover the physiological basis of different kinds of awareness. A second area of discovery was the discrimination of the two forms of consciousness that were to become the basis of his system. This occurred after Burrow had established himself as a successful practitioner of psychoanalysis and had written several papers in the orthodox Freudian mode. The discovery came when he allowed one of his analysands, Clarence Shields, to reciprocate in the analytic situation and analyze him. The two coanalyzed each other. Burrow admits that many patients had asked him to do this before Shields, but he had himself been analyzed, and he treated the request as a resistance. Burrow described what happened:

> What calls for more vital emphasis, however, is the fact that along with the deepening, if reluctant, realization of my intolerance of self-defeat, there came gradually to me the realization that my analyst, in changing places with me, had merely shifted to the authoritarian vantage ground I had myself relinquished and that the situation had remained essentially unaltered still. (Burrow 1927, xv–xvii)

It was out of this disappointment with the reversal of the analytic situation that Burrow began to focus on the "authoritarian," "I'm right" attitude as the source of conflict in human relations. Burrow and Shields entered a new phase in their dialogue. They sought to trace within each other the sources of each other's "authoritarianism and autocracy toward the other." From these investigations, which were later broadened to include group members, Burrow discovered that the autocratic attitude was so ingrained as to be a kind of human awareness, the normal everyday consciousness, which he labeled "ditentive" awareness. Ditentive consciousness was found to be associated with muscular tensions in the body, and the whole system represented the process necessary for one person to establish a personal identity "different" from all others. One's self-esteem appeared to be totally dependent upon this ditentive way of relating and interacting with others. It was an evaluative, distancing attitude of specialness and superiority that led persons to get into "ego" battles and try to depreciate each other as though the exaltation of the one depended upon the deprecation of the other. Yet, Burrow and Shields kept at it and after years of effort found that they had entered into a mode of relating altogether different from the ditentive mode. This they called the *cotentive* mode of awareness. In this mode they were not defensive toward each other, nor did they take each other for granted; they were much less tense and seemed to anticipate what the other was thinking. They could react to one another without conscious anticipation. They had discovered a bond of solidarity unmixed with familial affective bonds. Much of Burrow's career went into trying to scientifically verify the existence of cotentive consciousness, which he felt was the source of species awareness. Here are the results of Burrow's researches:

> There were: (1) A marked and consistent slowing of the respiratory rate in cotention as compared with ditention, the decrease in the rate in cotention being accompanied by an increase in the thoracic and abdominal amplitude of the respiratory movements. (2) A reduction in number of eye movements in cotention. . . . (3) A characteristic and consistent alteration in brain wave pattern (EEG) during cotention. This alteration consists of a reduction in alpha-time and a general diminution in cortical potential, which is most pronounced in the motor regions. (Burrow 1953, 395)

In the state of cotentive consciousness, each could relate smoothly with the other and say things that might otherwise be hurtful to the self-esteem of the "I" persona. Each could see himself from the other's point of view without injury or self-deception. The bond of phylic solidarity was a kind of love stripped of the grandiosity and posturing so often inseparable from human loving. It was a love that did not come from the individual but from the species or phyloorganism through the individual.

Burrow's fundamental insight was that man's natural self-love reaches its fulfillment as love of the species or phylum and that love of the phylum ensures the love of the neighbor and the self in "equilibrium." The psychoneuroses are due to self-love that has torn itself free of the phylum and been directed falsely toward a symbolic unity of the self and other rather than an actual unity. But without reflection and nourishment from the phylum, this love leads to pain, loneliness, and alienation and eventually turns into destructive energy as a will to dominate others. The deep religious metaphor in this view of human nature is clearly evident; the question rather is to pinpoint the exact source of religious inspiration.

The clearest analogy to Burrow's view of human nature comes from his own religious tradition. We need look no further than Augustine's *caritas* concept. Like Origen before him, Augustine tries to link together the Christian Agape concept with the Greek philosophic concept of divine love. As Nygren articulates, in Agape God loves man in his evil state in an unmotivated way (the election and incarnation depending upon God's inexplicable expansion of essence to touch the creature without any will or act on the creature's part). In the Greek concept of divine love, Eros, man seeks perfection out of the need of carnal presence and seeks to transcend out of will and motivation to a higher participation in spiritual presence of the Deity. In Augustine, *amor sui* ultimately becomes *amor Dei* but only after a period of anguished pursuit of substitutes that always prove unsatisfying and destructive to the life of the spirit. Thus, *amor sui* that is directed to objects other than God becomes *cupiditas* but when directed to God becomes *caritas*. Since man is radically dependent upon God, loving God is loving oneself as one's true self. Not realizing the radical dependence of one's nature upon God leads to loving of a substitute, namely, an earthly symbol or token of God. Therefore to truly love oneself is not to love oneself but to love only God, while not loving God is necessarily falsely loving oneself. In Augustine's words,

> For in some inexplicable way, it is a fact that he who loves himself and not God, does not love himself; and whoever loves God and not himself, does love himself. For he who cannot live of himself, will certainly die if he loves himself. Consequently, he does not love himself who loves himself to his own loss of life. But when anyone loves Him by whom he lives, he loves the more by not loving himself since he ceases to love himself in order to love Him by whom he lives. (Nygren 1969, 543)

For Augustine *caritas* always contains Eros since love is always motivated and acquisitive whether human or God's. God's love, like human love, is ultimately self-directed in that God loves Himself *in* his creature, not the creature's sinfulness per se. But Agape is also present since one's loving of oneself is kindled by God's loving of Himself in the creature, such that the person is not really loving the self after all, but God in the self. The upward movement of Eros and the downward movement of Agape meet in *caritas* that is itself most perfectly exemplified as love to neighbor. Love to neighbor becomes the test of whether *amor sui* is really *amor Dei* because no man truly loves another but loves God *in* the other. In other words, self-love can easily masquerade as love of God because of the ethereal nature of God's presence. It is much harder to pretend to love God in loving the neighbor because devotion to the neighbor is something of a trial at the outset and requires more sacrifice than an inwardly directed pretense of the love of God.

Let us now make some substitutions of terms to compare Burrow's system. Burrow's God is the principle of order embodied in the phyloorganism of the human species. He said he believed *only* in God. The human individual is radically dependent upon the phylum, so much so that the source of evil (neurosis) derives from a false apprehension of independence due to the evolutionarily recent capacity for symbolic manipulation (freedom). Because of this experience of freedom, natural human self-love uncouples from the phylum and is directed reflexively to the "I" persona. This corresponds to *cupiditas* in Augustine.

Ditentive consciousness is love directed to an object other than the phylum (God) and never finds satisfaction but always tension and conflict. Since the "I" persona is never fully gratified by its purely symbolic unities—such as nation, social group, traditional religion—there is continual movement back to the phylum (God). The breakthrough to cotentive consciousness is a final resting of affect in its true object, the phylum, where gratification is ultimately achieved. In other words, man loves himself but not his individuality (I persona); rather man loves the phylum in the self. Also the phylum loves itself in and through each individual. Thus individuals need to find the phylum in themselves while the phylum finds itself in them. There is a movement from the individual toward the phylum and from the phylum toward the individual, and that is why therapy should take place in groups, not dyads. The presence of several persons brings to pass the phylum that, as a group process, seeks out itself in each individual.

The group process that is phyloanalysis is always more than the sum of those individuals present. Cotentive consciousness represents the point at which the individual participates lovingly in the phylum in a concrete, gratifying way reminiscent of the Agape love feast of the early Christians. Much like the public confession of sins practiced by the early Church, the members of Burrow's group confess the sins of their respective "I" personae in common. Burrow's term for the presencing of the phylum is *solidarity,* a term we can interpret to be essentially identical to *caritas*.

What are the external evidences for this interpretation of Burrow's system? It is clear from Burrow's published letters that he was not consciously appropriating religious concepts. There was, however, a peculiar defense of Jesus and an admiration for him as a "thinker." In his numerous attacks upon religion, he frequently mentioned that Jesus had hit upon a hidden truth. For example, in a letter to a former patient dated March 26, 1928, he discussed religion in the following manner:

It is to make an image called "God" and place it in the sky, rather than make the true principle of life the internal organic integrity of man himself. Christ, the real religionist, knew better: "The kingdom of heaven is within you," he said. The pseudoreligionists, so many of them so-called Christians, look everywhere else than within them for the peace that surpasseth understanding. But still consulting their "understanding," they lose all touch with the clear heart of man and the principle uniting him in a common race life, and pursue superstitious images of good and bad. (Galt 1958, 202)

Burrow never used the word *love* in his scientific writing, but he seemed to be writing about love on every page. In a letter dated September 9, 1927, Burrow responded to the writer D. H. Lawrence, who had apparently called him to task on this very point: "But isn't it with religion as it is with love—love that cannot endure to hear its own name so much as whispered? 'They put their finger on their lip, the powers above. They love but name not love.' What man can adore and call it adoring" (Galt 1958, 186). With regard to his scientific writing style, Burrow admitted to Lawrence, "It *is* awful, and you have diagnosed me in no imprecise manner. The as yet unresolved conflict within me between science and art is the thunderous noise one hears on very page as I come laboring along" (Galt 1958, 187). The awkwardness of Burrow's style evidenced his internal struggle to avoid manifesting the deep artistic and religious impulses that threatened to emerge every time he took pen in hand. His letters are more natural and at the same time more expressive of these impulses.

Burrow represents the culmination of the psychiatry of the spirit; he supplied an entirely secularized scientific "theology" shot through with deep religious metaphors. We can define three phases. In phase one, psychiatrists took a strongly physiological and apparently materialist view of psychopathology to fight both religiously inspired therapeutics and nontraditional spiritualism. This was the competitive phase when psychiatry was fighting for its professional existence as a legitimate clinical science (1840–80). Phase two began in the late 1880s and lasted until the 1920s, when psychiatry, aided by psychoanalysis, became psychological and saw itself as part of a continuum with religious experience. Here cooperation with religiously inspired therapies was the order of the day. The view that consciousness constituted a continuum with "spiritual" life or phenomena was very popular among psychiatrists, who were often willing to entertain the possibility that spiritual disorders ranked within the broad spectrum of psychopathology. After the First World War, psychiatry, along with academic psychology, entered a phase of rapid growth, only to be drastically accelerated after the Second World War. Because of the dominance of putatively scientific ideas in the growth process, formal and thematic involvement with theology ceased; nevertheless, theological ideas continued to have an undercurrent influence in the "depth" part of the many depth psychologies that flourished in the twentieth century (Browning 1987).

References

Brown, N. O. 1959. *Life Against Death: The Psychoanalytic Meaning of History.* New York: Vintage Books.

Browning, D. S. 1987. *Religious Thought and Modern Psychologies.* Philadelphia: Fortress Press.

Bucke, R. M. 1901. *Cosmic Consciousness.* (Reprint) New York: Sutton, 1969.

———. 1878. "The Moral Nature of the Great Sympathetic." *American Journal of Insanity* 35, 11.

Burrow, Trigant. 1909. *The Determination of the Position of a Momentary Impression in the Temporal Course of a Moving Visual Impression.* Lancaster, PA: Review Publishing Co.

———. 1927. *The Social Basis of Consciousness.* London: K. Paul, Trench, Trudner and Co.

———. 1953. *Science and Man's Behavior: The Contribution of Phylobiology.* New York: Philosophical Library.

Clark, M. 1981. "The Rejection of Psychological Approaches to Mental Disorder in Late Nineteenth-Century British Psychiatry." In *Madhouses, Mad Doctors, and Madmen: The Social History of Psychiatry in the Victorian Era,* ed. A. Scull. Philadelphia: University of Pennsylvania Press.

Ellenberger, H. F. 1970. *The Discovery of the Unconscious: The History and Evolution of Dynamic Psychiatry.* New York: Basic Books.

Galt, W. 1958. *A Search for Man's Sanity: The Selected Letters of Trigant Burrow.* New York: Oxford University Press.

Hale, Nathan, Jr. 1971. *Freud and the Americans: The Beginnings of Psychoanalysis in the United States, 1876–1917.* New York: Oxford University Press.

Hammond, W. A. 1876. *Spiritualism and Allied Causes and Conditions of Nervous Derangement.* New York: G. P. Putnam's Sons.

Hoeldtke, R. 1967. "The History of Associationism and British Medical Psychology." *Medical History* 11 (January): 46–65.

Holifield, E. B. 1983. *A History of Pastoral Care in America: From Salvation to Self-Realization.* Nashville, TN: Abington Press.

Hyslop, J. H. 1907. "Objects of the Institute." *Journal of the American Society for Psychical Research,* (January).

———. 1919. *Contact with the Other World: The Latest Evidence as to Communication With the Dead.* New York: Century Co.

Ireland, W. W. 1885. *The Blot upon the Brain: Studies in History and Psychology.* New York: G. P. Putnam's Sons.

———. 1889. *Through the Ivory Gate: Studies in Psychology and History.* New York: G. P. Putnam's Sons.

Mason, Osgood. 1897. *Telepathy and the Subliminal Self: An Account of Recent Investigations Regarding Hypnotism, Automatism, Dreams, Phantasms, and Related Phenomena.* New York: Henry Holt and Co.

Muller, Anton. 1967. *Medizin und Okkultismus um die Jahrhundert wende (1875–1925)*. Zurich: Juris Druck.

Nygren, A. 1969. *Agape and Eros, Parts I & II*, trans. P. S. Watson. New York: Harper and Row.

Powell, R. C. 1979. "The 'Subliminal' versus the 'Subconscious' in the American Acceptance of Psychoanalysis, 1906–1910." *Journal of the History of Behavioral Science* 15: 155–65.

Schofield, Alfred. 1901. *The Unconscious Mind*. New York: Funk and Wagnalls.

Shortt, S. E. D. 1986. *Victorian Lunacy: Richard M. Bucke and the Practice of Late Nineteenth-Century Psychiatry*. London: Cambridge University Press.

Williams, J. P. 1985. "Psychical Research and Psychiatry in late Victorian Britain; Trance as Ecstasy or Trance as Insanity." *The Anatomy of Madness: Essays in the History of Psychiatry*, Vol. 1, ed. W. F. Bynum, R. Porter and M. Shephard, 233–54. London: Tavistock Publications.

Worcester, E., S. McComb, and I. Coriat. 1908. *Religion and Medicine: The Moral Control of Nervous Disorders*. New York: Moffat, Yard and Co.

PART TWO

Ethical Issues and Psychiatry

CHAPTER SIX

BETWEEN THE PRIESTLY DOCTOR AND THE MYTH OF MENTAL ILLNESS

Ian S. Evison, D.Min.

What should be the relationship of psychiatry to social ethics? Should psychiatry seek to be value neutral, to base its judgments wholly on scientific criteria? Or should psychiatry—must psychiatry inevitably—seek to promote a determinate view of the good person and the good society? Psychiatry has struggled with this problem since the beginnings of the profession in North America in the nineteenth century. Psychiatry has found itself involved in each great social conflict in the past century and a half. Before the Civil War, psychiatrists discussed whether *drapetomania,* slaves running away from their masters, was a mental disease (Cartwright 1851, 707). During the suffragette campaigns of the late nineteenth century, psychiatrists discussed whether the discontent of women was a form of "nervousness" that might be remedied by a "rest cure" (Gilman [1892] 1980). During the Vietnam war, psychiatrists discussed how to cure the "inappropriate" reluctance of soldiers to go into battle (Bloch 1969). And during recent revisions in the standard diagnostic manual, the DSM-III, psychiatrists have classified smoking as an illness and no longer refer to homosexuality as an illness.

During some periods, psychiatry has been confident that it finally has disentangled itself from social ethics, yet retrospectively it is hard to say that this was so. What is notable is the correlation between periods when psychiatry has been confident about its ethical neutrality, and periods when the nation has been complacent about the ethical virtue of existing social arrangements. Since every movement from abolition to women's liberation has turned up new insights about the ethical presuppositions of psychiatric diagnosis, the conclusion is unavoidable that the entanglement of psychiatry with ethics is permanent.

Yet it is an empty victory simply to force upon psychiatry the realization that judgments concerning mental illness have an ethical core. For psychiatry has at the same time a need to establish itself as independent of ethical entanglement. Nor is this drive based simply on Cartesian anxiety concerning relativism inherited from Western philosophic traditions (Bernstein 1983, 16–17). It also arises from the concrete exigencies of practice. Reliable and responsible ways to make difficult decisions need to be found.

Is there a third option beyond both the improbable claim to be ethically neutral and the impractical suggestion that psychiatry resign itself to relativism? Will psychiatry drown in indeterminacy if it lets go of the claim to be purely scientific? My aim in this paper is to describe such a "third option." To establish it, I propose to use practical theology and its reflection on the affirmations of ultimate concern of a community in terms of their implications for the goals, norms, and means of practice. In particular, I hope to show that, although the basic orienting goals of psychiatric practice cannot be determined by empirical technical reasoning, this does not mean that the ends must remain indeterminate: our choices concerning ultimate ends (*theo*) can be informed, if not determined, by reasoned discussion (*logy*). In this reasoned discussion, theological ethics plays a central role (Tracy 1977, 88).

A way to balance the ethical dependence and independence of psychiatry—I will argue—is to see the orienting goal of psychiatry as a minimum one of promoting "basic human functioning." A psychiatry that understood itself as in service of such a basic goal would be free from broader agendas of personal and social reform, and yet would have a solid base from which to develop limited self-critical and social-critical roles.

This paper is organized in three sections. In each I will bring into conversation representatives of the two tendencies in psychiatry that I have identified: Robert Lifton and Thomas Szasz, as representatives of activism and value-neutrality respectively. In the first section, I will sketch out an interpretation of the history of psychiatry broad enough to show how the historical arguments made by Lifton and Szasz are not simply contradictory, but rather are part of a larger whole. In the second, I will use the conversation between Lifton and Szasz to bring out the orienting world views of each. And in the third, I will add my own voice to the conversation as a mediation, arguing that each is partly right and that the profession of psychiatry should understand itself as serving the limited ethical end of *basic human functioning*.

The Social and Historical Context

The history of psychiatry has most often been written as an account of developing technologies of treatment; however, this view does not do justice to the complexity of the relationship of the professions to culture. The issues at stake are not narrowly technical. Lifton and Szasz each see part of this. The first task is to place their differing insights within a single larger history of the professions.

The psychiatrist who will serve in this paper as an example of activist psychiatry, Robert Lifton, found precedence for his ethically committed vision in the derivation of the word *professional*. Speaking of the struggle between ethically committed and ethically neutral visions of the professions, Lifton commented:

> One source of perspective on that struggle was a return to the root idea of profession, the idea of what it means to profess. Indeed, an examination of the evolution of these two words could provide something close to a cultural history of the West. The prefix "pro" means forward, toward the front, forth, out, or into a public position. "Fess" derives from the Latin *fateri* or *fass,* meaning to confess, own, acknowledge. To profess (or be professed), then, originally meant a personal form of out-front public acknowledgment. And that which was acknowledged or "confessed" always (until the sixteenth century) had to do with religion: with taking the vows of a religious order or declaring one's religious faith. But as society became secularized, the word came to mean "to make claim to have knowledge of an art or science" or "to declare oneself expert or proficient in" an enterprise of any kind. (Lifton 1976, 165–66)

There is truth in Lifton's observation of the religious origins of the professions. Law and medicine arose in the twelfth and thirteenth centuries as specialties among the clergy (Ullman 1975; Berman 1985). We can still see the faint religious imprint in the fact that the word *professional* carries connotations of responsibility and seriousness as well as technical competence, and in the respect that people in the professions, especially in the "learned professions" of ministry, medicine, and law, command in areas far beyond their technical competences.

Yet one must be careful. Lifton concluded that the idea of ethical neutrality is a later addition and a by-product of secularization. This is not so. The independence of the professions, if not their ethical neutrality in the modern sense, is as old as the dependence of the professions on the religious substance of the culture. The independence of the profession is rooted in the relationships of independence and dependence implicit in the covenanting between Yahweh and the people of Israel and in the covenanting of feudal lords and vassals in which suzerainty relationships were reaffirmed—relationships in which the vassals provided services to the lords in return for privileges. The professions by analogy were in service of God and society but had independent domains in which they were entitled to exercise stewardship.

This heritage has been mediated to us through the figures of the Prot-

estant Reformation who translated the substance of the medieval understanding of the relationship of the professions to society by the concepts
of *calling* and *vocation*. In the call is the origin of both a special dependence
upon God of the one called and the legitimation of certain independent
actions. The pervasive influence of these ideas has become well-known
through Weber's *The Protestant Ethic and the Spirit of Capitalism*. Calvin's
own summary in the *Institutes* captures the essentials:

> The Lord bids each one of us in all life's actions to look to his calling.
> For he knows with what great restlessness human nature flames, with
> what fickleness it is born hither and thither, how its ambition longs to
> embrace various things at once. Therefore, lest through our stupidity
> and rashness everything be turned topsy-turvy, he has named these vari-
> ous kinds of living "callings." Therefore each individual has his own post
> so that he may not heedlessly wander about throughout life. Now, so
> necessary is this distinction that all our actions are judged by it, often
> indeed far otherwise than in the judgment of human and philosophical
> reason. No deed is considered more noble, even among philosophers,
> than to free one's country from tyranny. Yet a private citizen who lays
> his hand upon a tyrant is openly condemned by the heavenly judge. (Bk.
> 3, ch. 10, sec. 6)

Secular occupations are "from God," and they imply a responsibility to
society as a whole, yet not—as Calvin took pains to explain—an unlimited
license to political activity. Also, contrary to the thesis that ethical neutrality is a by-product of secularization, it should be noted that Calvin gave
solidly theological reasons for the independence from politics of people in
secular callings.

In fact, so strong are Calvin's theological arguments against political
involvement that one might ask whether he was condemning it completely. Within the concept of a "vocation" or a "profession" there is always a dialectic between involvement and detachment, and while Calvin
stressed the detachment side of the dialectic, he did not destroy the dialectic itself. Calvin's statements against political involvement must be seen
against the background of the debacle of the peasant's revolt in Munster
in 1535, which raised the fear that the Reformation might lead to complete anarchy (Williams 1975, 378–81). When Calvin said cautionary
things about political involvement by Christians, he was concerned that if
involvement could be structured and limited, the possibility for both religious and political reform would be destroyed. He did not proscribe all
political activity but only the questioning of the ultimate grounding or
political organization of society.

The religious substance of the concept of calling in the professions
dissipated with the rise of professional schools associated with universities

in Paris, Berlin, and Bologna, and the general secularization of European culture in the seventeenth and eighteenth centuries. This resulted not in the loss of the wider responsibility of the professions, but rather in a transformation of it. For example, the privilege of wearing an academic robe implied a responsibility to the wider cultural heritage, transmitting, transforming, and applying the ethos of the culture in an evolving situation (Adams 1986, 269).

The rise of the professional association in Anglo-Saxon cultures caused an important development in the dialectic of professional involvement in and independence from the wider culture. Thomas Hobbes called voluntary associations of all sorts "worms in the entrails of the sovereign": they made possible organized dissent by providing independent centers of legitimation and authority. Yet the ultimate decision of our political system has been to allow and encourage such associations. They have been important vehicles for mediation and for making politically effective the involved yet detached nature of groups in society (Adams 1986, 276). The professional association is a further development in which voluntary associations representing professions receive quasi-governmental powers within certain spheres. In its special status, the professional association repeats the same dual identity: it is a private group, yet corresponding with its special privileges it has a special responsibility to society as a whole.

Although to be "professional" has always meant to have special technical knowledge (as the priest knowing the liturgy), this knowledge did not become what we think of as technical knowledge—empirically based and supported by massive technology—until comparatively recently. Nor was it seen as the exclusive source of legitimacy. A number of factors, including the explosive growth of science and technology in the later nineteenth and early twentieth centuries, contributed to an expanded understanding of a profession as a group of people defined by their technical ability to perform a task or provide a service. In fact this definition eclipsed the understanding of the broader cultural involvement of professions.

In Germany, the consolidation of the unified state and the concomitant development of a rationalized bureaucracy led to the understanding of the professions as serving particular limited duties in a larger structure. In England, development of laissez-faire mercantilism gave rise to an understanding of professionals as independent business people who dealt with clients on the basis of freely negotiated contracts. Thomas Szasz finds precedence for his views of value-neutrality in this era:

> Doctors and patients have come a long way since the nineteenth century, but we had better think twice before we conclude it has all been progress. It is of more than passing interest to note, in this connection, one of the

definitions of the word *profession* in the *Oxford English Dictionary.* "A profession in our country," wrote a British gentleman named Maurice in
1829, "is expressly that kind of business which deals with men as men,
and is thus distinguished from a Trade, which deals primarily for the
external wants or occasions of men." Until recently, this criterion applied
particularly to the practice of medicine and law, the relations between
practitioners and their clients being based on mutual respect and trust
and of course, the studied avoidance of coercion. (Szasz 1987, 129).

While there are problems with this interpretation, Szasz is correct to turn
to the era of the rise of British mercantilism for the antecedents to his
views, including his opinion that the professional has no social roles aside
from the services to individuals rendered in fulfillment of contracts (all
other activities being without contract and hence, in his view, coercive).

The American professions were massively influenced by their German
and British counterparts in the latter nineteenth and early twentieth centuries. The foreign impulses toward functionalism combined with domes-
tic impulses, most notably the increasing pluralization of society that was
occurring with massive immigration. Paul Starr has noted that the multi-
plication of nonstandard medical practitioners and the protection to incompetence provided by the anonymity of urban life led the medical
establishment to assert a right to a monopoly on care (Starr 1982, 18).
Further, in the increasingly pluralistic environment, ways were needed to
serve people that were not dependent on commonality of culture or even
language between professional and client. In medicine the triumph of the
functional view was marked by the publishing of the Flexner report in
1910, *Medical Education in the United States and Canada,* and the reorganization of the AMA in 1901.

The history of psychiatry in the later nineteenth and early twentieth
centuries is both an example of these developments and a reaction against
them. James Luther Adams, speaking from an acquaintance with Erikson
and Fromm, said that "the appearance of the psychiatrist is itself a sign of
the demand for professional men who are capable of a wider competence
than is suggested by the term 'specialty of function.'" Yet Adams immediately questioned whether "the average psychiatrist has the professional
training that fits him for his dealing with the basic questions of ethos
having to do with the very meaning of life" (Adams 1986, 273). While
the development of psychiatry can be interpreted as a reaction against the
functionalization of medicine, it is also an example of it. The development
of psychiatry testifies to the continued concern of the medical profession
for something more than the narrowly functional, and it is also an extension of the functional view into new areas.

While it is tempting to interpret the history of the professions as one
of inexorable increase in technical competence and functionalism, and to

project this inexorable increase into the future (Ramsey 1970, xvi), this view is simplistic. It suggests that the only ethical challenge of the professions is to decide how to use new technologies. The complexity of the ethical challenge was highlighted at a recent conference in honor of the Flexner report ("Flexner and the 1990's: Medical Education in the 20th Century", University of Illinois at Chicago, June 10–11, 1986). The picture of medicine that emerged was one in which the technology of medicine would continue to develop, but in which the development of medicine as a whole would not be technology driven. It was pointed out that, in spite of popular views to the contrary, no "cures" to major diseases have been discovered since the polio vaccine in the 1950s and that researchers on the major "killer diseases" of cancer and heart disease hardly speak in terms of discovering "cures."

Psychiatrists have realized that the high hopes for "cures" to the major mental illnesses that accompanied the introduction of antipsychotic drugs and the resulting sharp reductions in population of mental institutions in the late fifties were inflated (Freedman et al. 1975, 1921). The mentally ill homeless today on the nation's streets are a guilty reminder that deinstitutionalization was not cure, and even has led some to question whether it is correct to speak of "cures" to mental illnesses at all.

The impulses towards functionalism in medicine that characterized the "Flexner Era" seem to be spent. If they are, it will mean that economic and social factors will drive medicine as much as technological ones. Social and preventive medicine will attain new prominence. It will mean also a new rapprochement between technical reasoning about means of accomplishing specific ends, and practical moral reasoning about how it is good to live.

Works that search out the historical conditioning and the ethical presuppositions of science have multiplied in recent decades (e.g., Kuhn 1970). While these works perform the hermeneutical task of showing the ethical and religious components of "scientific" ideas, few take the additional step of critically showing how the ethical or religious ideas can be evaluated. This is a crucial omission, since one of the reasons that professions in the late nineteenth century began to claim to be "value-free" was that they despaired of the possibility of ethical discussion in a pluralistic society. The insight that our ideas must depend on ethical presuppositions without the demonstration that our practices can depend on them is a counsel of despair. It leaves only the options of fideism and nihilism.

Having provided a broad cultural interpretation of the changing fortunes of the ethical dimension of the professions, I must immediately point out that one cannot go directly from an understanding of the ethical dimension to practical decisions about what is to be done. The cultural situation is only one factor impinging on practice. The institutional roles of psychiatrists are evolving. Patient populations and the economics of psychiatric practice are changing. The technological base is developing. Yet, it is perhaps in such a complex situation that higher level orienting perspectives for this profession become the most important.

The Contemporary Debate between Activist and Value-Neutral Psychiatry: Robert Lifton vs. Thomas Szasz

Two contrasting visions for psychiatry have in recent years fought for dominance: ethical commitment and ethical neutrality. To explore these positions and to help develop a mediating option I will bring representatives of these two tendencies into conversation in this section: Robert Lifton on the side of activist psychiatry and ethical commitment, and Thomas Szasz on the side of value neutrality. Although these two figures are alienated from much of contemporary psychiatry, they represent ideal types who embody significant tendencies in the profession.

Within psychiatry there is a significant undercurrent of belief that tends toward the view that "neuroses of society" produce individual neuroses and therefore psychiatrists must to some extent take responsibility for "treating" society as well as the individual. The implications of this activist view would enlarge psychiatry to almost priestly dimensions, giving the profession a role in writing ethical prescriptions for the good society. On the other hand, some believe that social problems will be generated as long as individuals are unregenerated. Taken to its extreme, this view implies that the only route to changing society is through changing individuals, and further, that one should only work to change individuals in the sense of seeking to restore or promote an ethically neutral quality of health. Most psychiatrists avoid both these extremes and claim that their concern is with something much less grandiose than whether ultimately society causes individual problems or individuals cause social problems. Yet, in order to explore the issues that exist between the activist and the value-neutral positions, I have not chosen people who represent this middle view. Like the doctor who waited for her patients to get sicker so that diagnosis would be easier, I have chosen, rather, two extreme cases. Although my purpose in this section is to point out the philosophical issues between the different prescriptions for change in the psychiatric profession, I do not mean to imply that the position of either Lifton or Szasz is without empirical grounding or that the existence of a philosophic dimension to their thought ipso facto brings into question its validity.

Robert Lifton

Robert Lifton has become known as a psychohistorian. Many of his books have been studies of individuals caught up in the dynamics of history. If one looks at how he interprets the actions of a specific person, it is easy to see the connection between the judgments he makes and his much broader views about human action and responsibility. His broader philosophical and ethical commitments and his related thoughts about the role of psychiatry are exemplified in his involvement in the defense of Patty Hearst.

Patty Hearst appeared to Lifton as a bland wisp of a woman caught up in terrorism. For him the analogy to the victims of Chinese brainwashing during the Korean war was clear. The *New York Times* reported his testimony:

> Prisoners of the Chinese, he said, were cut off from their past to make them reliant on their captors. Dr. Lifton said that in Miss Hearst's case the bank robberies cut her ties to the past. But he also said that "there was no ideological conversion" although her compliance with orders was "absolute."
>
> Finally, the prisoners returning to Hong Kong seemed to be confused and to want to indicate some remaining tie to the behavior and thought pattern set by their treatment, Dr. Lifton said.
>
> It was in that connection that he sought to explain another thing that has been a problem for Miss Hearst's defense: the clenched fist salute she repeatedly gave immediately after her arrest.
>
> "That is the sort of thing that I described as the last act of compliance among those coming back from China." (February 28, 1976, p. 32)

Lifton clearly believed that his ideas about people caught up in the dynamics of history could lead to insights of more general applicability:

> In my work . . . I found that studying an extreme situation such as that facing the survivors of the atomic bomb can lead to insights about everyday death, about ordinary people facing what Kurt Vonnegut has called "plain old death." Our psychological ideas about death have become so stereotyped, so limited and impoverished, that exposure to a holocaust like Hiroshima, or My Lai, or the entire American involvement in Indochina, forces us to develop new ideas and hypotheses that begin to account for some of the reactions we observe. (Lifton 1976, 29)

At the furthest reaches of generality these "new ideas and hypotheses" imply that the best way to understand human action generally is *as caught up in history.* As Lifton expressed it, the theme of death and the continuity of life became in his later work his controlling image (Lifton 1976, 61). This image became a "new paradigm" for understanding life (Lifton 1976, 60).

Lifton asserted that, whereas in Freud's day the major psychological dynamics were repression and release of sexual energy, today the major dynamics are better understood in terms of the struggle of life against the forces of death (Lifton 1973, 20). He quoted Camus's character, the plague doctor, Dr. Rieux: "The task of life is to construct an art of living in times of catastrophe in order to be reborn by fighting openly against the death instinct at work in our history" (Lifton 1976, 116). Yet in stark contrast to the view of Camus, the struggle against the death instinct was not for Lifton a struggle of will, but of impersonal forces of life and death. The forces of life arise out of a mythic zone, which, quoting Eliade, he described as "the zone of the sacred, the zone of absolute reality" (Lifton 1976, 145). The true principle of life is the principle of Protean transformation (Lifton 1961, 316). If Lifton thought the individual will has any significance, he did not discuss it. When he described the My Lai massacre there were no actors present, only embodiments of social forces. There was no massacre, only an "atrocity-producing situation," a combination of elements that were "inevitably genocidal" (Lifton 1973, 109).

> In all, it is not too much to say that the illusions surrounding an aberrant American quest for immortalizing glory, virtue, power, control, influence, and know-how are directly responsible for the more focused My Lai illusion. (Lifton 1973, 66)

Likewise, Patty Hearst is a tragic figure because "given who she was and what had happened to her, there was really no other path she could have taken" (Lifton as quoted by Szasz 1976a, 11).

In this understanding, the task of the doctor and of the good person generally becomes more the cure of a sick society than the cure of individuals:

> As a giver of forms the insurgent survivor must perforce become a leader. Dr. Rieux, the central figure of *The Plague,* is called upon to provide both medical and spiritual therapy. His antagonist is not only the plague itself, but the more general evil the plague stands for—"the feeling of suffocation from which we all suffered and the atmosphere of dread and exile in which we lived." (Lifton 1976, 120)

The role of a professional is to pro-fess. Doctors who claimed to be ethically neutral but provide "curative" treatment for soldiers who refuse to fight in an unjust war were for Lifton paradigmatic examples of those who would use the forces of life for the purposes of death.

Psychotherapy must be more than a means of curing the individual. When Lifton led group therapy sessions for Vietnam veterans, their aim was not so much to help individuals as to create new social arrangements and rejuvenate old ones.

> The rap groups have been one small expression . . . of a much larger cultural struggle . . . toward creating animating institutions. Whether these emerge from existing institutions significantly modified or as "alternative institutions," they can serve the important function of providing new ways of being a professional and of working with professionals. (Lifton 1976, 161)

Like the stones the builders discarded, the Vietnam veterans became the cornerstone of the new society. "I want to raise the question of the significance of an important change undergone by a relatively small group of men for a larger change in human consciousness now sought from many sides" (Lifton 1976, 21).

Is this psychology or social philosophy? It is hard to say at what point this line is crossed, but it is also hard to avoid the resonances of this with such clear exemplars of social philosophy as John Winthrop's "City on a Hill." The Massachusetts Bay Colony, like the veterans' rap groups, was created as an "animating institution." It was created to regenerate Europe "weighed down with the weight of death." Both Lifton and Winthrop assumed that in a regenerated society individuals would be regenerated. Both ran into problems when this did not happen.

Looked at in historical perspective, Lifton's rap groups continue the communitarian theme in American social philosophy, which has been renewed in a myriad of forms from Brook Farm through the Owenite communities, the social settlement movement, the Pullman Community, the Great Society programs, and the communes of the sixties. In each there was the assumption that in the society was the salvation of the individual, and that the way to rejuvenate society was to create model institutions. All of these experiments ran into trouble over the fact that even in the most regenerate of social arrangements some people remained stubbornly unregenerate.

It is intriguing how Lifton, like many American communitarians, shares features with romanticism and its responses to Enlightenment rationalism. His reference to the Middle Ages as a time before rationalism (for Lifton before professional*ism*) had vitiated ability of the will to act with conviction, is reminiscent of romantic nostalgia for that era exemplified by Novalis's *Christianity and Europe* of 1799. Yet like Balzac in *The Quest for the Absolute*, Lifton does not denigrate the scientists but rather enlarges their role to almost priestly dimensions. The way Lifton emphasizes reason as symbol-making in the mythic realm, in contrast to discursive reason, also closely parallels the distinction Kant made and Coleridge developed between Understanding and Reason (*Verstand* and *Vernunft*). Further in common with romanticism, Lifton is deeply conscious that there is a dark and destructive side to what lies beyond consciousness (as shown in Schopenhauer's *The World as Will and Idea,* 1818). Patty Hearst is a tragic figure, not because of the terrible consequences of her choices but because she is helpless before forces greater than herself. Most basically, there is the affinity at the level of anthropology: for the romantics, the Enlightenment had made people the masters of their own fates at the price of emphasizing what Wordsworth termed the "inferior faculties" of reason, and at the price of cutting them off from access to the dimension of truth itself, the "principles of truth" (Baumer 1973, 203). Like Schopenhauer and Coleridge in their rebellions against Lockean and Humean empiricism, Lifton breaks out of rationalism at the price of reducing the function of the will to that of receptivity to the forces of the universe, thus losing a conceptual place for choice in his thought.

Thomas Szasz

Thomas Szasz is a perceptive critic of Lifton because his basic affinities of thought are precisely opposite. He agrees with Lifton that psychiatry hides its dependence on ethical presuppositions, but his view of what should be done about the problem is precisely opposite. Whereas Lifton proposes that psychiatry should become explicit about its ethical commitments, Szasz believes that any hope for psychiatry—and on the question of whether there is hope he has become ever more doubtful—rests in reestablishing psychiatry on a value-neutral basis. This opposition between Lifton and Szasz arises from diverse sources, starting with the fact that each takes different practical problems in professional practice as symptomatic of the problems of psychiatry in general, and ending with the fact that each draws upon a different stream of social thought and a different philosophic tradition. Whereas Lifton's orientation was towards the communitarian tradition of American social thought, and to romanticism, Szasz's orientation is towards individualism and the Enlightenment.

The task of sketching out the philosophic dimensions of Szasz's thought is both easier and harder than it was for Lifton. It is easier in that, while Lifton is rarely explicit or even conscious of how he draws on wider cultural resources, Szasz is both conscious and explicit. There is no need to conjecture about which philosophers he is indebted to. He tells us: Locke, Hume, and Mill (Szasz 1987, 354–55). However, the philosophic dimensions of Szasz's thought are also harder to trace than those of Lifton because, in spite of his voluminous writings, he rarely elaborates his own constructive proposals. Never an optimist, in recent years he has become bleakly cynical about the possibilities for change in psychiatry or society.

It is thus necessary to review the thinking of Szasz in two stages, first, to summarize his criticism of our representative of activist psychiatry, Lifton, and second, to review Szasz's constructive position from such hints of it as can be found in the nooks and crannies of his work.

Whereas Lifton developed his position by reflecting on the role of psychiatrists in such world-transforming dynamics as war, Szasz began to develop his position by reflecting on the role of psychiatrists in involuntary hospitalization of mental patients and, slightly later on, what he decided was the mirror problem, the role of psychiatrists as court witnesses. His observation was that involuntary hospitalization had become a means by which society or a person's family could control behavior that was bothersome but not illegal. Likewise, the insanity defense became a means whereby a person could be excused for actions that were illegal. Both practices make end runs around fundamental principles of democratic government—that a person only can be deprived of liberty by a finding of criminal guilt in a public trial, and that a person who performs a criminal act will be held accountable.

Especially at the time he wrote his original work on the myth of mental illness, Szasz was making observations on which there was broad, if not universal, accord both in the psychiatric profession and in the general public. What was controversial about Szasz's position was his generalizations of his more limited observations.

He arrived at his sweeping conclusion that mental illness is a "myth" by roughly this chain of reasoning: hospitalization for mental diseases has been subject to abuse, whereas hospitalization for physical diseases has not. Hence is it logical to look for the cause of the abuse in the distinction between mental and bodily diseases. What is the distinction? Szasz noticed that there is a fundamental difference between saying that someone has mental disease and saying she has liver disease. This distinction is revealed in the nuance of language. When it is said that a person's liver is diseased, the presumption is that an examination of the liver could be made and some physical anomaly found; the same cannot be said concerning a mental disease. It might be possible to perform an operation on a person's brain and find a physical anomaly there, but then it would not be mental disease but brain disease. In fact, it is in the space between mind disease and brain disease that Szasz located the possibilities for abuse. To say that a person has a "diseased mind" is, he argued, like saying there is a disease in the body politic. It is a metaphor expressing disapproval of actions that we judge to be wrong.

> Illnesses of the body reflect a general consensus on the definition of health. However, the behavior which people come to criticize and view as mental illness is simply a disagreement on whether or not such a behavior should be permitted. (Szasz 1983, 218)

Nor does it change the metaphorical nature of the judgment that a relationship can at times be established between mental diseases and physical diseases.

When a psychiatrist says that someone is mentally "ill," she is making a value judgment. Yet psychiatrists claim to make purely empirical judgments:

> [I hold] that contemporary psychotherapists deal with problems of living, rather than mental illnesses, and their cures stand in opposition to a currently prevalent claim according to which mental illness is just as "real" and "objective" as bodily illness. This is a confusing claim since it is never known exactly what is meant by such words as "real" and "objective." I suspect, however, that what is intended by the proponents of this view is to create the idea in the popular mind that mental illness is some sort of disease entity, like an infection or a malignancy. . . . In my opinion, there is not a shred of evidence to support this idea. (Szasz 1960, 116)

For psychiatrists and their patients to act as though mental disease is real disease is a double impersonation in which a patient pretends to be sick and a psychiatrist pretends to give treatment.

Szasz pointed out that belief in mental illness, or at least acting as if one believed in mental illness, can function as belief in myth—hence his well-known claim that mental illness is mythical. From this follow his radical normative claims about the practices of psychiatry: since they are based on claims concerning "mythical" illnesses, neither involuntary hospitalization nor the insanity defense are ever legitimate, and psychiatry can be made legitimate, if at all, only by reestablishing it on a value-free foundation.

In saying this, Szasz does not intend to argue that the phenomena referred to as mental illness do not exist. "While I have argued that mental illnesses do not exist, I obviously do not imply that the social and psychological occurrences to which this label is currently attached also do not exist" (Szasz 1960, 11). His point rather is anthropological (Szasz 1983, 207, 227). He wishes to "criticize and counter a contemporary tendency to deny the moral aspects of psychiatry (and psychotherapy) and to substitute for them allegedly value-free medical considerations" (Szasz 1960, 116). "The problem with the medical model is that it disguises moral matters as medical" (Szasz 1983, 221).

How is morality disguised as medicine? Supposedly mental disease causes a person to lose the capacity of moral responsibility, much as multiple sclerosis causes loss of muscle control. In actuality the direction of the logic is precisely the reverse:

> Critical consideration of the connections between mental illness and responsibility thus points to a relationship of profound negation: as death negates life, insanity negates responsibility. It is not so much, as is commonly believed, that insanity diminishes or annuls the mentally ill person's capacity for responsibility; instead it is rather that our idea of insanity itself negates our concept of responsibility. Although it appears as if nonresponsibility were a condition separate from insanity but sometimes caused by it . . . in fact nonresponsibility and insanity are essentially synonymous. (Szasz 1983, 269)

The problem caused by the negation of responsibility is not only, or even primarily, injustice to individuals; at a more profound level the harm is that all are diminished as human beings.

The logic of determinism does not—Szasz argues—admit of distinctions. If one chooses to view life according to the logic of determinism, all free will becomes an illusion. Szasz quotes Freud:

> Many people, as is well known, contest the assumption of complete psychical determinism by appealing to a special feeling of conviction that there is free will. This feeling of conviction exists; and it does not give way before a belief of determinism. (However) . . . what is left free by one side receives its motivation from the other side, from the unconscious; and in this way determinism in the psychical sphere is still carried out without a gap. (Szasz 1987, 243)

While psychiatrists may often think, like Freud, that they free people to love and to work, they instead promote a view of the human as determined. While claiming to extend the sphere of reason in human life, psychiatry extinguishes it in a revived doctrine of predestination.

Thomas Szasz's response to Lifton's testimony in the Hearst case began with this broadside:

> Dr. Robert Jay Lifton, professor of psychiatry at Yale University, testified (as he was quoted as saying in the *New York Times*) that Patty Hearst "came under the category that I wrote about in my book of the obviously confused about what had happened to her." In the style characteristic of the courtroom psychiatrist, he thus makes Hearst into a "case" about whose conduct he, the brainwashing expert, knows more than does the "patient" herself. Such psychiatric self-flattery is acquired at the expense of the patient's self-esteem, not to mention, in this case, her father's money. (Szasz 1976a, 11)

Lifton discussed a metaphorical disease, brain washing, as if it were a literal disease and so transformed a discussion of whether what Hearst did

was right or wrong into a discussion of whether she was sick or healthy.
Szasz commented:

> The crucial question becomes: What is "brainwashing"? Are there, as the
> term implies, two kinds of brains: washed and unwashed? How do we
> know which is which?
>
> Actually, it's all quite simple. Like many dramatic terms, "brain-
> washing" is a metaphor. A person can no more wash another's brain with
> coercion or conversation than he can make him bleed with a cutting
> remark.
>
> If there is no such thing as brainwashing, what does this metaphor
> stand for? It stands for one of the most universal human experiences and
> events, namely for one person influencing another. However we do not
> call all types of personal or psychological influences "brainwashing."
> We reserve this term for influences of which we disapprove. (Szasz
> 1976, 11)

In spite of this pointed criticism, Szasz was less concerned with the
specifics of Lifton's testimony than with the principle that psychiatrists
have no role in the courtroom. Such a role subverts the political system.
This same criticism applied equally to Lifton's conclusion that My Lai was
"an atrocity-producing situation," and to any conclusion that a person's
actions are caused by social forces. Lifton was able to uncover the "fact"
that actions are determined because he had assumed it.

However, Szasz's position was not simply a psychiatric version of law-
and-order politics. His point was more fundamental: it is dangerous to
excuse someone on the basis of lack of moral responsibility. This danger is
evident if we note the affinity between how Lifton excused Patty Hearst's
actions and how her father dismissed them—just as he dismissed the views
of Patty's mother and of women in general as childlike (Weed 1976).

Another plausible psychological interpretation of Patty's "conversion"
to that of her captors was that she wanted to force her father to take her
seriously. If this was so, Lifton's "defense" that she was not responsible for
her actions was a cruel extension of her father's and society's sexism. As
Szasz has said:

> That this psychiatric-psychoanalytic view on responsibility encourages
> lay people to be irresponsible and physicians to be paternalistic is ob-
> vious and requires no further comment. Perhaps because it is less ob-
> vious, people often do not realize that relieving a person of his
> responsibility is tantamount to relieving him, partly or entirely, of his
> humanity as well. The person who claims that he, not his brother, is
> responsible for his brother's welfare and happiness, stabs at the very heart
> of his brother as a person." (Szasz 1987, 245)

The insight has not been lost on oppressed groups that it is a short step from being excused on the basis of not being responsible for one's actions, to being dismissed as not fully human.

What has Szasz accomplished with his critique? Although he has not proven that action is free, he has refuted the opposing position advocated by Lifton. Thus, he has made two important contributions. First, he has shown, from a different, less sympathetic angle, what was said in my earlier discussion of Lifton's position: that in building his position Lifton must have drawn from sources other than empirical observation. I would not say that this fact invalidates Lifton's position, but I do agree heartily that Lifton did something other than deduce conclusions from evidence. However, I would put the case more positively, saying that in Lifton's position there is an interplay between empirical and philosophical perspectives. This does not mean that the involvement of psychiatrists in the judicial process, which Lifton advocates, is completely illegitimate, but we do need a discussion of whether such hybrid practical moral conclusions have grounds for legitimacy.

The second way in which Szasz's critique advances the discussion is to suggest the need for a second look at Szasz's own position. If he has not proven that actions are free on the basis of deductions from empirical evidence, then what is the source of this conclusion? It emerges that there is just as much of a dialectic between empirical observation and world view for Szasz as there is for Lifton. Whereas the communitarian stream of social thought and romanticism inform Lifton's work, individualism and Enlightenment rationalism mediated through laissez-faire perspectives inform Szasz.

It remains to investigate Szasz's own constructive position. Although this position appears only infrequently in his work, and hardly at all in his most recent publications, it is decisively important if we are to understand the commitments which lie behind his critiques. He presents himself as wanting simply to establish the truth by exposing falsehood, yet he is guided in decisive ways in his pursuit of these goals by broader visions of the good person and the good society.

Szasz's observation that specific actions are not determined shades into a more general conclusion: the world is a place in which actions are free.

> Man's actions represent free choices for which he is responsible, but for which he may rhetorically seek to avoid responsibility, most prominently through attributing behavior to literal and/or figurative gods. The traditional Judeo-Christian monotheistic god would be an example of the former, while physicians might be classified as the latter.
> The crucial moral characteristic of the human condition is the dual

experience of freedom of the will and personal responsibility. (Szasz 1983, 23–24)

Szasz seems blind to the fact that the *will* is "mythical" in the same sense he argued *mind* or *mental illness* to be. Luckily for him this does not mean that *free will* is necessarily an illegitimate concept, but only that it is philosophically rather than empirically based, and is connected with a broader philosophical point of view.

Szasz's understanding of action as free is connected with his understanding of the struggle of reason against irrationalism.

> Man's awareness of himself and of the world about him seems to be a steadily expanding one, bringing in its wake an ever larger burden of understanding. . . . This burden then, is to be expected and must not be misinterpreted. Our only rational means of lightening it is more understanding, and appropriate action based on such understanding. The main alternative lies in action as though the burden were not what in fact we perceive it to be and taking refuge in an outmoded theological view of man. (Szasz 1960, 117)

The hero of this world view is the person who takes on the burden of understanding, aware of her limits, content with the slow gains of reason, and steadfastly refusing blandishment of the "theological view of man" and its successors. For Lifton, the paradigmatic examples of human wrongdoing are the psychiatrists who use the forces of life to promote war. But for Szasz, the chief examples are the psychiatrists who are the successors to the historic opponents of free will: the theologians and priests.

Recently Szasz has become so cynical about the alliance of psychiatry and medicine with the forces of determinism and irrationalism that he rarely mentions his ideals for psychiatry. However, he did indicate his vision for the profession in his early works. In *The Ethics of Psychoanalysis* Szasz proposed a vision of psychiatry that he called "autonomous psychotherapy."

> I chose this expression [autonomous psychotherapy] to indicate the paramount aim of this procedure: preservation and expansion of the client's autonomy. To emphasize the nature of the therapeutic method, rather than its aim, the procedure could also be called "contractual psychotherapy"; the analyst-analysand relationship is determined neither by the patient's "therapeutic needs" nor by the analyst's "therapeutic ambition," but rather by an explicit and mutually accepted set of promises and expectations, which I call "the contract." (Szasz 1965, 7)

The contract for Szasz was not one feature of therapy, but rather its essence. The ability to keep a contract became for him both the goal of therapy and the definition of health:

> In large part, the analysis of the analytic situation is the analysis of the contract. A contractual agreement, by its very nature, may be broken in one of two ways: by underfulfilling or by overfulfilling one's obligations. These two types of contract violation correspond, roughly, to the characterological postures of the person who exploits and the one who allows himself to be exploited. To an extent, the former is typical of the so-called oral-demanding, or greedy, individual or of the sadist, and the latter, of the so-called mature, or generous person or of the masochist. (Szasz 1965, 191)

The ability to give fair measure—the ultimate commercial virtue—is the norm of health. Self-sacrifice—except as it is required to precisely fulfill contractual obligations—is not only a questionable good; it is positively a vice. By this extension of his logic, Szasz revealed that "ethically neutral" is not ethical neutrality. If Szasz wants psychiatrists to stand above the fray of moral disagreements, and above the efforts to improve society, it is so as to be more visible as a beacon pointing beyond them:

> Perhaps the relationship between the modern psychotherapist and his patient is a beacon that ever-increasing numbers of men will find themselves forced to follow, lest they become spiritually enslaved or physically destroyed. (Szasz 1961, 310)

"Autonomous" psychotherapy produces the prototype of the good person and the psychotherapeutic relationship is the norm for all relationships.

Szasz's image of the good person was also an image of the good society, since he presumed, as all advocates of *laissez-faire* must to remain consistent, that there is a preestablished harmony of interests:

> In a modern society, based more on contract that on status, the autonomous personality will be socially more competent and useful than his heteronomous counterpart. Moreover, and very significantly, autonomy is the only positive freedom whose realization does not injure others. (Szasz 1965, 22)

If only each person would act autonomously, the best result would be achieved for all. To accept the notion that one person can hurt another by pursuit of self-interest is, Szasz concluded, like accepting the notion that "a sadist is one who refuses to hurt a masochist" (Szasz 1965, 23).

This is the Enlightenment as it filtered through Locke, Hume, and

Mill, and even more directly into the American experience through Emerson. The standard of good becomes the good inside, and doing anything other than realizing this is betrayal:

> Nothing is at last sacred but the integrity of our own mind. . . . On my saying, "What have I to do with the sacredness of traditions, if I live wholly from within?" my friend suggested—"But these impulses may be from below, not from above." I replied, "They do not seem to me to be such, but if I am the devil's child, I will live then from the devil." No law can be sacred to me but that of my nature. (Emerson 1899, 47–48)

When developed to this point, autonomy is more than a good. It has swallowed up the good.

The social ideal of *laissez-faire* individualism has traveled a crooked course from the eighteenth century, when it was the battle cry of the middle class against aristocratic privilege, to the nineteenth century, when it reversed its meaning to become the battle cry of the robber barons against social legislation. The dictum that each is entitled to the fruits of his labors came to mean whoever has got it must deserve it. Emerson's "Self-Reliance" became William Graham Sumner's succinct answer to the question of what social classes owe to each other: nothing (Sumner [1883] 1986). Not only is social activism not morally obligatory, it is a disruption of social laws, what Szasz called "coercion," and what Sumner called "social meddling." Whereas Lifton's ideal of the professional was someone who pro-fesses, Szasz's ideal is of a professional who at all costs avoids doing so.

Lifton's and Szasz's views of the relation of professionalism to ethics are two parts of an earlier dual concept. Robert Lifton's understanding of the professions, as committed to sustaining and transforming the ethical vision of culture, is a distant relative of the view that callings are from God and of the understanding expressed in such customs as the wearing of academic robes by professionals. Thomas Szasz's understanding of the professions as independent from ethics is similarly related to theological understandings of the independence of those who practice a calling within an appointed domain of stewardship. There is a family resemblance between Calvin's view that we each serve God best by sticking to our individual callings, and Szasz's view that society profits most when each person sticks to a policy of noninterference.

Furthermore, these differing views of the professions are rooted in differences in basic anthropology. In *The Nature and Destiny of Man*, Reinhold Niebuhr has shown how romantic understandings of the human as determined and rationalist understandings of the human as free are byproducts of the breakup of classic theological understandings of the human as self-transcending. This basic theological understanding originates in an Augustinian concept of the human as made in the image of God. Paul Tillich, also drawing heavily on this Augustinian heritage, described determinism and free will as a basic polar opposition in the ontological structure of the human. As Tillich described it, free will and determinism, or freedom and destiny, exist in dialectical relationship. Destiny is a structured aspect of myself and my environment that makes me who I am. It is the concreteness out of which decisions arise. Freedom, on the other hand, is the structure of destiny made real (Tillich 1951, 182–86).

Yet this view contains a danger. To say that two divergent tendencies in the understanding of the relationship of ethics to the professions are the "broken halves" of a classic theological understanding of calling or vocation points prematurely to a normative solution. Even if the two tendencies were once held together in classical theological formulations, this does not mean that they can be, or should be, again. It still needs to be argued that those theological concepts meet contemporary demands, particularly the demand that they be compatible with radical pluralism.

The reasons for this go beyond the fact that arguments based on the authority of a particular religious tradition are unlikely to succeed in a public forum. There are theological objections to any proposal that replaces the present with the past. History moves forward, not only chronologically but also theologically. Lifton and Szasz have done more than move away from theological understandings of vocation; they have advanced those understandings—and have done so for compelling reasons. Given this, can classic traditions of reflection still serve as guides?

Solution

Can a theological concept help guide our understanding of the relationship between ethics and the professions? In the 1820s, de Tocqueville observed that in America a distinguishing feature of public life was the way theological, and explicitly Christian, presuppositions guided public discourse: "Christianity reigns without obstacles, by universal consent; consequently, everything in the moral field is certain and fixed, although the world of politics is given over to argument and experiment" (*Democracy in America*, [1835, 1840] 1969, 292, as quoted in Bellah 1986, 80).

Yet, in spite of what de Tocqueville said, the question of the proper role of such concepts is perennial. A generation ago John Dewey, John Courtney Murray, and Walter Lippman all argued the need for a public philosophy which, if it were not quite a public theology, would be at least informed by particular cultural traditions. As Bruce Kuklick has argued, neither Lippman nor Dewey quite managed to do public philosophy without doing public theology (Bellah 1986, 82), and, of course, Murray did not argue that one should try. Although Lippman, Dewey, and Murray disagreed on the substance of a public theology, Murray's statement of the need for one speaks for all three.

> And if this country is to be overthrown from within or from without, I would suggest that it will not be overthrown by Communism. It will be overthrown because it will have made an impossible experiment. It will have undertaken to establish a technological order of most marvelous intricacy, which will have been constructed and will operate without relations to true political ends; and this technological order will hang, as it were, suspended over a moral confusion; and this moral confusion will itself be suspended over a spiritual vacuum. This would be the real danger resulting from a type of fallacious, fictitious, fragile unity that could be created among us. ("Return to Tribalism," *Catholic Mind,* January 1962, as cited in Neuhaus 1984, 85)

The issue has surfaced again recently, first in Solzhenitsyn's Harvard speech, and then in Richard Neuhaus's *The Naked Public Square.* Yet there remains the suspicion that those who have been most strident in their criticisms have not understood fully the legitimate claims of pluralism. This is certainly true for Solzhenitsyn, whose own view of public life is both theocentric and Christocentric.

There is a group who would argue that "public theology" is an oxymoron. Or, rather, there are two groups who have historically opposed the concept of a public theology. Channing first observed that the extreme secularists and the extreme religionists come together to support the notion that if an issue is not resolvable by narrowly empirical means, then it is not amenable to rational discussion at all (Channing 1849, vol. 3, 66). William James similarly observed the affinities between narrow empiricists and supernaturalists (James [1902] 1925, 19).

Does theology have a place in public discussion? Szasz stressed the human capacity for choice; Lifton stressed what lies outside the human choice. Each criticized religion for including in its understanding of the human that part of the dual understanding that he excluded. Tillich commented that in the contradiction between free will and determinism, reason looks into its abyss. Whether to view the human as a creature of reason or as a creature of vitality cannot be decided by theoretical reason or reduced to narrowly empirical terms.

A characteristic of classic theological understandings of the human is that they have held together free and determined aspects of the human spirit. Even when the human capacity for choice has been emphasized least, voluntaristic elements have been retained in theological discussion. There has rarely, if ever, been a time without general agreement that human beings must be recognized as responsible. This has not been simply a political necessity of a ruling power. It has also been an insight held most tenaciously when the church was most oppressed. The reason for this is one that Szasz accurately recognized: to be "understood" in the sense of being held to be not responsible is also to be dismissed, or regarded as not fully human.

In affinity with Lifton, an appreciation of the limitations of the will has also been part of classic theological understandings. The human capacity for choice is limited first by physical limitations and by habit, but more profoundly we are limited by internal divisions of the will that the apostle Paul referred to when he said, "what I would, that I do not; but what I hate, that I do" (Romans 7:15).

Whatever the ultimate foundation of religious truth, a proximate norm for it must be that it accord with common human experience. The further limits of religious truth may be beyond rational discussion; yet there exists an arena of discourse that is authentically theological, but about which broadly empirical public discussions and evaluations are possible.

While no imposition of the understandings of a particular religious tradition can or should be made, it may be possible for the concept of the professions to be renewed by allowing itself to be instructed by both tendencies of the classic theological concept of calling. Such an understanding of the professions would borrow its form from the theological concept; yet its content would be independently justifiable as a mediation between such poles of thinking as are represented by Lifton and Szasz.

Psychiatry should not seek either to "base itself wholly on science" or to serve expansive visions of individual and social good, but should rather serve the admittedly ethical but limited goal of *basic human functioning*. Basic functioning is a basement concept on which can be built the more expansive ideas of virtue. It contains a rudimentary view of what it is to be a good person, but only in the minimal sense of a person whose actions could be discussed as good or bad. It is a goal defined formally as that norm which, when violated, brings into question the humanness of an action, not its morality, and materially as the community consensus refined by reflection and critique.

A psychiatry which served the goal of basic human functioning would not claim to be based purely on science, but it would still be scientific in a number of respects. It would include reasoning about how to achieve the end of adequate functioning, and about whether a person corresponds to the minimum concept of adequate functioning. Furthermore, it would retain the asceticism often characteristic of science in that it would hold itself back from direct participation in debates about more complete understandings of the nature of the good person and the good society. Psychiatry has been accused of a poverty of ends. In the understanding I am proposing, psychiatry would make this fault a virtue, taking a "vow of poverty" concerning ends, practicing an ascetic attitude concerning larger visions of individual and social good, and making use of only that which is necessary for practicing its own vocation.

Yet this understanding of psychiatry could also be instructed by Lifton's side of the concept of calling. It could say, when asked to treat a soldier who would not fight, that it could serve the larger end of combat effectiveness of the unit only by serving the narrower end of basic functioning. To the extent that soldiers who were capable of basic functioning still chose not to fight, psychiatry would have no role in convincing them to change their minds. Likewise, psychiatry could not say anything about the metaphysical validity of religious beliefs, but would be able to say that particular religious practices undermined the capacity for basic functioning. Thus, although such a psychiatry could not follow Lifton in his larger demand that psychiatry help build the good society, it could contribute to a social good greater than the sum of its contribution to the adequate functioning of individuals.

Such an understanding of the role of psychiatry as serving a limited but authentically moral end, is in keeping with its position as a profession. A profession organizing itself into a voluntary association, such as the American Psychiatric Association, occupies a mediating function in society (Adams 1986, 268). Unlike a political party or a religious denomination, a professional association has a fiduciary responsibility to society as a whole. Because of the fact that it is a private organization, not directly regulated by the government, and yet has a larger public role, one could argue that it rightfully should be conservative in the ends it chooses to serve. Such an end as adequate functioning is one that would allow psychiatry to serve both its narrower and its larger roles in society.

In the specific case of Patty Hearst, psychiatry would be able to testify concerning how her actions corresponded to a norm of adequate functioning. However, it could not make the kinds of global claims that Lifton made at the trial. It would need to recognize that in entering the courtroom it had entered an area beyond its fiduciary responsibility. Such a position in fact corresponds to the emerging self-understanding of the profession. The American Psychiatric Association has endorsed the position that psychiatrists should not be allowed to testify about " 'ultimate issues' such as whether or not the defendant was, in their judgment, 'sane' or 'insane', 'responsible' or not. . . ." (American Psychiatric Association 1982, 13). Even Szasz has suggested that within such bounds there may be a place for psychiatric testimony (Szasz 1983, 146).

The suggestion I make that adequate functioning become the governing norm of mental health has precedent in the American context. Richard Cabot, in a 1908 article entitled "An American Type of Psychotherapy," proposed a moral component to psychiatry that could be established on the basis of a broad social consensus; this is not altogether different from the concept of adequate functioning I propose (Cabot 1908, 7). His proposal did not win the day then, but may bear reconsidering now.

References

Adams, James L. 1986. *Voluntary Associations: Socio-cultural Analyses and Theological Interpretation*. Chicago: Exploration Press.

American Medical Association. 1983. "The Insanity Defense in Criminal Trials and Limitations of Psychiatric Testimony." Report G of the Board of Trustees.

American Psychiatric Association. 1982. *American Psychiatric Association Statement on the Insanity Defense*.

Baumer, Franklin L. 1973. "Romanticism." In *Dictionary of the History of Ideas*, 198–204. New York: Scribner's.

Bellah, Robert N. 1986. "Public Philosophy and Public Theology in America Today." In *Civil Religion and Political Theology*, ed. Leroy S. Rouner. Notre Dame, IN: University of Notre Dame Press.

Berman, Harold. 1985. *Law and Revolution: The Formation of the Western Legal Tradition*. Cambridge: Harvard University Press.

Bernstein, Richard J. 1983. *Beyond Objectivism and Relativism*. Philadelphia: University of Pennsylvania Press.

Bloch, H. Spencer. 1969. "Army Clinical Psychiatry in the Combat Zone—1967–1968." *American Journal of Psychiatry* 126, 3 (September): 289–98.

Cabot, Richard C. 1908. "The American Type of Psychotherapy." *Psychotherapy* 1, 1: 5–13.

Calvin, John. 1966. *The Institutes of the Christian Religion* (1559). Volume 1. Philadelphia: Westminster Press.

Cartwright, Samuel A. 1851. "Report on the Diseases and Physical Peculiarities of the Negro Race." *New Orleans Medical and Surgical Journal*, May, pp. 691–715.

Channing, William E. 1849. *The Works of William E. Channing*. Boston: George G. Channing.

Emerson, Ralph Waldo. 1899. *Essays: First Series*. Philadelphia: Henry Alemus.

Flexner, Abraham. 1910. *Medical Education in the United States and Canada*. Bulletin no. 4. New York: Carnegie Foundation for the Advancement of Teaching.

Freedman, Alfred M., Harold I. Kaplan, and Benjamin J. Sadock, eds. 1975. *Comprehensive Textbook of Psychiatry*. Second edition. Baltimore: Williams and Wilkins.

Gamwell, Franklin I. "Religion and Reason in American Politics." *Journal of Law and Religion* 2:325–42.

Gilman, Charlotte Perkins. 1892. "The Yellow Wallpaper." *New England Magazine*, January, pp. 3–20.

———. 1980. *The Charlotte Perkins Gilman Reader*. New York: Pantheon Books.

Ingleby, David, ed. 1980. *Critical Psychiatry: The Politics of Mental Health*. New York: Pantheon.

James, William. 1922. *Pragmatism: A New Name for Some Old Ways of Thinking*. London: Longmans, Green and Co.

———. 1925. *The Varieties of Religious Experience* (1902). New York: Longmans, Green and Co.

Kuhn, Thomas. 1970. *The Structure of Scientific Revolutions*. Chicago: University of Chicago Press.

Kuklick, Bruce. 1977. *The Rise of American Philosophy*. New Haven: Yale University Press.

Laor, Nathaniel. 1982. "Szasz, Feuchtersleben, and the History of Psychiatry." *Psychiatry* (November): 316–24.

———. 1984. "The Autonomy of the Mentally Ill: A Case Study in Individualistic Ethics." *Philosophy of Social Science* 14: 331–49.

Lifton, Robert Jay. 1961. *Thought Reform and the Psychology of Totalism: A Study of Brainwashing in China*. New York: Norton.

———. 1961. *History and Human Survival*. New York: Random House.

———. 1967. *Boundaries: Psychological Man in Revolution*. New York: Random House.

———. 1973. *Home from the War: Vietnam Veterans, Neither Victims nor Executioners*. New York: Simon and Schuster.

———. 1976. *The Life of the Self: Toward a New Psychology*. New York: Simon and Schuster.

———. 1979. *The Broken Connection: On Death and the Continuity of Life*. New York: Simon and Schuster.

Maxim, Jerrold S. 1986. *The New Psychiatry*. New York: Mentor.

Neuhaus, Richard. 1984. *The Naked Public Square; Religion and Democracy in America*. Grand Rapids, MI: Eerdmans.

Niebuhr, Reinhold. 1941. *The Nature and Destiny of Man: A Christian Interpretation*, Volumes 1 and 2. New York: Scribner's.

Ramsey, Paul. 1970. *The Patient as a Person*. New Haven: Yale University Press.

Rouner, Leroy, ed. 1986. *Civil Religion and Political Theology*. Notre Dame, IN: University of Notre Dame Press.

Schleiermacher, Friedrich. 1966. *Brief Outline on the Study of Theology*. Richmond, VA: John Knox Press.

Starr, Paul. 1982. *The Social Transformation of American Medicine*. New York: Basic Books.

Sumner, William Graham. 1986. *What Social Classes Owe to Each Other* (1883). Caldwell, ID: Caxton Printers.

Szasz, Thomas. 1957. "Commitment of the Mentally Ill: Treatment of Social Restraint?" *Journal of Nervous and Mental Diseases* 125: 293–307.

———. 1960. "The Myth of Mental Illness." *American Psychologist* 115: 113–18.

———. 1961. *The Myth of Mental Illness: Foundations of a Theory of Personal Conduct*. New York: Harper and Row.

———. 1963. *Law, Liberty, and Psychiatry: An Inquiry into the Social Uses of Mental Health Practices*. New York: Macmillan.

————. 1965. *The Ethics of Psychoanalysis: The Theory and Method of Autonomous Psychotherapy.* New York and London: Basic Books.

————. 1973. *The Manufacture of Madness: A Comparative Study of the Inquisition and the Mental Health Movement.* Frogmore, St. Albans: Granada Publishing Ltd.

————. 1976a. "Mercenary Psychiatry." *New Republic,* March 13, pp. 10–12.

————. 1976b. "Some Call It Brainwashing." *New Republic,* March 6, pp. 10–123.

————. 1977. *The Theology of Medicine: The Political-Philosophical Foundations of Medical Ethics.* Baton Rouge: Louisiana State University Press.

————. 1978. *The Myth of Psychotherapy: Mental Healing as Religion, Rhetoric, and Repression.* Garden City, NY: Anchor Press.

————. 1983. *Thomas Szasz: Primary Values and Major Contentions,* ed. Richard E. Vatz and Lee S. Weinberg. Buffalo: Prometheus Books.

————. 1987. *Insanity: The Idea and Its Consequences.* New York: Wiley.

Tillich, Paul. 1951. *Systematic Theology: Volume I.* Chicago: University of Chicago Press.

Tocqueville, Alexis de. 1969. *Democracy in America.* 1835, 1840. New York: Doubleday Anchor.

Tracy, David. 1977. "Revisionist Practical Theology and the Meaning of Public Discourse." *Pastoral Psychology* 26, 2 (Winter): 83–94.

Ullman, Walter. 1975. *Law and Politics in the Middle Ages.* Ithaca, NY: Cornell University Press.

Weed, Steven. 1976. *My Search for Patty Hearst.* New York: Crown.

Williams, George. 1975. *The Radical Reformation.* Philadelphia: Westminster Press.

CHAPTER SEVEN

ETHICAL PROBLEMS FOR PSYCHIATRY AND SOCIETY: THE ROLE OF A PUBLIC PHILOSOPHY FOR PSYCHIATRY

Daniel J. Anzia, M.D.

Psychiatrists are double agents. They serve not only their patients, as do all physicians, but also the interests of society. This reality has been acknowledged and discussed by knowledgeable observers of the psychiatric profession such as sociologist David Mechanic (1981). Thomas Szasz (1974, 259–61) has clearly elucidated this double-agent role, and he decries as immoral actions of psychiatrists and society that result in involuntary, noncontractual treatment or confinement. Nevertheless, practicing psychiatrists must accommodate and come to terms with this dual allegiance in their day-to-day work. In fact, from my experience, it seems a reasonable hypothesis that many, if not most, psychiatrists have been comfortable with this double-agent role, probably by virtue of their training and socialization in the values of the profession as a whole. For example, working with the family and school of an adolescent patient, or acting on the need for involuntary hospitalization of a suicidal or threatening paranoid adult, all the while balancing the duty to maintain the patient's confidentiality as much as possible, seem to be tasks accepted as "part of the job" by most psychiatrists.

Certain clinical situations bring this double-agent role into clear focus. Situations that require the psychiatrist to function as a moral arbiter or the agent of society's moral judgment often make the practitioner uncomfortable, and should. Although the profession has not become convinced that it must define its own proper role in such situations, it is actively struggling with the issues involved. However, it may not be able to delineate its role without the thoughtful contributions of other professions and society as a whole. This book addresses the problem from the position of the faith traditions. In contributing to both the process and product of a public philosophy of psychiatry, it may help the profession and society clarify the kind of enterprise psychiatry is and ought to be, and what its roles, its boundaries, and its relations with other professions are and ought to be.

In this essay I will use clinical examples to illustrate some types of questions a public philosophy for psychiatry might address. The clinical examples will involve two kinds of situations in which psychiatrists may be troubled by their double-agent role: (1) assessment and definition of patient competence to consent to or refuse medical treatment, and (2) times when psychiatrists must assume responsibility in some way for the actions of their patients.

It is not my intention to analyze the relationships of these two problems to each other in this essay, although ways may be seen in which they are connected in our beliefs about what it means to be a human person. Rather, I use them as two different examples to support the thesis that psychiatrists, their patients, and the community could benefit from a clarified public philosophy.

Autonomy and Competence

In the flourishing of the discipline of medical ethics in the last few decades, and in the development of the law during that same period, one of the central problems has been the conflict between individual autonomy and traditional medical paternalism. When an individual's self-determination opposes the medical wish to treat a patient for the person's own good, whose will shall prevail?

Robert Veatch (1984) has restated his conviction that "the case is overwhelming that autonomy takes moral precedence over paternalism. Respecting the patient's autonomy always takes precedence over benefitting the patient against the patient's autonomous will" (p. 38). He notes that this overwhelming triumph of autonomy is limited in its impact on the pressing problems of the 1980s, which largely concern such communal issues as distribution of limited resources. Such problems require the development of a social ethic less focused on the individual's desires and preferences and more on the common good (pp. 38–40).

I'm inclined to agree with Veatch about the need to turn our attention; for psychiatrists and their patients the problems of fair distribution of resources are already vexing and require increased attention. But in the day-to-day practice of psychiatry, situations continue to arise around autonomy and paternalism. Families, nurses, other physicians, lawyers, judges, and even patients have not all had the opportunity or inclination to be convinced by the "overwhelming case" in the literature of medical ethics. Those who are inclined to override stated preferences of patients "for the patient's benefit" may find an avenue that is left open to them by even the most ardent advocates of the primacy of individual autonomy. This avenue is to question the competence of the patient.

Unfortunately, the exact relationship between autonomy and competence is not clear. The concepts have developed historically alongside of and somewhat independently of each other. Yet they are often found in tandem, and their meanings may be confused. I will consider briefly the history of the concept of competence, then turn to some clinical examples and the questions of competence raised in them. This discussion will lead back to a more detailed consideration of the relationships of competence, autonomy, and the views of human personhood at stake.

Competence: The Concept

Beauchamp and McCullough (1984, 117 ff.), in a most informative discussion of competence, point out that the concept has accrued layers of meaning connected in various ways because medicine, law, psychiatry, and philosophy have had competing theories of competence related to their special interests. Nevertheless, the idea ranging across these theories is that competence is the ability to perform a task, though as used in the professions it is clearly not simply a synonym for ability (Culver and Gert 1982, 53–54).

As a legal concept, competence has a long history (Gutheil and Applebaum 1982). In both its general and specific senses, it is tied to the concept of guardianship. That is, if someone is incompetent to perform specific tasks, a guardian should be appointed to perform them.

The general sense of competence is linked to the ability to manage the ordinary affairs of life. Gutheil and Applebaum define competence as "that state, described in many of the statutes governing guardianship procedures, determined by the ability to handle all one's affairs in an adequate manner" (p. 215). This ability has commonly been defined vaguely in both statute and common law. This vagueness has allowed considerable flexibility for the judiciary to determine whether an individual is incompetent and therefore in need of guardianship.

From Roman times, through the ages of feudalism and monarchy, the traditional role of the guardian was to assume responsibility for the *property* of those who were unable to manage it for themselves. Only in modern law has the responsibility of the guardian for the *person* of the incompetent individual been recognized. The responsibilities for the property and person have often been tied together, though they need not be.

Prior to the last several decades, many persons were held to be generally incompetent simply because they were hospitalized in mental or psychiatric institutions. This often led to a sweeping loss of rights unrelated to the particular mental difficulties of the individual. In more recent decades the due process of individual hearings, with evidence presented by both sides before a court, has become the standard setting for deciding questions of competence and incompetence.

The specific senses of competence in the legal tradition are defined in relation to particular acts: competence to stand trial, to manage one's finances, to enter a contract, or to write a will, for example. Recent developments in the law have included possibilities of limited guardianship that correspond with these notions of specific competence or incompetence. It has been recognized traditionally, for example, that incompetence to handle finances might be best addressed by a limited guardianship for that function only. For specific incompetence to consent to or to refuse medical treatment, limited guardianship for this task alone has been given some consideration, though currently it is rarely used. States that have adopted limited guardianship statutes still most frequently appoint "standard" guardians.

As we noted earlier, competence has also been a medical and psychiatric concept. This is true, at least in part, because the practical application of the legal concept has involved physicians. Gutheil and Applebaum (1982) note that while the final determination of legal competence or incompetence is made by the judge, it "is the clinician who usually decides if a judicial determination of competence is warranted and, in many cases, it is the clinician's assessment that serves as the basis, often the sole basis, for the judge's decision" (p. 215).

In the past, the clinician involved has often been the family physician, licensed to practice medicine "in all its branches." But in the modern evolution of medicine, physicians have tended increasingly to delegate this clinical role to a specialist, the psychiatrist, or even to a subspecialist, the forensic psychiatrist.

Now let us consider two clinical situations faced by a rather typical general hospital psychiatrist, which will focus some of the issues at hand.

CASE 1

Mr. Jones is a thirty-two-year-old man who required emergency admission to the hospital for acute renal failure. On admission he was stuporous and obviously very ill. His blood chemistries were dangerously abnormal due to his kidney failure. He underwent peritoneal dialysis as an emergency procedure; it corrected the chemical abnormalities and returned him to clear consciousness and a sense of relative well-being within days. He now told his doctors and nurses that his religious beliefs required him to trust in the healing power of faith and prayer; he did not want further treatment in the hospital but wished to be discharged. Since his kidney function had not returned (though it might), his physicians saw this decision as posing a clear danger to his life, and so they asked a psychiatrist to evaluate the patient.

In the interview with the psychiatrist, the patient described his beliefs and practice as those of a fundamentalist Christian. He believed that the Bible teaches that faith and prayer can heal, and that believers should not seek help from physicians except as a last resort; such a necessity indicated that one's faith was simply not strong enough. He had finally been encouraged to come to the hospital by his wife and pastor, but he now saw his partial recovery as another opportunity to reassert his faith and give God the opportunity to heal him. He understood the seriousness of his illness, what the doctors were advising and why; he was clear and consistent in his reasons for refusing the recommended treatment. He had no wish to die and showed no sign of mental disorder. His wife, also a member of the same faith community, supported his decision.

Why had psychiatric consultation been requested in this case? Several possible reasons are pertinent to our inquiry.

First, some physicians respond to treatment refusals of this nature with a sense of outrage or indignation, feeling that such a clearly "wrong" choice is surely incompetent and should not be allowed, or at least they should not have to participate in it. They may seek to distance themselves from acquiescence, placing the problem in someone else's hands *by questioning the competence* of the patient. This is especially likely if the physician believes that a doctor's overriding duty to the patient is to promote the patient's best interests as the physician sees them.

Second, consultation may be requested not because incompetence is presumed, but because physicians believe that in such a serious matter competence should be certified, and that certifying competence involves empirical observations best performed by an expert. Two appropriate questions for the psychiatrist might be: (1) Does the patient clearly understand the facts: the expected course of the illness if not treated, the risks of refusal, the treatment alternatives and their expected risks and benefits? (2) Is there any disorder of mental functioning or emotional state that could be interfering with the patient's reasoning or hindering the capacity to make a free choice in the matter? The psychiatrist is presumably trained and experienced in examining reasoning and emotions. Determining whether there are impediments to fully rational and free choice is an empirical role for the psychiatrist; however, as we shall see, it is far from "value-free."

Third, the psychiatrist may be consulted because it seems to the doctors that the patient is choosing death when death is not inevitable. There is a tendency to equate choosing death with suicide, and the psychiatrist is the professional who is supposed to handle suicide. Is this patient's choice suicidal, and can we do anything about it? The psychiatrist's questioning of the patient revealed that the patient was not choosing to die, nor did he wish to die. The distinction between suicide and accepting one's natural death is equivalent to the distinction between not attempting to prolong life and actively seeking to end it, which enters into the debate on euthanasia. In this case, the patient was neither seeking nor even ready to accept death as inevitable or desirable.

If the patient were actively seeking to die, and this act of leaving the hospital were the method of "suicide," would the law allow intervention to prevent it? Involuntary hospitalization to prevent the infliction of harm on oneself is generally allowed by law only if this danger is the result of a mental disorder. This condition in the law should prevent involuntary hospitalization from being used to interfere with behavior that is dangerous but the product of free personal choice, such as sky-diving, mountain climbing, cigarette smoking, providing medical treatment to victims of bubonic plague, or health-jeopardizing adherence to religious beliefs. In the case of Jones, signs of mental disorder were absent, and so the law would not allow involuntary hospitalization, much less involuntary treatment. (Developments in common law have asserted the right of even involuntarily hospitalized patients to refuse particular treatments. Incompetence to decide about hospitalization does not necessarily imply other kinds of incompetence.[1])

Do death wishes alone constitute evidence of a mental disorder? If one so defined the situation, the law might allow intervention to prevent this danger to the self. It is just such a definition of mental disorder, however, that would be assailable as a rationalization to justify social control, rather than connected with treatment. (It is reminiscent of the definition of dissent against the state as mental disorder in the Soviet Union.) Whether psychiatrists should be allowed or even expected to interfere with dangerous choices is an important question for a public philosophy for psychiatry.

Perl and Shelp (1982) have noted that consultations such as in the case of Jones are not unusual for psychiatrists in a general hospital setting, and that physicians and others may request them when they find themselves in moral dilemmas. There is a dilemma with Jones. Should we respect his apparently autonomous choice, or are we to pursue his best interests as we see them because this is our duty or mission? The predominant answer in the medical ethics literature and the law is that such paternalism cannot be justified. However, there is also a seeming consensus that situations of reduced autonomy and diminished competence may allow "weak" paternalistic intervention (Beauchamp and Childress 1983; Veatch 1981; Engelhardt 1986). I believe that questioning competence is frequently used either to justify paternalistic intervention or to avoid confronting a moral dilemma: How ought we to balance conflicting duties? In this situation we also face a more fundamental ontological question: How truly autonomous are human beings?

CASE 2

Mrs. Green, a forty-five-year-old woman, was brought to the emergency room on a bitterly cold January night. A passerby had found her unconscious, lying in the snow, without a coat. She was suffering from serious hypothermia from exposure to cold. Following vigorous emergency treatment, she regained consciousness and began talking rapidly and excitedly about how she had received a special mission from God to save mankind. She had not been sure how to do this until voices had told her that God wanted her now. She had been wandering, trying to determine where to go, before she lost consciousness. Her husband supplied the additional information that she had been in an excited state for four days since being laid off from her job. She had slept no more than a few hours on any night since and not at all for forty-eight hours. She had been easily irritated, and had accused him of being an agent of Satan when he tried to get her to the family doctor.

No evidence of ongoing illness or injury was found, and the psychiatrist was called to evaluate the patient, who demanded to be released from the hospital.

This sort of issue is common in psychiatric practice. Though the matter is seldom couched in terms of competence, it does involve a question of competence, the competence to consent to or refuse admission to a hospital for psychiatric treatment.

This problem has both empirical and moral aspects. In this case the patient is refusing consent. The empirical questions that will enter into assessment of whether the patient may be hospitalized involuntarily include whether the patient has a mental illness, whether as a result of the mental illness the patient is likely to harm herself or others in the near future if not hospitalized, or whether the patient is able to provide for her basic physical needs.

In this case, recent events and numerous signs and symptoms are consistent with the diagnosis of mania, though other diagnostic possibilities exist. It is reasonable for the psychiatrist to conclude that she has a mental disorder. She has already demonstrated the danger that she poses to herself in this state; she was near death from exposure. She was also not providing for her basic needs for adequate clothing and shelter; in some states this would be sufficient justification for involuntary hospitalization even if she had not reached such a dangerous degree of exposure.

This patient meets the legal criteria for involuntary hospitalization under even the most limiting state law. Many manic patients present a more marginal or questionable fit to the criteria of dangerousness. They may be creating personal or family havoc because their judgment is colored by their elated or irritable moods; they may be squandering their own or their families' assets in an orgy of spending or travel; or they may get into fights because of their irritability. These behaviors are distinct from their normal personality characteristics and are often viewed by them later with puzzlement, disbelief, guilt, and shame. And yet there may be no clear evidence that they are likely to harm themselves or anyone else or that they will fail to meet their own basic needs—at least until they have already begun to do so or have actually done so. The psychiatrist may face the decision of whether to interpret the law broadly and admit the patient, or to stand by, with effective treatments available, hoping that the patient will seek help voluntarily.

There is another important question to be addressed. If a patient's competence to refuse hospitalization is questioned, should her competence to voluntarily consent be questioned as well? In reality, one seldom questions the competence of a patient who agrees to recommended psychiatric hospitalization, though Lidz et al. (1984) have shown, in the most thorough empirical study to date of informed consent in psychiatric settings, that such consents are often far from ideal. In medical settings, too, doctors are much more likely to question the competence of a patient who opposes recommended treatment than one who complies. Even noncompliant decisions are not so troubling when there are alternative choices that are relatively equal in the professional's view—for example, two treatments of roughly equal effectiveness or a choice between no treatment and an uncomfortable or burdensome protocol with little likelihood of success. But when a patient rejects a treatment that is clearly the most effective, physicians are likely to find the decision troubling and to question the patient's competence to decide.

The tendency to question the patient's competence to refuse but presume competence to consent might be seen as a cynical manipulation or rationalization. As James Drane (1984) has argued, however, it could also represent a more complex moral sensitivity. We will examine this further.

Competence: Tests and Standards

While the law has traditionally been vague in its definitions of competence and incompetence, speaking of the incompetent person in general terms such as "one who is so affected mentally as to be deprived of sane and normal action" (Gutheil and Applebaum 1982, 215) scholars of psychiatry and ethics have given increasing attention to the criteria used to determine competence in different situations.

Roth, Meisel, and Lidz (1977) have enumerated five tests for competence to consent to treatment, which are set at various levels of stringency.

1. Evidencing a choice: Only the patient who does not directly evidence a preference, either verbally or behaviorally, is to be considered incompetent.
2. "Reasonable" outcome of choice: Only the patient who fails to choose what a hypothetical "reasonable" person would choose should be considered incompetent.
3. Choice based on "rational" reasons: If the patient's choice can be demonstrated to be the product of a mental illness, the patient is incompetent.
4. The ability to understand: Competence is determined by the *ability* to understand and appraise risks, benefits, and alternatives. Decisions need not be rational in process or outcome.
5. Actual understanding: The patient's actual understanding, not an abstract ability to understand, is the deciding factor.

Choosing which test to apply can obviously affect the result. By the first standard, evidencing a choice, neither of our patients would be considered incompetent. By the "reasonable choice" standard, Jones might be considered incompetent, whereas by the "ability to understand" and "actual understanding" standards he would probably be considered competent. Roth et al. discuss in detail the technical, legal, and moral advantages and disadvantages of each test, then state:

> In effect, the test that is actually applied combines elements of all the tests described above. However, the circumstances in which competence becomes an issue determine which elements of which tests are stressed, and which are underplayed. Although, in theory, competence is an independent variable, that determines whether or not the patient's decision to accept or refuse treatment is to be honored, in practice it seems to be dependent on the interplay of two other variables: the risk/benefit ratio of treatment and the valence of the patient's decision, i.e., whether he or she consents to or refuses treatment. (Roth et al. 1977, 282–83)

They thus acknowledge the role professional and societal values play in the choice of empirical standards. In fact, they conclude by saying that

> the search for a single test of competence is a search for a Holy Grail. . . .
> In practice, judgments of competence go beyond semantics or straight forward applications of legal rules; such judgments reflect social consid-

erations and societal biases as much as they reflect matters of law and medicine. (Roth et al. 1977, 283)

Which roles do we as a society wish to assign to judges, lawyers, psychiatrists, and others in determining not only that correct judgments are made according to standards, but which standards are used? Diverse interest groups may contribute their voices to the debate on such a public policy question. Psychiatry as a profession may have a unified or disjointed stand. Analysis of the ethical dimensions of these competence issues may help us more clearly understand what the professional values at stake may be.

Competence: Moral Aspects

Judgments of patient competence or incompetence, as we have already seen, are not simply factual. My argument is that they are moral judgments with a purpose: to justify the beneficent interventions of others or their forbearance from intervening.

Beauchamp and McCullough (1984, 105–32) have presented a most helpful and scholarly reflection on the relationship of reduced autonomy and diminished competence. They argue that the concepts are frequently confused, because they are frequently associated, but that they are, in fact, distinct. They do acknowledge, however, that "the language of reduced and substantially reduced autonomy has emerged largely from philosophical ethics and contemporary medical ethics. It has parallels, however, in the language of competence and incompetence in medicine and law" (p. 117).

Beauchamp and McCullough's discussion is set in the context of their consideration of two models of the moral responsibility of physicians (pp. 22–51). The *autonomy model*

> takes the values and beliefs of the patient to be the primary moral consideration in determining the physician's moral responsibilities in patient care: If the patient's values directly conflict with medicine's values, the fundamental responsibility of physicians is to respect and to facilitate a patient's self-determination in making decisions about his or her medical fate. (p. 42)

The *beneficence model* takes as the fundamental moral responsibility the promotion of goods for patients, as medicine sees those goods, and the prevention of harms, as medicine sees those harms. The authors view both models as having normative force for physicians; adopting one exclusively would result in the sacrifice of significant values.

After presenting these models, they present a detailed analysis of medical paternalism in which they argue that debate over "justifiable paternalism" is often not a debate about paternalism in the strict sense, because what is being contemplated is not interference with a patient who is substantially autonomous.

> The problem of medical paternalism should thus be reconceived as a set of problems about determinations of autonomy and competence, eventuating in questions about how to justify diagnostic and therapeutic interventions in cases where a patient is at a level of questionable or reduced autonomy and in need of medical care. (p. 103)

The authors then explain, in detail, what they mean by reduced autonomy and diminished competence, drawing largely on the analysis by Roth et al. (1977) previously discussed. While they do point out differences between these notions, there is also considerable overlap. Both autonomy and competence, for example, have to do with abilities to marshal knowledge, understand, and reason through. The exact relation, in the final analysis, between reduced autonomy and diminished competence is not completely clear. They speak of competence diminished because capability for autonomous decisions has been significantly reduced (Beauchamp and McCullough 1984, 126). I would pose it the opposite way: the patient's capacity for autonomous decisions is reduced because competence has been diminished. The explanation for our opposite inclinations may be, as they have themselves pointed out (p. 117), that I am more attuned to the language of competence from medicine and the law, while as professional ethicists they are more attuned to the language of autonomy.

In the end, I believe this quibble matters little. I thoroughly agree with them that the ultimate outcome, the "intentionality" of judgments of reduced autonomy or diminished competence, is the justification of the intervention or nonintervention of the physician and other caregivers. So, Beauchamp and McCullough (1984) warn, "a commitment to one or more of the tests of competence previously discussed inevitably carries some form of value commitment regarding justified intervention" (pp. 125–26). The choice of which test of competence to employ will reflect one's leaning toward the autonomy model or the beneficence model.

Reconsider the case of Jones: an evaluator who favored the autonomy model might choose Roth's standard 1, evidencing a choice, or standard 4, the ability to understand; in either case, Jones would be considered competent. An evaluator inclined to the beneficence model might prefer standard 2, the reasonable outcome of choice. Since Jones did not choose what the "reasonable" person would be expected to choose, he could be considered incompetent.

It is important to realize that it is not simply a matter of which model the physician or psychiatrist leans toward. The law itself does not specify a single standard to which judges are bound; the final competence determination of the court will reflect which model the judge leans toward. It is probably fair to say that the Anglo-Saxon law tradition favors the autonomy model more strongly. The Hippocratic medical tradition favors the beneficence model.

Let me now attempt to illustrate some of the difficult or painful situations encountered by the psychiatrist, who may be more or less aware of the moral nature of competence questions.

First, the psychiatrist encounters those who favor the beneficence model in an extreme way. These are likely to be other physicians (but may be nurses or other medical professionals) or beleaguered family members. These people seek to have the patient treated regardless of the patient's wishes, and they question the competence of noncompliant patients. They at least are puzzled, and more often dismayed or angry, if the psychiatrist says that the patient is competent to decide. "What do you mean he can just walk out?" "How can you as a physician let someone do this to himself?" "Aren't you going to do something?" "Don't you care?"

Second, the psychiatrist encounters those who favor the autonomy model in an extreme way. Examples might be civil liberties lawyers, "watchdog" groups, or other family members (even in the same family with those discussed above). These people seek to have the patient's wishes carried out regardless of the consequences. They are disinclined to see incompetence except at the extremes, such as coma. They at least are scandalized, and more likely furious or horrified, if the patient is detained or someone questions the patient's competence. "What do you mean you can keep him against his will? We're calling a lawyer." "You can't get away with this." "Who gave you the right to play God?"

Third, the psychiatrist who recognizes the value of both models must move in favor of one or the other in particular cases. A psychiatrist who believes this choice should be determined by the nuances of reduced autonomy or diminished competence will inevitably be faced with patients in whom these reductions are of unclear degree. Jeffrie Murphy (1979) writes,

> The real problem that will face us, then, is what to do in the borderline cases. When in doubt, which way should we err—on the side of safety or on the side of liberty? It is vital that we do not adopt analyses of incompetence or patterns of argument that obscure the obviously moral nature of this question. (p. 174)

If the psychiatrist errs on the side of safety, she will override some autonomous choices; if she errs on the side of liberty, she will sometimes fail to protect someone who is not really autonomous or competent from the harmful effects of a bad decision. Is there a way to prevent, or at least minimize, these errors?

James Drane (1984), focusing on informed consent, has proposed a helpful model in which the standard of competence to be applied would depend on the dangerousness of the medical decision. He is attempting to lay the groundwork for a consensus on a *procedure* that would protect the values of both the autonomy model and the beneficence model. He proposes three "sliding" standards:

1. The least stringent standard of competence would be applied to "those medical decisions that are not dangerous and objectively are in the patient's best interest" (p. 926). This would include consent to recommended and needed treatment, even when patients are quite ill and cognitively impaired. What is required by this standard is that the patient is *aware* of the general situation and *assents* to this reasonable expectation. This corresponds most closely to test 1 of Roth et al., but contains test 2, the "reasonable outcome," as well.

2. The next, more stringent, standard would be applied in chronic illness, if the treatment is more dangerous or of less definite benefit, or if there are real treatment alternatives. Here the requirement would be that the patient "must be able to understand the risks and outcomes of the different options and then be able to choose a decision based on this understanding" (p. 926). This standard combines tests 4 and 5 of Roth et al.

3. The most stringent standard would be used "for those decisions that are very dangerous and fly in the face of both professional and public rationality" (p. 927). This would come into play with refusals of vitally needed, effective treatment. What would be required here is appreciation of the implications (the highest degree of understanding), and a subjectively critical and rational decision that can be verbally stated and argued. This standard also combines tests 4 and 5 of Roth et al. but adds the requirement of the ability to argue rationally, the most demanding demonstration of ability to understand and actual understanding.

Of note is that different standards might apply for consenting than for refusing consent. This runs counter to the views of Roth et al. (1977), who argue for symmetry of standards. Drane (1984, 927) justifies this as attempting to minimize harm, that is, appealing to the values of the beneficence model. However, he argues that the sliding standard attempts to *balance* the values of maximum autonomy and maximum benefit for patients. Drane's proposal deserves attention as a helpful step toward addressing the conflicts between the autonomy model and the beneficence model in a way sensitive to real clinical situations.

The responsibility for participating in the determination of an individual's competence, whether in the general or specific sense, raises issues for a public philosophy for psychiatry and for medicine in general. The notion that the determination of competence or incompetence is simply empirical is incorrect; there are too many possible standards full of moral implications applied by many people with differing moral points of view. The ways in which it is most reasonable to draw professional boundaries in this task are not clear; the issue is a weighty matter for public philosophy. Finally, such cases raise the fundamental ontological question of how truly competent, and thus autonomous, any human being is. Let us approach this question from another direction.

Freedom and Responsibility

Two cases will illustrate another problem that could be addressed in the development of a public philosophy for psychiatry—the problem of the relationship between the freedom and responsibility of the patient and the professional responsibility of the psychiatrist.

CASE 3

James was a twenty-seven-year-old man brought to the hospital by his family because they had become frightened by his behavior. James had told them that he had been hearing voices that made fun of him, and that his thoughts were being stolen from him and broadcast through the television. A week before his admission to the hospital he had grabbed a kitchen knife and threatened suicide. He had denied problems when his family and the family doctor had tried to convince him to go to the hospital, and they had finally had to ask the police to bring him in after he had driven off in a family member's car.

James's problems were not entirely new. He had previously been treated by a psychologist and a psychiatrist, and he had taken both antipsychotic and antidepressant medication. His father had died of a heart attack a year earlier. James had decreased his social activity after his father's death and complained of being abandoned by his friends.

James's mother and older brothers and sisters had felt intimidated in recent weeks by his threatening behavior. Their wishes at the time of admission were that we "teach him that he cannot demand anything he wants and get it, and teach him to be nicer to others and to use proper eating manners and hygiene."

The family was also concerned about James's drinking, which he himself denied. But they also felt guilty for his troubles and were quick to defend him against criticism. It became clear that his father had not taken good care of himself, had been overweight, and had smoked excessively despite doctors' advice following earlier problems with chest pain. When he had pain he frequently told James and other family members they were "killing" him.

As the hospitalization went on, the family became critical of the doctors and staff for not giving them the answers they needed. These complaints were registered despite intensive therapeutic efforts directed toward both James and his family.

The staff found itself struggling with the issue of its therapeutic responsibilities. Were its responsibilities those James and his family were all too eager to define? Patients may require a lot of services, many of which are not readily available elsewhere, and which may really be good for the patient. Should providing these services be the responsibilities of hospitals, their doctors, and their staffs by default?

Is James capable of better functioning? Should he be expected to grow "in wisdom and age and grace," or should his inaction, helplessness, and even boorishness be accepted by his family and others around him? It is all too easy for us humans to blame others for the evils that befall us or that we ourselves create. There seems to be an innate tendency, which we may use adaptively or maladaptively, to what the psychodynamic tradition calls denial and sees as an unconscious defense against anxiety. We all use it at times, even without the kind of role model that James had in his father, a man who never took responsibility for himself, instead blaming others for his problems or denying their existence altogether.

How much responsibility should be attributed to James? Attributing all or most of the responsibility to him may be callous. If, in fact, he suffers from a serious brain disease or malfunction (as evidenced by his psychotic episodes), he has little power to correct it without some treatment from "outside" (the responsibility of the psychiatrist). On the other hand, attributing no responsibility to James would mean the loss of all therapeutic leverage. If he were in no way responsible, there would be no personal agent to whom to appeal for cooperation in the treatment. All intervention would have to be done *to* him and not *with* him, as if James were not a person at all.

A case from the courts illustrates another aspect of the problem of patient responsibility and the responsibility of health professionals—one that is all too real a consideration in the daily practice of psychiatry as in the rest of medicine. That is, a physician's concern for legal ramifications sometimes rivals concern for the best interests of the patient.

CASE 4

A young woman was injured when her car was struck by a vehicle that a young man drove through a red light at fifty to sixty miles per hour. To witnesses, he appeared intoxicated. Five days earlier he had been released from a state hospital, where he had received treatment for a psychotic condition. He had emasculated himself in his psychotic state and had been involuntarily committed for a period of treatment. During this time (about two weeks) the doctor formed the opinion that the psychosis was caused by the drug phencyclidine ("angel dust"), which the man had taken. The psychosis cleared and the patient was judged to have returned to normal personality and behavior. However, the doctor noted his potential dangerousness and unpredictability, especially if he were to use "angel dust" again or quit taking his antipsychotic medication.

A jury found the doctor liable for the young woman's injuries in a malpractice action, despite her having been a chance victim. On appeal the state supreme court affirmed the verdict, ruling that the therapist had a duty to protect any person foreseeably in danger, rejecting other courts' reasoning limiting potential liability to readily identifiable victims.[2]

When something bad happens as a result of the actions of a patient, who shall be held responsible? Why does a person's receiving the help of a physician make the physician responsible for what the patient does subsequently? Is consulting a physician a way to escape responsibility for one's own actions?

We are ambivalent as a society about the answers to questions such as these. We are increasingly strict with drunk drivers because we realize that they can kill people. We extend this responsibility to tavern owners and even private citizens who serve them liquor. But we do not blame the drunk drivers' families or doctors who have tried to get them to stop drinking.

On the other hand, we have increasingly held mental health professionals responsible in tort for the dangerous acts of their patients. This began in earnest with the Tarasoff definition of the duty to warn an identified victim if it is not appropriate or possible to seek civil commitment of the patient[3] (Mills et al. 1987). This responsibility has now been extended in the Tarasoff case to a responsibility to protect unidentifiable potential victims not from the acts of a patient with an ongoing mental disorder but from the unintentional acts of an ex-patient who voluntarily ingests a dangerous drug when no longer under the supervision of the physician.

We may wish to hold psychiatrists responsible for preventing dangerous actions of patients who have active, serious mental disturbances that can be expected to respond to treatment. I might include in such a group aggressive psychotic patients, currently intoxicated patients, or even those whose current physical addiction makes it difficult to stop their current use of the drug causing their loss of control. But to hold psychiatrists responsible for preventing no longer addicted patients from ever again ingesting a dangerous drug would lead to indefinite deprivation of liberty for many people who have never harmed anyone and never would. Are we really ready for the kind of preventive detention this seems to require?

We are also ambivalent about the responsibility of patients for criminal acts and use of the insanity defense. The legal system and juries continue to find defendants not guilty by reason of insanity (though rarely in comparison to the number of cases). But there is considerable public opinion that such a defense should not be allowed, or that, if such verdicts must be allowed, psychiatrists should act as jailors sensitive to the public's fears and moral judgment.

Further analysis of this issue is beyond the scope of this essay. Rather we must look at the general moral issues raised by these cases.

Responsibility: Moral Aspects

These cases reflect the ways in which patients, their families, and mental health professions can be caught in our societal indecision around the question of how much responsibility to attribute to patients and how much to those who care for them as patients. I believe that the answers to these questions have implications far beyond those of therapeutic strategies or the tort liabilities of physicians. The implications are centrally related to our notions of human personhood: human autonomy and freedom, human moral responsibility.

A public philosophy for psychiatry would profitably include many perspectives on freedom and responsibility. I will briefly look at three: one from the history of psychiatry, one from the law, and one from literature.

A PSYCHIATRIC PERSPECTIVE

Freud's discoveries about psychic determinism undoubtedly raised new doubts about cherished beliefs in human freedom. Freud's writings contain some ambiguity about how he viewed the relationship of psychic determinism to human responsibility (Moore 1984). It was, after all, the determinism of mental processes that Freud was asserting most strongly, not a total determination of human action. He seems to have concluded that the existence of the unconscious in mental life does not absolve one of responsibility. For example, he wrote about moral responsibility for dreams:

> Obviously one must hold oneself responsible for the evil impulses of one's dreams. What else is one to do with them? Unless the content of the dream (rightly understood) is inspired by alien spirits, it is part of my own being. If I seek to classify the impulses that are present in me according to social standards into good and bad, I must assume responsibility for both sorts; and if, in defence, I say that what is unknown, unconscious and repressed in me is not my "ego," then I shall not be basing my position upon psycho-analysis, I shall not have accepted its conclusions—and I shall perhaps be taught better by the criticisms of my fellow-men, by the disturbances in my actions and the confusion of my feelings. I shall perhaps learn that what I am disavowing not only "is" me but sometimes "acts" from out of me as well.
>
> It is true that in the metapsychological sense this bad repressed content does not belong to my "ego"—that is, assuming that I am a morally blameless individual—but to an "id" upon which my ego is seated. But this ego developed out of the id, it forms with it a single biological unit, it is only a specially modified peripheral portion of it, and it is subject to the influences and obeys the suggestions that arise from the id. For any vital purpose, a separation of the ego from the id would be a hopeless undertaking.
>
> Moreover, if I were to give way to my moral pride and tried to decree that for the purposes of moral valuation I might disregard the evil in the id and need not make my ego responsible for it, what use would that be to me? Experience shows me that I nevertheless do take that responsibility, that I am somehow compelled to do so. (Freud 1925, 133)

Freud saw psychoanalysis, in its action of striving to bring to consciousness that which is unconscious, as freeing the individual from compulsion or ignorance, and enabling greater responsibility. In "On Psychotherapy" (1905, 266), he wrote:

> If, however, you will look at the matter from our point of view, you will understand that the transformation of this unconscious material in the mind of the patient into conscious material must have the result of correcting his deviation from normality and of lifting the compulsion to which his mind has been subjected. For conscious will-power governs only conscious mental processes, and every mental compulsion is rooted in the unconscious. Nor need you ever fear that the patient will be harmed by the shock accompanying the introduction of the unconscious into consciousness, for you can convince yourself theoretically that the somatic and emotional effect of an impulse that has become conscious can never be so powerful as that of an unconscious one. It is only by the

application of our highest mental functions, which are bound up with consciousness, that we can control all our impulses.

A LEGAL PERSPECTIVE

An extremely helpful analysis of the psychiatric and legal notions of responsibility has been done by law professor Michael Moore in *Law and Psychiatry: Rethinking the Relationship* (1984). Moore examines philosophically how psychiatry and the law view human persons, human action, and human responsibility.

Moore's most general concern is "how we do and should think of ourselves" (p. xi). The theme important to him is "a view of what persons are like: a view that we are responsible for who we are and what we do because we have the capacities rationally to will our fate in this world. Such a view entails ultimate metaphysical faith in our reason and its power to control our actions" (p. xi).

Moore's comparison of the legal and psychiatric views of causation and responsibility includes dissection of the psychiatric (psychodynamic) concept of the unconscious and its causal implications. Does acknowledgment of the explanatory power of the unconscious as causally related to human behavior necessarily imply that persons are not morally responsible? Moore's ultimate philosophical conclusion is to reject this hard determinist position on the ground that determinism and responsibility are not inconsistent (p. 360 ff.). He argues that we humans have causal powers to change our world even though the exercise of these causal powers may be fully determined by other factors. We have the capacities to reason practically and to perform complex actions to change things in the world to suit our wants. It is the presence of these capacities that we see as constituting our autonomy and as the source of our responsibility for our actions. (An interesting feature of his argument is that it does not require seeing ourselves as free or having "free will.")

Moore rejects the attempt to reconcile the notions of the unconscious and of responsibility through a kind of partial or "selective" determinism, in which degrees of freedom are also active. He claims that this ultimately does not make sense. "It makes sense to say that we are determined or that we are free, but to speak of being partly determined or partly free makes as much sense as speaking of being partly pregnant" (p. 365). "If common sense believes that there can be a little bit of causation, then it is wrong— wrong because this is inconsistent with our more basic metaphysical ideas of what kinds of causal relations exist" (p. 358).

I disagree. It seems to me that it can be sensible to understand freedom and determinism as dimensional, not categorical, concepts. (Moore's use of Morse's (1982) description of this as "impure common sense" (p. 1030) seems rhetorical.) We may well disagree because we have different metaphysical ideas of what kinds of causal relations exist. The degrees to which freedom and determinism each seem to be causally active depend on circumstances and also on our point of view. Looked at from the therapist's perspective, through the scientific instrument of clinical observation, much (some say all) of the patient's action seems determined by preceding events and forces. On the other hand, the patient has the experience of choice, of freedom, with which we can identify because of our own experience of freedom, and which we can infer as contributing to the explanation of actions. These two points of view are also not inevitably isolated from each other. The patient whose self-understanding is increasing through treatment will identify determining factors in himself. It can be seen as the goal of therapy that the determining forces will be lessened, freeing the person for more truly autonomous personhood, whether through self-understanding in psychotherapeutic treatment, through learning in behavioral treatments, or through the salutary effects of psychotropic medication on brain function.

While we might come to the conclusion by somewhat different philosophical means, I can agree with Moore (1984, 283) in seeing human beings as rational and autonomous agents with moral responsibility. I also endorse his concluding statement: "In this fight about a radical rethinking of who we are, both law and psychiatry are on the same side in defending an intentional conceptualization of persons as rational and autonomous agents. On this issue both, to my way of thinking, are on the side of the angels" (p. 425).

Moore's work is an excellent contribution to the development of public philosophies for both law and psychiatry. He takes an important area of common interest and does serious philosophical analysis and argumentation. In the process he contributes to a greater understanding by each profession of itself, of the other, and of their relations. In the final analysis he sees the psychiatric and legal views of persons as more alike than different and not incompatible (pp. 424–25).

A LITERARY PERSPECTIVE

As an example of a powerful literary vision of these issues of freedom and responsibility, recall the story of the Grand Inquisitor told by the atheist brother Ivan to his religious brother Alexey in *The Brothers Karamazov*. The Grand Inquisitor indicts Jesus who has appeared in Seville at the height of the Inquisition: "I tell Thee that man is tormented by no greater anxiety than to find some one quickly to whom he can hand over that gift of freedom with which the ill-fated creature is born. . . . Instead of taking possession of men's freedom, Thou didst increase it, and burdened the spiritual kingdom of mankind with its sufferings forever" (Dostoyevsky 1950, 302). Jesus remains silent. At the conclusion of the tale Alexey responds to Ivan: "Your poem is in praise of Jesus, not in blame of Him— as you meant it to be. And who will believe you about freedom? Is that the way to understand it?" (p. 309).

It is painful for human beings to be burdened with the gift of freedom and responsibility, but ennobling to us. It is consistent with respect for persons, and with therapeutic work as a psychiatrist, to see our responsibility to our patients as both to recognize their autonomy and to foster their assumption of responsibility. This seems to me to be truly beneficent care.

Conclusion: Public Philosophy in a Pluralistic Society

The development of a fuller public philosophy requires many more contributions. Like Moore's analysis these contributions will need to look at our fundamental beliefs about the ontology of the human person, our moral duties and the warrants we see as grounding them, and the convictions we have, if any, of the purpose or direction of human life. Such fundamental concepts are operative in our convictions about what professionals should be and do, whether we are within the professions or outside them. An analysis of the shared and divergent views of psychiatry and the world faith traditions on these matters could be extremely rich, and the present volume only hints at this richness.

Engelhardt (1986, 37–49) points out that in our modern pluralistic society we no longer have a universally acceptable final arbiter for ethical disputes when values and principles conflict. What must remain is respect for the autonomy of moral agents, and commitment to persuasion rather than coercion.

While no one faith tradition can enforce its point of view, I am certain that the faith traditions will have volumes to speak about rationality and responsibility, about respect for persons and autonomy, about beneficence and care. The concept of autonomy bears close relationship to philosophical and religious concepts of freedom and responsibility. The faith traditions may use different language and different stories to tell us about these things. They may speak in terms of sin, salvation, and redemption. Similarly, the concept of beneficence bears close relationship to religious concepts about the human condition, human needs, relationships, and care. The faith traditions may speak in terms of original sin, covenant, charity, and virtue. It is a challenge for a public philosophy to understand the shared meanings of these different languages.

R. M. Hare (1981) points out how difficult it is for the physician to reflect critically and thoroughly. Reflection is seldom if ever possible in the heat of the clinical situation, when the need for guidance is greatest. Reasoned ethical reflection at a distance can help us form guides for ourselves to use when we have little time to reflect. Such reflection is also important for lawyers and judges, religious leaders, concerned patients and families, and the community as a whole. No one is competent to see from all important points of view. Such reflection, exchange of ideas, and persuasion will contribute to a more refined sense of what we should be as professionals, and perhaps a more comfortable resolution of the conflicts of being "double agents." The result may be a greater clarity for both professional and society about how to balance the interests of our individual patients and our broader community in our professional service.

Notes

1. Rogers v Okin, 478 F Supp 1342, 1364 (D Mass 1979); Rogers v Commissioner of Mental Health, 390 Mass 498 (1982); Rogers v Okin, 634 F 2d 650 (1st Cir 1980); and Rennie v Klein, 476 F Supp 1294 (D NJ 1979); Rennie v Klein, 653 F 2d 836 (3rd Cir 1981).

2. Petersen v State, 100 Wn2d 421, 671 P 2d 230 (Wsh 1983).

3. Tarasoff v Regents of the University of California, 118 Cal Rptr 129 (Cal 1974), and reargued 17 Cal 3d 425, 551 P 2d 334, 131 Cal Rptr 33 (1976).

References

Beauchamp, T. L. and J. F. Childress. 1983. *Principles of Biomedical Ethics.* New York: Oxford University Press.

Beauchamp, T. L. and L. B. McCullough. 1984. *Medical Ethics: The Moral Responsibilities of Physicians.* Englewood Cliffs, N.J.: Prentice-Hall.

Culver, C., and B. Gert. 1982. *Philosophy in Medicine: Conceptual and Ethical Issues in Medicine and Psychiatry,* 53–54. New York: Oxford University Press.

Dostoyevsky, F. 1950. *The Brothers Karamazov,* trans. Constance Garnett. New York: Random House.

Drane, James F. 1984. "Competency to Give an Informed Consent: A Model for Making Clinical Assessments." *Journal of the American Medical Association* 252:925–27.

Engelhardt, H. T. 1986. *The Foundations of Bioethics.* New York: Oxford University Press.

Freud, S. 1905. "On Psychotherapy." In *Complete Psychological Works,* standard edition, Vol. 7, 257–68. London: Hogarth Press, 1953–1981.

———. 1925. "Some Additional Notes on Dream-Interpretation as a Whole." In *Complete Psychological Works,* standard edition, Vol. 19, 133. London: Hogarth Press, 1953–1981.

Gutheil, T. G. and P. S. Applebaum. 1982. *Clinical Handbook of Psychiatry and the Law,* 215–32. New York: McGraw-Hill. I am indebted to this work for several points in the discussion of the legal concept of competence.

Hare, R. M. 1981. "The Philosophical Basis of Psychiatric Ethics." *Psychiatric Ethics,* ed. S. Bloch and P. Chodoff, 31–45. Oxford: Oxford University Press.

Lidz, C. W., A. Meisel, E. Zerubavel, et al. 1984. *Informed Consent: A Study of Decisionmaking in Psychiatry.* New York: Guilford Press.

Mechanic, David. 1981. "The Social Dimension: The Psychiatrist as Double Agent." In *Psychiatric Ethics,* ed. S. Bloch and P. Chodoff. Oxford: Oxford University Press.

Mills, M. J., S. Sullivan, and S. Eth. 1987. "Protecting Third Parties: A Decade after Tarasoff." *American Journal of Psychiatry* 144:68–74.

Moore, M. S. 1984. *Law and Psychiatry: Rethinking the Relationship.* Cambridge: Cambridge University Press.

Morse, S. 1982. "Failed Explanations and Criminal Responsibility: Experts and the Unconscious." *Virginia Law Review* 68:971–1084.

Murphy, Jeffrie G. 1979. "Incompetence and Paternalism." *Retribution, Justice, and Therapy: Essays in the Philosophy of Law.* Boston: D. Reidel.

Perl, M., and E. E. Shelp. 1982. "Psychiatric Consultation Masking Moral Dilemmas in Medicine." *New England Journal of Medicine* 307:618–21.

Roth, L. H., A. Meisel and C. W. Lidz. 1977. "Tests of Competency to Consent to Treatment." *American Journal of Psychiatry* 134:279–84.

Szasz, Thomas. 1974. *The Myth of Mental Illness.* New York: Harper and Row.

Veatch, Robert M. 1981. *A Theory of Medical Ethics.* New York: Basic Books.

———. 1984. *Autonomy's Temporary Triumph.* Hastings Center Report, October.

CHAPTER EIGHT

THE RISE AND DECLINE OF PSYCHOSURGERY: HISTORICAL FACTORS AND ETHICAL ISSUES

Douglas E. Anderson, M.D.

When one mentions psychosurgery, people often think of the frontal lo-botomized patient-prisoner in the novel (Kesey 1962) and movie *One Flew Over the Cuckoo's Nest*. An uneasiness accompanies conversations about the topic, both at the thought of people who would tamper with the mind and concerning those who require such drastic and intrusive measures. Even more disconcerting are questions of mind control and po-litical uses of psychosurgery. In fact, practiced in evolving forms since 1935, psychosurgery is part of the larger story of the "social transforma-tion" of American medicine (Starr 1982). It is also a history of scientific achievement. Through several of the various branches of the psychosur-gery story, basic and fundamental insights into human brain function have been gained. As in all neuroscientific discovery, only small bits of knowl-edge accrue, revealing a partially developed, theoretical image of the brain's functions and mechanisms. Even then, to summarize these findings is to notice several possible interpretive levels.

As the story of psychosurgery is a social history and a history of sci-ence, it is also the history of an ethical debate. The boundaries of this debate are frequently difficult to perceive. The debate sometimes deterio-rates into legal and political manipulations, and representatives of "sci-ence" itself at times indulge in fictional speculation by inflating the importance of specific experimental findings or techniques. Additionally, the language of the debate is imprecise and/or technical. The terms *psycho-surgery, mental illness, informed consent,* and *therapy,* for example, are used in an extraordinary number of ways and have various definitions.

Fairly severe limitations are inherent in an analysis of psychosurgical history. Presuppositions underlie the perspectives of historians and of those who have taken part in the history. It is especially important to ac-knowledge this in light of the disparity that exists in psychiatric thought today. There are those who feel the whole of modern technical medicine is fundamentally mistaken in its intention and method (Illych 1976). Additionally, some within psychiatry have come to the conclusion that mental illness itself is a myth (Szasz 1974). The perspective, then, from which this paper is written begins with the following presuppositions:

1. Human beings can suffer from physical disease, illness, and malady.
2. Persons can also suffer from mental anguish, psychic pain, and thought disorder which can be categorized, when appearing in certain behavioral constellations, as mental illness, madness, insanity, etc. For the most part, pathology at the cellular level remains unknown or incomplete.
3. The human has a spiritual essence in that there exists a mystery of "being"—a mystery that will neither be fully penetrated by scientific method or discovery nor be fully accessible by rational thought. That is to say, although people may perceive a progressive encroachment upon the "spiritual essence" of human existence by advances in scientific description, this perception is fallacious. Scientific descriptions may become more detailed but they will never quantify the fundamental mysteries of the mind—its beauty, paradox, and awe-inspiring qualities. The mind-body problem is not contained wholly within the province of science or rational thought.
4. The history and philosophy of medicine have been characterized, for the most part, by care of and commitment to those who suffer with disease, illness, and malady. This tradition centers on treatment or therapy rendered through various diets, habits, rituals, medicines, and techniques. The incorporation of complex technologies into modern therapy has brought with it new problems that require attention. Where the technology is part of an experimental protocol, the issue is that of carefully distinguishing between therapeutic and nontherapeutic human experimentations. Further, the relationship—the contract or covenant—between experimenter and subject must be carefully defined. Here, past errors and abuses in conduct have helped to form present-day ethical guidelines and legislation regulating research. While one can describe these developments as they pertain to psychosurgery, they are far from completed stories; they reflect the roles of changing popular opinion and cultural mores as well as careful ethical thinking.
5. Abuse and neglect of the mentally and psychologically infirm are not only of the past but still plague us at all levels of society. There remain perversions of therapy, such as the misdiagnosis and institutionalization of political dissenters in several countries. American reformers in psychiatric therapy have failed to address the problems

of deinstitutionalized mental patients, who frequently are identified as "street people". However, that physicians in general have intended to help patients will be assumed. No attempt will be made to determine the extent to which other motivation governed their actions, unless it is obvious and stated (as in nontherapeutic research). Starting with these presuppositions, the purpose here is not to defend psychosurgery but to place the psychosurgical story in the perspective of the traditions from which it grew.

Perhaps one must look at prehistory for the first seeds of thought pointing the way to a crude but effective therapeutic procedure through the human skull. It is a remarkable fact that humans actually performed craniotomies—surgical procedures through the skull—in prehistory. Skull specimens operated upon in the presence of fracture and with evidence of subsequent healing demonstrate at least occasional success in treating the malady from which the patient suffered. Archeologists conclude, from several lines of evidence, that the procedures were surgical rather than magical. These skills were lost to civilization and were regained only recently, in the latter half of the nineteenth century.

The modern era of neurosurgery, heralded by the advent of general anesthesia (1846) and spurred by successes such as the first removal of a spinal cord tumor by Victor Horsley in 1887, took off in the early 1900s. Harvey Cushing at Johns Hopkins University provided an example of an extraordinary clinician-diagnostician, a superb and pioneering neurosurgeon and neuroscientist, who to this day is admired and respected by those who practice neurological surgery. This is not to say that neurosurgery was not confounded by postoperative complications, frequent failure, and dying patients. But during the early 1900s promise was finally seen in the neurosurgeon's ability to operate through the skull to resect benign tumors, clip aneurysms, relieve pain, and, in general, to treat brain disease by surgical means. The idea of clinician as technician (May 1983) certainly found firm footing in this era, as the attempts and successes of surgical therapy brought an expanded role for surgery in American medicine in general.

However, the development and state of psychiatry during the latter half of the nineteenth century was entirely different. It was not the beneficiary of scientific advances such as Lister's (1867) work on antisepsis, Roentgen's work in diagnostic X-ray (1895), and the like. While psychological-psychiatric theory was being advanced, little success was seen in therapy. Those most severely afflicted with mental illness, the "mad" or "insane," had been the subjects of a sweeping campaign for reform in the early 1800s. Bolstered by therapeutic optimism, the establishment of state-supported mental hospitals was seen as "rescuing the mad from maltreatment, neglect, and inhumanity and ushering in a golden age of kindness, scientifically guided treatment, and cure" (Skull 1983:329). The visions of a "technical, objective . . . environment that provided the best possible conditions for recovery" (p. 330) proved ephemeral; instead, by the late nineteenth century, the "public asylums . . . had become mammoth institutions, huge custodial warehouses in which the conditions of the patient's existence departed further and further from those in the outside world" (p. 331). One found "patients in the prime of life sitting or lying about, moping idly and listlessly in the debilitating atmosphere of the wards, and sinking gradually into a torpor, like that of living corpses" (Mitchell 1894).

In the midst of this era, in 1890, Gottlieb Burkhardt, superintendent of the insane asylum in Prefargier, Switzerland, attempted a radical new therapeutic measure. The animal experiments of F. L. Goltz in 1881 and 1884 led Burkhardt to believe that removal of 2–5 grams of brain tissue from various regions of the brain (left temporal, parietal, frontal lobe) would be a tactic useful in "sedating" certain patients. Four operations were required on the first patient, "who eventually recovered sufficiently to live at peace with her fellow patients" (Freeman and Watts 1942). Burkhardt operated on a total of six "very excitable" patients. However, the entire thrust of his work was opposed by the medical-psychiatric community. Except for operations performed by the Russian surgeon Puusepp in 1910 and reported in 1914, no further attempts at surgical psychiatric therapy were made until 1935. Puusepp attempted operations only on unilateral frontal-parietal connections of an "insane" patient, with negligible results.

At the second International Neurological Congress in 1935 at London, experimental work with animals again provided impetus to reconsider the murky and deep relationship between brain and behavior. Fulton and Jacobsen, researching the role of frontal association areas in the chimpanzee brain, observed a calming effect on behavior when the frontal lobes of the brain were removed. Egaz Moniz, a Portuguese neurologist, who is recognized as the father of psychosurgery, was in attendance. Already a proponent of a theory implicating "abnormal synaptic connections" in psychosis, Moniz thought that ". . . to cure these patients we must destroy the more or less fixed arrangements of cellular connections that exist in the brain, and particularly those which are related to the frontal lobes" (Freeman and Watts 1950:xvi). Convinced of this basic premise, Moniz and Almeida Lima, a neurosurgeon, performed the first operations on patients in Europe in 1935. Six cylindrical cores were made in the frontal lobes. "All of the patients survived and of the first twenty reported, seven were recovered, seven were improved, with the best results obtained in the agitated depressions, while the schizophrenics were for the most part unaffected" (p. xvii). It appears that "the criteria for successful outcome were limited to reducing or eliminating certain affective and behavioral symptoms regardless of negative psychological effects" (Kucharski 1984). Initially, apparent success with the operation was encouraging enough for Walter Freeman (a neurologist) and James Watts (a neurosurgeon) to perform the first procedure in the United States in 1936, at George Washington University on a sixty-three-year-old woman with "agitated depression." Their operation, which became known as "frontal lobotomy," consisted of severing most of the connections between the frontal lobes and the rest of the brain. They had no difficulty in finding patients who had failed to respond to traditional therapy, which in 1935 included, among other techniques, insulin shock and early attempts at electroconvulsive therapy.

Patients who consented to this drastic, new, and frightening operation not infrequently consented in the belief they would surely die during the operation. Most of the surgeries were performed under local anesthesia, and extensive conversations with the patients were recorded during the procedures to monitor the effects of various surgical maneuvers. Lucidity of the patients during early parts of the operation was sometimes concretely reflected in their answers to interrogation. One patient when asked "what is going through your mind at this point?" replied, "A knife." It was found early in their experience that, in order for the operation to be successful in the long term, a sudden change in mental state characterized by "confusion, disorientation, lethargy," . . . and sometimes conditions akin to "catatonia" was necessary at some point in the operation. This would then signal the end of the procedure, at which time the patient was brought back to his or her room. This "state" would last sometimes only minutes, and other times for extended periods. It would usually be accompanied by incontinence and a lack of "motivation" for almost any activity and would gradually give way to a return of "normal" functioning. Occasionally, a return of the symptoms that prompted the operation would be seen as well. In these cases it was not uncommon to consider and perform a second "more extensive" operation. The specific diagnoses of patients most likely to improve with the operation were, of course, unknown. However, it was found that at least three categories of patients improved. Those categories included patients with (1) intractable agitation, (2) intractable depression, or (3) obsessive-compulsive disorder. Several reports cited patients who returned to their professions and homes. However, the prevailing notion that "society can accommodate itself to the most humble laborer, but justifiably distrusts the mad thinker" was clear from the tenor of postoperative analyses (Freeman and Watts 1950:xix). The constellation of postoperative side effects—those mental and psychological changes that accompanied, but were not a part of, the desired therapeutic effect—affected patients to widely varying degrees. The imprecision of the lesion sites, the various "diagnoses—illnesses" for which the patients were operated, and the premorbid personality of the patients were all potential variables involved in this disparity. However, certain consistencies were observed. "Case 56 six weeks after prefrontal lobotomy . . . showed marked inertia for a considerable period after operation and was rather irritable and tactless. Her preoccupations and hallucinations disappeared" (p. 122). Besides "inertia," or lack thereof, other common side effects included euphoria, restlessness, hunger, weight gain, and disturbance in sphincter control "rarely lasting longer than two weeks" (p. 123). Intelligence tests revealed little in the way of postoperative change. Personality "profiles" (such as Rorschach ink blot and several other psychometric tests) revealed "less response perseveration, less self reference, and a shift of attitude (with regard to) the experiment from one of high affect or pained constraint and reluctance to one of apathy" (p. 170).

Whereas a cautious approval of frontal lobotomy was occasionally heard for those "cases where the chances of remission were remote" (*JAMA* Editorial, 1941), others attacked the concept of frontal lobotomy on both ethical and scientific methodological grounds. Not only did the procedure seem intuitively and unnecessarily "meddlesome" (*Medical Record* Editorial, 1940), but the results on certain patient groups, especially schizophrenics, did not seem to warrant further clinical trials. From 1936 to 1944, frontal lobotomy gathered slow support, and by 1944, Ziegler reported 618 cases performed in this country (Ziegler 1944). The appearance in 1942 of the book *Psychosurgery* by Freeman and Watts, which presented knowledge about the function of the frontal lobes in animals and humans along with detailed clinical information on frontal-lobotomized patients, added momentum to the process of incorporating frontal lobotomy into mainline medical/psychiatric practice. Freeman and Watts, however, did not use a control group. Nor did they assess and compare carefully the relationship between diagnosis and outcome or between lesion size or site and outcome. Several other ambiguities lessened the scientific impact of their work.

One of the first major clinical trials with frontal lobotomy in the 1940s was a rare prospective, controlled, cooperative study performed over several years by six hospitals of the United States Veterans Administration (Bull et al. 1959). This study included 373 patients, 97 percent of whom were schizophrenics—the group known from anecdotal case reports to benefit *least* from frontal lobotomy. Fifty percent of the patients, functioning as controls, were matched in advance to patients who would undergo either standard frontal lobotomy or a less extensive operation known as "bimedial lobotomy." Careful preoperative and postoperative examinations with neuropsychological evaluations were cited along with five-year follow-up examinations. The final report (issued in 1959) concluded that "the community adjustment of lobotomized patients, regardless of the type of operation, was better than that of their matched controls" (p. 217). Although this appears to be the most carefully controlled study, other important studies did not corroborate these findings and concluded that lobotomy was not of significant therapeutic value (Robin 1958).

While studies of the therapeutic value of the frontal lobotomy for the most part provided momentum for psychosurgical practice, other studies provided direction for the refinement of the frontal lobotomy. The classic representative of this type of study, the Columbia-Greystone project, was designed to ascertain the relationship between disrupted brain tissue and subsequent behavioral changes. In essence, what was defined loosely as frontal lobotomy was actually several different and inaccurate cuts through portions of the frontal lobes of the brain. This information, when correlated with behavioral changes, would direct refinement of the original frontal lobotomy to more specific and focused sites of destruction (Mettler 1949). This information would not be incorporated for several years into psychosurgical practice. Instead, a more "convenient" way of performing frontal lobotomy was introduced in 1948.

Fiamberti published a technique of transorbital leukotomy (Fiamberti 1948). This technique entailed the introduction of a sharp "trocar" in the potential space between the upper eyelid and the eyeball (orbit). It was then thrust through the thin bones of the orbital roof into the inferior or lower portions of the frontal lobe. The trocar would then be manipulated to sever the brain tissue of this region of the frontal lobes on both sides. This procedure became known as "ice pick" surgery because of the similarity between the operating instrument and an ice pick. While this development cannot be considered a technical refinement in terms of smaller lesion size, less postoperative morbidity, or side effects, it did lessen the need for a lengthy in-patient hospital stay and allowed for the procedure to be performed in the physician's office.

Freeman's early decision to adopt this procedure was opposed by his neurosurgical collaborator Watts. Nevertheless, by 1949 one-third of all lobotomy procedures were performed by this method, Freeman having personally amassed about 400 cases in 1947–1949.

In 1949, the United States Public Health Service documented the performance of nearly eight thousand operations in the United States. In Great Britain and Wales, a study summarizing the results in 1942–1954 on an astounding 10,365 patients was published (Tooth and Newton 1954).

Important technical refinements, the principal aim of which was to decrease the number and magnitude of unwanted side effects while maintaining the therapeutic result, were advanced by several investigators. Poppen noted the importance of the medial (closest to the midline) and basilar (lower) portions of the frontal lobes (Poppen 1948). Scoville further refined the lesion site. Renamed "bifrontal tractotomy," this procedure would become one of the standard psychosurgical procedures of the 1960s and 1970s (Scoville et al. 1951). Wycis in Great Britain reported success with lesions in the thalamus of the brain and introduced stereotaxic technique, whereby one introduced long wire probes or electrodes into deep brain sites and created precise electrolytic lesions (Wycis and Speigel 1949). The end of the first era of psychosurgery, so dominated by the frontal lobotomy, culminated in the award of the 1949 Nobel Prize to Egaz Moniz.

After intense postwar psychosurgical activity, a rapid decline in the number of operations for psychiatric disorders occurred. This decline was due in part to the synthesis of chlorpromazine by Charpentier in 1950 and its subsequent use in the treatment of several psychiatric behavioral syndromes. In short, drug therapy became an alternative to surgical therapy in most cases. The second major cause of the decline of frontal lobotomy was the continuing problem of undesirable and unpredictable side effects.

Psychosurgery from its inception was the subject of emotional yet confined controversy. Although Freeman felt his procedures were meant "to relieve mental disorder and pain," others characterized frontal lobotomy as "partial euthanasia" (Solomon et al. 1949).

The controversy was fed by the widening scope of psychosurgery. First, there was the rapid extension of this technique to other patient populations, including children (Freeman and Watts 1945). Second, the lobotomy was performed on institutionalized patients in state mental hospitals (Elfeld 1942:81; Mackay 1948). Third, frontal lobotomy was used in attempts to treat drug addiction (Mason and Hanby 1948). This natural extension of the "new psychiatry" to well-known refractory psychologic disorders was symptomatic of a strong therapeutic urge on the part of clinicians and also of a "vision of growth without conflict" (Starr 1982:337) for medical-scientific authority.

In addition, patients and families demanded effective and potent therapy for their own or their loved one's condition after more traditional means had failed. Lay news journals and magazines contributed to the optimism and assured a wide-eyed readership. *Life* magazine in 1946 contended that the "superego was to be found in the frontal lobes."[1] In fact, the frontal lobes became known scientifically as "the uncharted provinces of the brain." Many neuroscientists came to believe that the frontal lobes (particularly the premotor regions) might not even be "accessible to meaningful scientific analysis" (p. 425). This has been countered by recent progress which, while probably only scratching the surface, is both considerable and awesome in its complexity. What became clear in 1950 was that the "seat of intelligence" was not in the frontal lobes, as conventional IQ tests were not adversely affected, and in some cases improved, following frontal lobotomy psychosurgery (Hebb 1939; Black 1976). Unfortunately, the side effects observed clinically were sometimes disturbing. A frontal lobotomized patient might demonstrate "poor judgment to everyday life, not only because of changes in personality but also because of an inability to organize everyday activities, and reduced flexibility and inventiveness in their approach to new problems."[2]

Given these clearly disadvantageous side effects, clinicians in the late 1940s refined and attempted to improve on the lobotomy. Smaller, more restricted lesions in the basilar, medial frontal regions were devoid of the more flagrant bipolar manifestations of (1) "frontal release" (disinhibition) or (2) the more familiar "cowlike" inertia that afflicted some who underwent frontal lobotomy. Thus, while there was a decline of psychosurgical activity in the mid-1950s, there was a persistent strand of surgical activity spurred by the availability of these less damaging techniques and by the persistence of intractable psychologic syndromes. While there were occasional reports addressing ethical issues, there did not seem to be a major public forum for debate, nor was there extreme concern that "sacred" boundaries were being violated as long as therapy was being rendered and persons benefitted (Robinson 1946; 1949).

Psychosurgery of the 1950s and 1960s

The second era of psychosurgery began in the late 1950s and early 1960s, well after the introduction of the first therapeutic psychoactive drugs. Instead of diagnoses, specific behavioral patterns having the "common denominator of excessive and futile emotional responses" (Sweet 1982) were most responsive to the evolving psychosurgical procedures. A significant change in surgery of the second era was that it became directed at several sites in the brain generally considered to be elements in the theoretical construct of the "limbic system."

The concept of the "limbic lobe" in the brain was proposed and described by French neurologist and anatomist Paul Broca in 1878. It was conceived of originally as "a ring of grey matter bordering the hemisphere against the central parts of the brain and arranged in a circular manner around the interventricular foramen" (Brodal 1981:689). The central brain structure in this "lobe" was the hypothalamus. The functions of this complex but very small brain region (weighing 4.5 grams) would prove to be especially important in the visceral (heart, lungs, gut), homeostatic (hunger, thirst, temperature regulation), and "emotional" integration of experimental animals and of the human being.

While many contributed to the development of "limbic system" theory, the following several scientists were instrumental in key developments of the theory as it applied to psychosurgery. First, in 1928, Bard demonstrated a condition known as "sham rage." Animals in which much of the brain (all of the cortex) was removed, leaving the hypothalamus and lower brainstem structures intact, would demonstrate severe expressions of rage with concomitant "hair erection," scratching, biting, and snarling to even very mild stimuli. Bard also showed that removing the posterior or hindmost part of the hypothalamus would abolish the rage response entirely (Bard 1928).

Second, Papez, in 1937, postulated the existence of a "system" of brain structures that might "constitute harmonious mechanism which may elaborate the functions of central emotions and participate in emotional expression" (Papez 1937). The theory of the "limbic system" and experiments surrounding its development suggested the presence of "centers" specific for the "control" of certain behavioral or emotional responses. Third, Nobel laureate Walter Hess employed a technique of electrically stimulating deep brain sites to define a topography of the hypothalamus based on behavioral responses. He defined discrete regions of the hypothalamus that, when stimulated, would elicit "affective-defensive" reactions and rage, insatiable hunger, sympathetic response (pupillary dilatation, sweating), sleep, etc. (Hess 1955). As further delineation of brain interconnectivity proceeded in the 1950s and 1960s, the brain structures composing this "system" concurrently increased steadily. This has continued unabated into the 1970s and 1980s, resulting in a decrease in the theoretical value and usefulness of the "limbic system" concept. Indeed, the limbic system appeared to be "on its way to including all brain regions and functions" (Brodal 1981:752). In earlier interpretations of the theory, small hypothalamic "centers" were thought to control complex behavioral processes. Now this is not widely accepted. Nevertheless, it is still clear that quite small and discrete brain regions are essential for certain distinct behavioral functions. Several scientists used electrical stimulation of the brain (ESB) to "map" the behavioral functions of various brain regions. Perhaps the most dramatic discovery in this field was that of a "pleasure center" deep within the brains of experimental animals. The animals could be taught to stimulate their own "pleasure centers" by pressing a lever, creating an "addiction to end all addictions" (Olds and Milner 1954). Delgado demonstrated the antithesis of the "pleasure center" and described an "aversive" center in the brain of the cat, which, when stimulated, could "motivate" more rapid learning (Delgado et al. 1954:587).

In 1956, Delgado reported on the development of the "stimoceiver" for the "radio transmission and reception of electrical messages to and from the brain in completely unrestrained [animal] subjects" (Higgins et al. 1966). This technique utilized chronically implanted deep-brain electrodes to detect abnormal electrical activity, such as is seen in seizure disorders or epilepsy with conventional scalp electrodes or electroencephalography. These electrical signals were analyzed by a remote computer, which signaled and activated another set of deeply placed brain electrodes. These electrodes were placed in a portion of the brain that would, when stimulated, send inhibitory or "calming" signals to the abnormal region of the brain. This work supported the idea that "direct communication could be established between brain and computer, circumventing normal sensory organs" (Delgado 1969:92). In 1968, a report of "intracerebral radiostimulation and recording in completely free patients" was published (Delgado et al. 1968). Theories were born in response to these quite remarkable research findings. One theory ascribed a central role to pleasure and reward systems of the brain in conditions such as schizophrenia. In a related theory, anhedonia, or the inability to experience pleasure, was postulated as the source of psychic chaos. Additionally, theoretical interest in the role of focal (confined to a particular brain region) seizure activity in pathological behavioral syndromes grew in straightforward response to the observation that various behaviors could be stimulated using (nonphysiological) ESB. However, ESB, which first appeared to be a powerful research tool, proved to be both methodologically and ethically a "therapy" with more peril than promise.

In 1969, Jose Delgado published the book *Physical Control of the Mind* The title was and is, to say the least, challenging and provocative. Although not the first, Delgado was one who forcefully brought "science"—and that term here is used loosely—face-to-face with religion, philosophy, politics, and sociology. The language he used in his book makes the point fully clear. Brain systems of reward ("pleasure centers") and punishment are spoken of as "heaven and hell within the brain" (p. 90). He also referred to "electrical stimulation of the will." He believed humanity to be

on the verge of a process of mental liberation and self-domination which is a continuation of our evolution. [This process has an] experimental approach based on the investigation of the depth of the brain in behaving subjects. Its practical applications do not rely on direct cerebral manipulations but on the integration of neurophysiological and psychological principles leading to a more intelligent education, starting from the moment of birth and continuing throughout life, with the preconceived plan of escaping from the blind forces of chance and of influencing cerebral mechanisms and mental structure in order to create a future man with greater personal freedom and originality, a member of the psychocivilized society, happier, less destructive, and better balanced than present man. (p. 223)

An attempt to cover all of the difficulties inherent in this prediction—from methodological to ethical—is beyond the scope of this paper. However, the impact on psychosurgical history can hardly be underestimated. First, the language has shifted from that of therapy rendered to individuals suffering from illness, malady, and disease, to that of "control" of the will with "a new factor in the constellation of behavioral determinants" (p. 215). It is immediately clear that this shift in language is overwhelmingly problematic even if Delgado advocated the use of ESB as an experimental tool only. Valenstein (1973) correctly pointed out that "there is good reason to suspect that brain stimulation, like drugs, would seriously weaken the conception of the self as a determiner of one's own destiny. . . . The belief that anyone could adjust in this world if a spontaneous orgasm followed by detached mental calmness was programmed in at 10, 2 and 6 o'clock seems ludicrous" (p. 173). Furthermore, what Delgado postulated (in 1969) is no less than "neurobioelectrically" defining the "will" within the brain. A fallacy exists in suggesting that a biochemical-bioelectrical definition of the "will" either exists, is imminent, or definitely will be developed simply because "will" is part of mental process. This is not to argue that "will" is not an emotional-perceptual-cognitive process that "occurs" within the brain. Further, there is certainly no evidence to suggest that this definition could be developed via brain-stimulation techniques.

Finally, it is interesting to note that while ESB has found only very limited use in the treatment of psychiatric syndromes (e.g., chronic cerebellar stimulation in the treatment of affective disorder) (Heath et al. 1980), it has found a limited place in a closely related field, that of the neurosurgical treatment of intractable movement disorders and intractable pain (Cox and Valenstein 1965). If an electrode is placed in a region of the brain stem known as the "periventricular grey" matter, electrical stimulation will result in the release of endogenous "opioids" (neurochemicals that are some thirteen times more potent than morphine) and will effectively relieve intractable pain in certain patients. The discovery of two of the endogenous opioids, enkephalins and endorphins, was as recent as 1975. They represent members of the larger family of brain peptides, which act as neuromodulators or neurotransmitters and are involved in the regulation of several brain systems, including pain perception (enkephalins and endorphins and others), and memory formation (ACTH, MSH, B-endorphin) (Krieger 1983). Research in this area is in its scientific infancy. The distinction between neurosurgery for intractable pain and affective disorder will be commented upon later in the paper. ESB also continues to be a useful research tool in the laboratory. It is successfully employed in the study of stress and anxiety states, epilepsy, and other disorders (Liebman 1985; Gloor et al. 1982).

Violence and the Brain

The focus of much of the lay interest in ESB was on its potential application to violent patients or individuals. Indeed, if one subject within the history of psychosurgery could be said to have aroused the most emotional response, it has been the treatment, therapy, even the investigation of violent behavior. Narabayashi in Japan was first to introduce the procedure of stereotaxic amygdalotomy (see below) for the treatment of patients with "severe hyperactive or destructive behavioral problems" (Narabayashi et al. 1963). Narabayashi's patient population was initially confined to patients who were feebleminded, classified as idiots or imbeciles due to trauma, encephalitis, or other prior maladies. Most but not all had temporal lobe epilepsy as well. The operations, however, were performed specifically for the intractable violent behavioral disorder. The procedure was found to be successful (and not simply sedative) in about two-thirds of the patients. Neurosurgical procedures performed during the 1950s and 1960s for the treatment of epilepsy or, in Narabayashi's series, behavioral manifestations "related" to clear diagnoses of temporal lobe epilepsy, were not seriously questioned, on either ethical or clinical grounds.

Stereotaxic (geometric system organization) is a term that refers to a surgical apparatus and technique that enables one to place long "needles" or probes into deep brain sites accurately and reproducibly, for the purpose of biopsy or destruction of small spherical or elliptical regions of tissue. The amygdala is located roughly in the innermost portion of the temporal lobe in a complex arrangement with structures important for memory (hippocampus of the temporal lobe). The amygdala was found to be integral in the manifestations of emotions, especially violent behavior, by several investigators, including Woods, who found vicious sewer rats could be tamed following removal of the amygdala (Woods 1956). It was found also to be a brain structure that is exceptionally sensitive to injury and susceptible to seizure activity (more than almost any other brain site). Thus, the connection between brain-injured, seizure-prone patients and violent behavior was postulated and developed.

Epilepsy was described by Hughlings Jackson "basically as an intermittent derangement of the nervous system due presumably to a sudden, excessive, disorderly discharge of cerebral neurons" (Adams and Victor 1981:209). Epilepsy with a focus in the temporal lobe already had been known to give rise to emotional and complex subjective psychic experiences. Wilder Penfield and others had shown the utility of surgical therapy for certain cases of epilepsy where medical therapy had been ineffective (Penfield and Jasper 1954). In addition, Gloor (1960) demonstrated the possibility that "behavioral abnormalities between temporal lobe epileptic attacks are found much more frequently in patients with psychomotor epilepsy than in any of the other types" (Gloor 1960). It was suggested that this may be due to a continuous state of irritation by the seizure focus in the brain without an actual seizure taking place.[3] The extension of stereotaxic amygdalectomy and other procedures to "episodically violent patients who have focal disease of their limbic brain without signs or symptoms of epilepsy" was on the horizon (Mark et al. 1972). Prior to this prediction, public perception about the nature of psychosurgical practice had already taken a turn from positivist scientific revelation[4] to a picture of sinister, punitive techniques of control and mind domination. Ken Kesey's novel (1962) *One Flew over the Cuckoo's Nest* depicted frontal lobotomy (which had not been performed widely in the United States since 1954) as having no significant relationship to therapy. The "martyrdom" of human freedom and dignity occurring at the hands of physicians and nurses as depicted in the novel and the movie was read and seen by a public at the edge of a crisis of faith. Without elaborating on the profound changes that were occurring throughout the United States, it is safe to say that "medicine, like many other American institutions, suffered a stunning loss of confidence in the 1970's" (Starr 1982:379). What was once considered expanding (even if meddlesome) scientific and clinical knowledge was now seen by some as a gross manifestation of political and social prejudice.

The publication in 1970 of Mark and Ervin's book *Violence and the Brain* appears to have heightened the emotional intensity of the psychosurgical debate. It warned of the potential for controlling violence on a large scale. The authors postulated the use of techniques such as Delgado's "stimoceiver" to monitor hypothetical "brain triggers" of violence or, in other words, seizure foci in the amygdala. The problems with this theory lay in the facts that (1) temporal lobe epilepsy was associated with a much lower incidence of violence than anticipated, (2) mechanisms to detect seizure foci in the amygdala were too invasive and too insensitive, and (3) there was no voluntary patient population for experimental trial.

In 1970, funds were appropriated from the Justice Department to begin a study of violence in society. A proposed Center for the Study of Life-Threatening Behavior was never established due to public opposition. Although Vernon Mark was later quoted as saying the book *Violence and the Brain* was written to stimulate interest in the research and investigation of violence, such research was clearly interpreted as an ominous trend by *Ebony* magazine, which in February 1973 published the article "New Threat to Blacks: Brain Surgery to Control Behavior." It was also interpreted as a symptom of a larger malady afflicting American medicine, "therapeutic relentlessness" (Hamberger 1973:83).

Many psychosurgeons, however, believed that, although negative public opinion was gathering momentum, there were extremely violent individuals with brain abnormalities that, while subtle, could be defined and treated. Using sleep electroencephalographic (EEG) recordings, olfactory stimulation, and intraamygdaloid recordings, Andy and Jurko showed that in "psychomotor epilepsy, the amygdala is in a state of relatively greater excitability in patients showing explosive and aggressive behavior than in those who do not show these behavioral features" (Andy and Jurko 1975). At the Fourth World Congress of Psychiatric Surgery held in Madrid in 1975, the surgical procedures applied to violent states and "pathologic aggressiveness" included posterior hypothalamotomy, amygdalotomy, and multitarget limbic surgery. The targets in the limbic surgery were the mesial (innermost portion of the) amygdala, the substantia innominate (another group of cells in the "limbic" circuitry), and small targets in the cingulum (an interior ridge of association fibers connecting other parts of the limbic system). One study performed on fifty-two patients with diagnoses of schizophrenia ($n = 33$) and "episodic dyscontrol" syndrome ($n = 19$) was conducted, using independent psychiatric evaluators and control groups. Results were reported on the basis of evaluations (qualitative and quantitative) of personal happiness, ability to function productively in society, and the presence or absence of psychotic recurrences. The patients who underwent operations were severely impaired, and "had been ill for considerable periods of time and had tried multiple psychotherapeutic modalities before undergoing surgery" (p. 476). Patients operated in this series for violence and aggression (sixteen of nineteen showed modest to marked improvement) did not improve as greatly as those with schizophrenia. Follow-ups were from six months to six years.

Sano had earlier reported excellent or good results with "rage" behavioral abnormalities in 95 percent of his cases (forty-three patients) who had received bilateral-stereotaxis lesions of the posterior hypothalamus (Sano et al. 1970). His results prompted a shift away from the restriction of targets to only the amygdala regions. The posterior hypothalamus also was the site of unilateral lesions for the treatment of four imprisoned men convicted of multiple violent rapes in the Federal Republic of Germany (Diekmann and Hassler 1975). Each operation, it is reported, was performed "at the request . . . of the patients during their detention" (p. 452). The operations were accompanied by preoperative and postoperative psychological testing, with two patients unoperated and used as controls. Each of the four patients reported postoperative reductions in "sexual drive." Improvements were noted in their concentration abilities, whereas visual memory in some cases deteriorated. Weight gain was seen in two of the four patients. Acute affective changes—"overall subjective improvement in mood"—were not consistent two years following surgery; instead, anxiety, "lack of control," and neurosis reappeared in three of the patients (p. 455). In addition, "similar long-term conditions prevailed in changes of sexuality." It was noted in conclusion that "the immediate postoperative effects are modified over time, and this development process determines whether the therapeutic goal is reached or not" (p. 456).

In the United States, a similar experiment in 1972 had been planned to compare surgical lesions in the amygdala with a trial of the drug cyproterone acetate on male hormonal production and behavior. Candidates for surgery would first have microelectrodes placed into the temporal lobes of their brains in an attempt to detect seizure activity. If seizure activity was found, the small region (five to eight cubic millimeters) would be destroyed with electric current. If no seizure activity was found, the protocol would be discontinued.

Eighteen years prior, Lewis Smith had been committed to a state maximum security institution for "criminal sexual psychopathy" after confessing to murder and rape. In November of 1972 he was transferred to a hospital/clinic to participate in this study of uncontrollable aggression. Smith, a candidate for the surgery, had signed informed consent, and the procedure was reviewed and approved by a community panel of three: a priest, a lawyer, and an accountant. Gabe Kaimowitz (1980) took legal action "to bar the use of institutionalized persons as human subjects for medical research, and particularly for psychosurgery" (p. 505). Kaimowitz felt that prisoners could not "decide when to go to the bathroom much less go for a walk or exercise rights of protest while under state control. How then [could] a prisoner voluntarily, knowingly, and competently consent to participate as a subject in state-funded and directed research to permanently alter his behavior" (p. 511). The court held that an involuntarily committed individual could not be competent to render an informed consent on the basis of "the very nature of his incarceration . . . the deprivation stemming from involuntary confinement."[5] This controversial decision has itself spawned a literature, much of it arguing "that [to say] the involuntarily committed as a matter of law, are so different from the rest of society that they cannot consent, or even have a guardian to do so, is absolutely antithetical to their best interests and inconsistent with the moral and political foundations of their basic civil rights" (Shuman 1977).

A National Commission for the Protection of Human Subjects of Biomedical and Behavioral Research, formed in 1972, found that "with the exception of the Kaimowitz Court, there is agreement that the competence of an institutionalized patient to give informed consent is not necessarily inadequate."[6] Annas et al. (1980:300) point out that if the chance for release is the coercive element behind consent to psychosurgery, then it may also be viewed as such in relation to other, more generally accepted forms of [psycho] therapy. Involuntary commitment could therefore be considered to coerce all decisions to engage in therapy, thereby making all such decisions invalid.

But, for most, the Kaimowitz decision emphasized the importance of limiting inducements for participation in psychotherapeutic research to those that could only possibly be related to the results of research. At present, some feel that any potential benefit to a participant in medical research constitutes coercion, and if stated as such, is unethical. However, the decision also prompted concerns on the opposite philosophic pole from those of Gabe Kaimowitz. As M. Hunter Brown (1974) wrote:

> I have a special concern for involuntary patients held in our state mental hospitals and state prisons. Often they cannot procure needed treatment and face an eternity behind walls and bars for a crime of illness. Much of their plight relates to semantics concerning informed consent and could be solved by a neutral ombudsman in each state. Excessively vigilant civil libertarians guarantee that the captive patient can spend the rest of his natural life in confinement with the comfort of knowing that no one took advantage of his legally manufactured incompetence to consent.

The consensus among neurosurgeons, physicians, and ethicists today seems to be that "experimental surgery" or clinical trials of accepted but unusual therapies are not appropriately performed in penal institutions, or at least it is prohibitively difficult to do so. Procedures for the syndrome now known as "Intermittant Explosive Disorder 312.34"[7] are extremely rare in the absence of an obvious temporal lobe disorder. Investigations and research into the understanding and nature of violent behavior have been severely hindered. As Louis West states, "It's as though the coin that says 'violence' on the one side says 'control' on the other; as though people believe that trying to prevent or even study violence would necessitate controlling society."[8]

The National Commission

In 1972 a national commission made up of eleven professionals from several medical and related disciplines was directed to study and recommend policies that should govern the use of psychosurgery.[9] The issues the commission cited as being especially controversial included (1) underlying scientific justification, (2) obtaining informed consent, (3) the question of brain inviolability, (4) the use of psychosurgery as a social or political tool, and (5) the categorization of psychosurgery as an accepted therapy rather than an experimental one.

Among its findings were estimates of the extent of psychosurgical practice in the United States and Great Britain. Compared to estimates "that 40,000 prefrontal lobotomies [had been] performed in the United States, the majority of them in the decade following 1945"[10] the reported number of psychological cases (none of which was prefrontal lobotomy) for the three years 1971–1973, was 1242 (corrected for those surgeons not responding to a questionnaire). Surgeons in the United Kingdom during the same period were performing psychosurgical procedures at approximately twice the rate of U.S. surgeons. Interestingly, four American surgeons (of a total of fifty-nine performing psychosurgery) performed nearly 50 percent of the surgery in 1973.

While the literature reviewed (152 articles reporting clinical psychosurgical series) was considered largely subjective, descriptive, and woefully lacking in objective test results, general agreement was noted regarding the type of patients most likely to improve following psychosurgery. Those patients were noted (again) to have severe depression, severe anxiety, or obsessive-compulsive neurosis. Patients with severe thought disorder were "less likely to improve." There was disagreement over the benefits achieved in schizophrenics, violent-aggressive individuals, and paraphiliacs (sexual deviants). A careful literature search and correspondence with active psychosurgeons revealed that minorities were grossly underrepresented in clinical series and that only seven psychosurgical procedures had been performed on children in the years from 1970–1976.[11]

The commission also directed an "independent evaluation of psychosurgical patients to be conducted by a team of psychologists, psychiatrists, neurologists, and social workers."[12] The patients ($n = 27$) in this study, all with illnesses of long standing, received one or more of the following psychosurgical procedures: (1) orbital undercutting (lower, inner frontal lobe fibers severed), (2) bilateral cingulotomy (a gyrus situated on the inner bank of the cerebral hemisphere), (3) prefrontal "sonic" lesions (ultrasound used to sever the anterior frontal lobar fibers). Eight patients served as nonoperated controls.

The results were surprisingly good. Seventy-eight percent of patients experienced "moderate improvement" to "very favorable" outcomes. Further, there were "no significant psychological or cognitive deficits attributable to psychosurgery . . . with the exception of an impairment of perseveration when shifting from one card category to another (Wisconsin Card Sorting test)."[13]

The commission's recommendations, published in 1977 and based upon much investigation and review, can be summarized as follows:

1. All psychosurgery should be performed in hospitals that have institutional review boards. The commission further cited "studies [which] appear[ed] to rebut any presumption that all forms of psychosurgery are unsafe and ineffective."[14]

2. Psychosurgical procedures on patients voluntarily residing in a mental institution should be allowed, with the provision that a National Psychosurgery Advisory Board approve the procedure as one of documented benefit "in the treatment of patients with the same disorder who are not so situated."[15]

3. Prisoners, involuntarily confined patients, and incompetent persons should be protected against coercion into either psychosurgical procedures or research involving the same by court review for each case, review by the Psychosurgery Advisory Board, legal guardianship (if necessary), removing any promise of lessened sentence, and submission to all other documents regarding experimentation on "mentally infirm" individuals.

4. Psychosurgery on children is not supported by any data available, but guidelines should allow for the possibility that a new therapy might prove advantageous for certain intractable conditions (if so defined).

5. A national psychosurgery registry should be established.

6. Research into the safety and efficacy of specific psychosurgical procedures should be carried out.

7. Compliance with the other recommendations should be forced, if necessary, through various means suggested by the commission.

8. National legislation should be passed to assure compliance with the regulations.

The commission's recommendations were approved unanimously except for one dissension from recommendations 2 and 3 and an abstention from recommendation 6. The dissenter disagreed with the extent of protection afforded voluntarily committed patients in institutions, suggesting prior court review of all psychosurgical procedures in voluntarily committed patients.

Conclusions

Psychosurgery is still performed in several countries, including Great Britain and the United States. Older techniques, along with the therapeutic climate in which they were practiced, have been supplanted. The procedures performed are more specific, less dangerous, and are associated with fewer side effects. Procedures employing new technology or creative ap-

plications of complementary technologies are emerging. Extremely min-
ute deep-brain lesions are possible without the use of the scalpel and drill,
through sharply focused high-energy irradiation (Gamma camera). The
location of the lesions can be tested with a variety of new noninvasive
imaging technologies such as nuclear magnetic resonance (Leksell et al.
1985).

Long-term follow-up evaluations of patients who first received the
restricted surgical procedures has recently been reported. Ballentine described 198 psychiatrically disabled patients with a mean followup of 8.6
years, all of whom had undergone stereotaxic cingulotomy. Stability in
postoperative improvement (completely recovered or functioning nor-
mally on medicines), followed and confirmed over at least five years, occurred in 36 percent of the patients. An additional 26 percent were
"markedly improved" but still had varying degrees of psychiatric disability
requiring treatment (Ballentine et al. 1987).

Many feel that psychosurgery is underutilized at present in the United
States. Few neurosurgeons have taken the initiative to attempt it in recent
years. However, a study showed that over 75 percent of British psychiatrists felt there were patients in their practices for whom psychosurgery
seemed appropriate (Snaith et al. 1984).

Progress thus has been significant in the technical aspects of psychosurgery—neuroscientific understanding of the brain and mental illness.
However, in some ways progress has brought more complexity than enlightenment. Modern medical science has not provided immediate answers or uncomplicated therapies for people who are mad or insane.

In response, a wide spectrum of therapeutic strategies has developed
throughout the history of psychosurgery. One school of thought suggests
that "disease," organic and pathological, is not compatible with, and does
not exist in, the mind, because it is nonorganic and spiritual. Another
school predicts that the definition of mind will be learned by accurately
describing the brain processes that bring it into being. As these processes
become accessible to scientific inquiry, so too will the bioelectric, biochemical, and cellular aberrancies that bring about madness.

The first school in its most extreme form claims that to seek relief for
existential or spiritual difficulty through technological means is a fundamental mistake (Szasz 1983b:289–90). Not only psychosurgery but all of
biotechnical psychiatry, psychoanalysis, and other modern psychotherapies are seen as mistakes. In regard to all of them, "everything worked and
nothing worked" (p. 290). Psychiatry with its various therapies is like so
many "religions with various branches and types" (p. 290).

The second school, in its most extreme form, seeks scientific-techno-
logical solutions to problems such as violence that are traditionally within
the province of social institutions. The view that "crime is crime and dis-

ease is disease" (Szasz 1983b:290) becomes open to serious question and is supplanted by an equally inflexible notion: "If behavior is in the chemistry, we are convinced it is not in the will" (Veatch 1973). As a result, the diagnosis of "mental illness" appears as a legal strategy in present-day courtrooms (Szasz 1983a).

Psychosurgery has adopted the radical stance that it is a duty to attempt to unlock the biological secrets of the diseased brain and mind for the purpose of therapy. The doctor's precept, *primum non nocere* ("first do no harm"), is viewed in the context of patient-prisoners "who had lost even the memory of hope"—a condition akin to terminal disease (Mitchell 1894).

However, it has become clear that therapy cannot always depend upon demonstrating a causative relationship between a deranged neuronal circuit and a mental symptom or syndrome. While it is obvious that a malignant brain tumor may cause death, it is not so obvious whether a temporal lobe tumor or seizure focus may cause repetitive violent or bizarre behavior. Causation is now construed as multidimensional, and it may be understood as "immediate," "intermediate," or "ultimate." Such distinctions must be employed in evaluation of the causes of all psychopathic syndromes. They concern not only the temporal dimension of causation but also myriad psychosocial, genetic, drug-related, and other factors and their interrelationships.

For such violent behavior as murder or rape, some might define the ultimate cause as simply "evil." If however, one discovers a temporal lobe tumor or scarred brain tissue (intermediate cause) producing seizures (immediate cause), which in turn are apparently causing the deviant behavior, is evil reduced to disturbed electrochemical processes? This is, in my estimation, a fallacy that confuses proximal (immediate) and ultimate levels of causation. Stated differently, the language used to describe events is not easily transferable across disciplinary boundaries. To address chemical and physiological causes of behavior (if they can be defined) is not necessarily to deny discussion of other meaningful dimensions of causation.

It so happens that even the most immediate causes for aberrant behavior are for the most part not yet accessible to neuroscientific methods. However, psychosurgical procedures, in their most refined forms, have addressed not causation, but structures necessary for the specific manifestations of certain affective illnesses. It is interesting to note that many psychoactive drugs also act by inhibiting the behavioral manifestations of mental illness.

Recent evidence suggests that over 20 percent of patients with severe depression do not recover over a two-year period with conventional therapy (including electroconvulsive therapy) (Keller et al. 1984). Since the major affective disorders (depression and manic depressive illness) afflict some 8 million to 14 million Americans each year, a significant number of persons might benefit from psychosurgical treatment of these diseases. Psychosurgery suffers from its association with mind control, punitive or oppressive behavior modification, and destruction of the personality. This one-sided view denies the oppression of mental illness and the personal meaning of suffering.

Notes

1. Quoted in *Psychiatric Quarterly,* Suppl. 20: 307–310, 1946.

2. W. Penfield, A. R. Luria, and J. M. Fuster, quoted in B. Milner and M. Petrides. *Trends in Neuroscience 7* (November 1984): 11.

3. The term *subictal* refers to a state of brain irritation less than that required for a complete seizure or ictal event.

4. See Editorial Comment: "Marvels of brain surgery," *Psychiatric Quarterly* Suppl. 20:307–310, 1946.

5. Quote from "Appendix," *Research Involving Those Institutionalized as Mentally Informed* (Washington, D.C.: National Commission for the Protection of Human Subjects of Biomedical and Behavioral Research, 1976).

6. Ibid.

7. See *American Psychiatric Association: Diagnostic and Statistical Manual of Mental Disorders,* 3d ed. (Washington, D.C.: APA, 1980).

8. Quoted in the *Journal of the American Medical Association 254* (Aug. 9, 1985):721.

9. See "Report and Recommendations—Psychosurgery: the National Commission for the Protection of Human Subjects of Biomedical and Behavioral Research," DHEW Pub. No. (OS)77–0001 (Washington, D.C.: U.S. Government Printing Office, 1972).

10. Ibid., p. 25.

11. Ibid., p. 30.

12. Ibid., p. 31.

13. Ibid., p. 40.

14. Ibid., p. 60.

15. Ibid., p. 63.

References

Adams, R. D., and M. Victor. 1981. *Principles of Neurology.* New York: McGraw Hill.

Andy, O. J., and M. Jurko. 1975. "The Human Amygdala: Excitability State and Aggression." *Neurosurgical Treatment in Psychiatry, Pain, and Epilepsy,* ed. W. Sweet et al., pp. 417–27. Baltimore: University Park.

Annas, G. J., L. H. Glantz and B. F. Katz. 1980. *The Psychosurgery Debate,* ed. E. Valenstein. San Francisco: Freeman.

Ballentine, H. T., A. J. Bouckoms, E. K. Thomas, and I. E. Giriunas. 1987. *Biological Psychiatry* 22: 807–19.

Bard, P. 1928. *American Journal of Physiology* 84: 490–515.

Black, F. W. 1976. *Journal of Clinical Psychology* 32: 366–72.

Brodal, A. 1981. *Neurological Anatomy.* Oxford: Oxford University Press.

Brown, M. H. 1974. *Appendix: Psychosurgery.* The National Commission for the Protection of Human Subjects of Biomedical and Behavioral Research, US-DHEW Publication No. (OS)77–0002 p.I.

Bull, J., C. J. Klett, and C. J. Gresoch. 1959. *Journal of Clinical Experimental Psycho-pathology* 20:205–17.

Cox, V. C., and E. S. Valenstein. 1965. *Science* 149: 323–25.

Delgado, J. M. R. 1969. *Physical Control of the Mind.* New York: Harper and Row.

Delgado, J. M. R. et al. 1968. *Journal of Nervous and Mental Disease* 147: 329–40.

Delgado, J. M. R., W. W. Roberts and N. E. Millner. 1954. *American Journal of Physiology* 179:587–93.

Diekmann, G., and R. Hassler. 1975. *Neurosurgical Treatment in Psychiatry, Pain, and Epilepsy,* ed. W. Sweet et al. Baltimore: University Park.

Elfeld, P. 1942. *Delaware State Medical Journal* 14: 81–83.

Fiamberti, A. M. 1948. *Archives psicol. neur., Milano* 9:445–47.

Freeman, Walter and James Watts. 1942. *Psychosurgery.* London: Bailliere, Tindall and Cox.

———. 1945. *American Journal of Psychiatry* 101: 739–48.

———. 1950. *Psychosurgery.* Springfield, IL: Charles C. Thomas.

Gloor, P. 1960. "Amygdala," *Handbook of Physiology* Vol. 2, ed. J. Field, H. W. Magoun and V. E. Hall, 1395–420. Washington, D.C.: American Physiological Society.

Gloor, P. et al. 1982. *Annals of Neurology* 12: 129–44.

Hamberger, J. 1973. *The Power and Frailty: The Future of Medicine and the Future of Man.* New York: Macmillan.

Heath, R. G., R. C. Llewellyn and A. M. Rouchell. 1980. *Biological Psychiatry* 15: 243–56.

Hebb, D. O. 1939. *Journal of General Psychology* 21: 73–87.

Hess, W. R. 1955. *Archives of Neurology and Psychiatry* 73: 127–29.

Higgins, J. W., G. F. Mahl, J. M. R. Delgado and H. Hamlin. 1956. *Archives of Neurology and Psychiatry* 76: 399–419.

Illych, Ivan. 1976. *Medical Nemesis.* New York: Pantheon.

Journal of the American Medical Association. Editorial. 1941. *JAMA* 117:534.

Kaimowitz, G. 1980. "My Case Against Psychosurgery." *The Psychosurgery Debate,* ed. E. Valenstein. San Francisco: Freeman.

Keller, M. G. et al. 1984. *JAMA* 252: 788–92, 10 August.

Kesey, K. 1962. *One Flew Over the Cuckoo's Nest.* New York: Viking Press.

Krieger, D. 1983. *Science* 222 (December):975–85.

Kucharski, Anastasia. 1984. *Neurosurgery* 14:765–72.

Leksell, L., T. Herner, D. Leksell, B. Persson and C. Lindquist. 1985. *Journal of Neurology, Neurosurgery and Psychiatry* 48 (January):19–20.

Liebman, J. M. 1985. *Neurosci. Behav. Review* 9 (Spring):75–86.

Mackay, G. W. 1948. *Journal of Mental Science* 94: 834–43.

Mark, V. H. and F. Ervin. 1970. _Violence and the Brain._ New York: Harper and Row.

Mark, V. H., W. H. Sweet, and F. R. Ervin. 1972. _Psychosurgery,_ ed. E. Hitchcock, L. Laitenen and K. Vaernet. Springfield, IL: Charles C. Thomas.

Mason, T.H. and W.B. Hanby. 1948. _JAMA_ 136 (17 April):1039–40.

May, William. 1983. _The Physician's Covenant._ Philadelphia: Westminster Press.

Medical Record. Editorial. 1940. _Medical Record_ 151:335–36.

Mettler, F. A. 1949. _New York State Journal of Medicine_ 49 (1 October):2283–86.

Mitchell, S. W. 1894. "Address before the American Medico-Psychological Association. Philadelphia." _Journal of Nervous and Mental Disorders_ 21:413–37.

Narabayashi, H., T. Nagao, Y. Saito, M. Yoshida and M. Hagahata. 1963. _Archives of Neurology_ 9:1–16.

Olds, J. and P. Milner. 1954. _Journal of Comparative Physiology and Psychology_ 47:419–27.

Papez, J. W. 1937. _Archives of Neurology and Psychiatry_ 38: 725.

Penfield, W. and H. Jasper. 1954. _Epilepsy and the Functional Anatomy of the Human Brain._ Boston: Little, Brown.

Poppen, J. L. 1948. _Digest of Neurology and Psychiatry_ 16: 403–8.

Robin, A. A. 1958. _Journal of Neurology, Neurosurgery and Psychiatry_ 21:262–69.

Robinson, M. F. 1946. _Journal of Abnormal and Social Psychology_ 41: 421.

———. 1949. Editorial. _New England Journal of Medicine_ 241 (10 August): 248–49.

Sano, K., M. Ogashiwa and B. Ishijima. 1970. _Journal of Neurosurgery_ 33: 689–707.

Scoville, W. B., K. Wilke and A. Pepe. 1951. _American Journal of Psychiatry_ 107:730–38.

Shuman, S. 1977. _Psychosurgery and the Medical Control of Violence._ Detroit: Wayne State University.

Skull, Andrew. 1983. In _Mental Illness: Changes and Trends,_ ed. Philip Bean. London: Wiley and Sons.

Snaith, R. P., D. J. E. Price and J. F. Wright. 1984. _British Journal of Psychiatry_ 144: 293–97.

Solomon, H. C., W. Freeman, et al. 1949. _Digest of Neurology and Psychiatry_ 17: 423–31.

Starr, Paul. 1982. _The Social Transformation of American Medicine._ New York: Basic Books.

Sweet, W. 1982. "Neurosurgical Aspects of Primary Affective Disorders." _Neurological Surgery,_ ed. Youmans. London: Saunders.

Szasz, Thomas. 1974. _The Myth of Mental Illness._ New York: Harper and Row.

———. 1983a. "Mental Illness as Strategy." _Mental Illness: Changes and Trends,_ ed. P. Bean. Chichester: Wiley.

———. 1983b. _States of Mind,_ ed. J. Miller. New York: Pantheon.

Tooth, G. C. and M. P. Newton. 1954. "Leukotomy in England and Wales 1942–1954." _Great Britain Ministry of Health, Report on Public Health,_ 104. London: Queen's Printing Office.

Valenstein, E. S. 1973. _Brain Control._ New York: Wiley.

Veatch, R. 1973. *Hastings Center Studies* 59:70.

Woods, R. 1956. *Nature* 170: 869.

Wycis, H. I. and E. A. Speigel. 1949. *Proceedings of the Royal Society of Medicine* 42 (suppl.):12–13.

Ziegler, L. H. 1944. *Archives of Neurology and Psychiatry* 51:202–3.

PART THREE

Religion and Psychiatric Practice

CHAPTER NINE

RELIGIOUS EXPERIENCE AND THE BIOPSYCHOSOCIAL MODEL

Donald M. Jacobson, M.D.

To understand the religious experience of patients it is necessary first to inquire about this experience if it is not spontaneously reported. Several authors have written about the taking of a religious history (Robinson 1986) and seminars have been offered on this topic (Van Dooren 1987). Clinicians are becoming more open to discussing such traditionally taboo topics as sexuality. Physicians are urged to explore their own feelings about sex and to overcome their prejudices and their need to impose conformity to traditional standards. Psychiatric practitioners, however, often ignore religious experience when taking a clinical history. They may do so because they misinterpret religious experience as a purely intrapsychic event, downplaying the other systems levels at which it influences our lives. Aside from the conceptual difficulties, the major reason for this omission may be that the traditional medical and psychiatric establishments often have not encouraged such exploration, assuming that it should be left to the clergy.

Religion is undoubtedly important in the lives of many people. It is important to explore the context, content, and meaning of patients' religious experiences and how they reflect their views of themselves and their world. Therapists perhaps also should address the lack of a religious paradigm or an atheistic stance, which could imply pseudo-independence, unresolved rebellion, or disavowal of major existential anxieties. Many individuals raised within a religious context may give up religion to adhere to the beliefs of a social peer group when they are older. In such persons faith and religious beliefs may be latent or unconscious and suppressed by cultural influences.

In a practitioner raised in a particular religious paradigm and perhaps expected to transfer to an atheistic stance as part of scientific training, inherent systems conflicts and loyalty conflicts may eventually surface. If these conflicts are not recognized and integrated, the clinician will be apt to avoid them in his or her own life and unlikely to pursue them in the lives of patients. Clinicians who have unresolved anger about their own families or denominations may generalize and displace it onto corporate religious experience in general, which is then devalued.

I encourage a longitudinal systems evaluation prior to deciding clinically whether a religious experience contains pathological elements or should be treated. Lack of a theistic focus itself may be as pathological as a neurotic religious focus—or even more so. The Reverend Ruth Barnhouse, M.D., stated that "even the most devout atheist has in his or her lack of belief in God an implicit image of that God that is rejected" (Barnhouse 1986). Both presence and absence of faith can be addressed in therapy and can often provide considerable data about a person's internal object relations and sense of self as well as about relationship patterns.

Some authors have addressed the issue of healthy versus pathological religion. In clinical practice, we may encounter a patient whose religious group has methods we would view as pathological, but the patient does not exhibit an impact from them. At other times we encounter individuals from supposedly healthy religious backgrounds who develop religious pathology. Religious experience can only be evaluated from a full systems perspective and with considerable knowledge of home life, interpersonal relationships, cultural background, family upbringing, and religious experience through life.

Not all religious experience has its primary origin in the psyche, and when evaluating change in religious experience, we must not assume that all religious pathology has been induced by a pathological religion or a deep-seated unconscious conflict. Etiologies of psychiatric illness can be biological, psychological, social, or a combination of these factors. Primary psychological issues can also affect religious experience and spill over into biopsychosocial spheres (e.g., a Vietnam veteran suffering from post traumatic disorder loses his faith when his ideal world is shattered and withdraws from social and religious activities when plagued with depression, anxiety, flashbacks, and psychosomatic health problems).

Religious experience is as varied as other experience. It is not an isolated intrapsychic event. The experience also has social and interpersonal components and in fact may be a person's primary social support. For people without families, organized religion may provide one of the only avenues of social interaction and protection from isolation. For them it may be psychotherapeutic. This major psychosocial support may even occur within the context of an unhealthy religious paradigm.

Many aspects of psychotherapy are present in religious services. They are a holding environment with consistency of time, place, liturgy, and leaders. Further, corporate worship provides a group therapy experience in which the commonality of human experience is addressed and in which self-definition and self-esteem are potentially enhanced. Regular encounters with members of a parish can be psychotherapeutic, and formal counseling is carried out by many clergy. In addition, organized worship can provide a forum in which people of all ages can interact and support each other. Given that most other organizations are collections of people based on age, profession, gender, etc., the intermingling of people of different ages, social backgrounds, genders, and races to celebrate and sacramentalize life events such as marriage, birth, and coming of age can provide a sense of continuity and sanctity of life that would be difficult to obtain otherwise.

The Biopsychosocial Model

The biopsychosocial model is the current paradigm presented by the DSM-III and the DSM-III-R published by the American Psychiatric Association as a model for organizing clinical data to refine syndromes and to aid further research (American Psychiatric Association 1980; 1987). With the development of general systems theory (von Bertalanffy 1968), literature about therapies other than traditional individual psychotherapies has increased. It is now recognized that psychopathology can be caused by multiple system stresses, not just neurotic fixations or conflicts.

Modern psychiatry has advanced considerably beyond the purely psychoanalytic view it espoused earlier in the century. There have been rapid advances in biological psychiatry (Berger and Brodie 1986) as well as in family (Nichols 1984) and group psychotherapy (Yalom 1985). One result has been an attempt to integrate these into a single usable model to help evaluate and treat patients. The biopsychosocial approach of Engel (1977) provides a way of thinking about the multitude of factors that make up a person's life and experience, and helps organize and conceptualize pathological experiences and processes (Miller and Miller 1985; Knall 1985; Matteson and Kim 1985). This model expands the traditional biomedical model and supplements traditional psychoanalysis with further data.

One can see outlined in figure 9.1 the multiple systems that are involved in our lives. A time axis outlines the developmental sequence, beginning with conception, progressing through death, and continuing into a possible afterlife. As a faith issue for an individual, the afterlife is a component of the system and can affect how that person interacts by the meaning that it implies. Likewise, God's possible presence is also noted in the system. The systems range from subatomic particles, through the various organic constituents comprising the person, and on up through higher levels of interaction including the two-person level, three-person level, family, community, and so on through the biosphere.

There is an intrapsychic mapping of the systems. We interact with systems not only in actuality but also as perceived. All these systems, both intrapsychic and actual, interact with each other over time. Each system is also a component of a higher system. Whether the biosphere is also a component of a higher system is unknown, as is the extent of possible subdivisions of subatomic particles. The existence of God or the extent of

Figure 9.1: An Expansion of Engel's Biopsychosocial Model (1977)

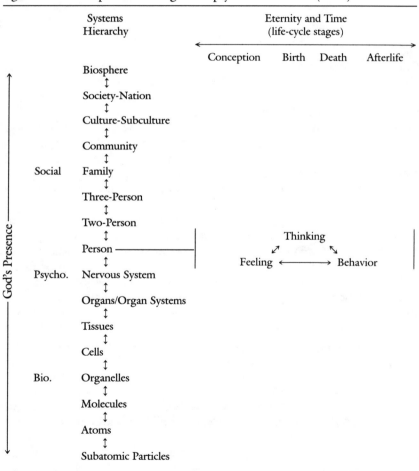

God's responsibility for the total system is a matter of personal interpretation.

The stability of the system is a function of the stability of its component parts and their ability to withstand stress both at their own level and from other levels. Disruption of the homeostasis or equilibrium may be initiated at any level from atom to nation or world. Whether the disturbance is contained at the level in which it started depends on the coping ability of the affected system. Also, changes in a level may influence a distant level but not closer levels, except perhaps secondarily through feedback loops. For example, if the government cuts social security benefits, an individual may be affected initially, and then the family subsequently, as the individual gathers in other resources or seeks support in relationships. At the person level, perceived change in the meaning attached to actual change may lead to additional subtle or even severe distortions that spill over into other systems.

Systems interact by positive or negative feedback. A positive change at one level may have negative consequences at another as the system reintegrates. For example, a job promotion may improve social status but also cause personal stress.

In dealing with such systems, the term *cure* is overly simplistic. To cure may be to remove a symptom, but this result alone may prove inadequate if stresses at other levels, real or perceived, are not identified and resolved so that the total system regains relative stability. For example, marital stress may trigger depression in one partner. That individual may enter treatment and respond well to antidepressant medication. However, the spouse may be unable to deal with the newly gained psychological strength of his or her partner and may become stressed, anxious, or depressed. Intervention may be needed at the marital or family level as well as the individual level. Rather than talk about "cure," we need to aim toward restabilization, readjustment, improved coping, or reestablishment of homeostasis or equilibrium so that the system can better tolerate change.

Strengthening of lower or higher levels may reinforce a level through positive feedback. A defect at a biological or nervous-system level can be positively or negatively influenced by events at the individual or two-person levels. For example, many multiple sclerosis patients are advised by their physicians to reduce stress. Likewise, psychotherapy may help a person with an organic condition, such as temporal lobe epilepsy, to improve relationship skills, and this may lessen the psychopathology (Blumer 1977). Social treatments of schizophrenia recently have been studied intensely, although a biological basis is assumed (McFarlane, Beels et al. 1983).

Along the vertical axis we can see the multiple levels that influence the individual, including when, where, and to whom he or she is born, and with what genetic or biological endowment. Along the horizontal axis we see that the individual must pass through many life stages and that conditions at any level can have an influence. Cumulative biological endowment and experience determine the expectations that the individual develops when the system is stable, and perhaps also the configuration that the system will take when stressed. Aspects of external reality are mapped onto the intrapsychic realm throughout a person's development, though childhood and adolescence are critical. This is not a true mapping of all facets of external reality. The person's perceptual and cognitive distortions and biases color the mapping process. Further, people are not merely passive recipients of life. They influence life and so alter the course of their fates. This perception represents a considerable turn away from the linear causality theories of early analytic thinking. This new way of thinking is called *circular causality*. It is manifested in the intrapsychic realm in internal object relations (Ogden 1983).

In using systems thinking in treating an individual with religious pathology, we begin by looking at the total system in which the person is enmeshed. To look only at the intrapsychic issues would be misleading. To look only at a single level would be misleading because each functions differently in isolation. For example, a parishioner might discuss in psychotherapy a relationship with God when he could be addressing implicitly the transference relationship with the counselor (Schwaber 1985). Relationships within this system are also interactive (Gill 1982).

General systems theory implicitly assumes that there is no noninteractive psychotherapy relationship. The analytic blank-screen technique must be seen as actually interactional—that is to say, one cannot do nothing. The silent analyst also influences the patient.

Family therapists working in this field see the identified patient as the one who is presented as ill by the family, when the pathological unit is rather the family itself. To treat the identified patient, the family may need to be treated (Nicholas 1977). Sometimes this may be the only treatment necessary. In older analytic thinking, the identified patient was often treated without addressing the problems of the larger family system. However, by utilizing the concepts of multiple and circular causality, the patient brought in by a family can learn how the family contributes to his or her difficulties and vice versa. The logic is of circular rather than linear causation. In an older therapy, unconscious early childhood conflicts would have been addressed, whereas in general living systems theory the family is addressed. This is not to say that all identified patients are patients because of family pathology. It would be reductionistic to view all adolescent patients as merely suffering from family conflicts. Indeed, it is this narrow view of the new theory that has led some therapists to erroneously assume that children and adolescents cannot suffer from organically based conditions (Poznanski 1985).

A Broadened Evaluation of Religious Experience

Having presented an outline of the biopsychosocial model, I will show how it can broaden our concept of religious experience. I will then give brief examples of the multiple levels to be evaluated.

In our evaluation of religious experience we will attempt to understand the origins and evolution of this experience, whether it is age and subculture appropriate, and whether it is stable or has changed markedly or perhaps pathologically. We will examine the levels at play including the group, the individual, and even the biological level. We are biological beings vulnerable to illness, and our central nervous systems are extremely delicate. A number of central nervous system illnesses affect mood and personality and hence religious experience. There is a biology of faith and religion, just as there are a psychology and a sociology. Alterations in religious experiences secondary to central nervous system disturbances would be a fertile area of research. Temporal lobe epilepsy causes hyperreligiosity and deepens affect. Depression causes a loss of affect and a subsequent loss of faith and desire for religious experience. It is important for religious communities that have opposed the use of psychotropic medication to be aware that such medications can often normalize a person's religious experience.

We have in this century experienced the societal use of the atomic level to cause severe destruction. Disruption at the atomic level can totally destroy life and obliterate religious experience. This has influenced the religious faith of those born since Hiroshima. On the level of meaning, one encounters individuals who have changed religious denominations due to the stance of a denomination on nuclear disarmament. I add this to show how a change in religious experience can be caused by an actual or perceived disruption.

On the molecular level, patients with electrolyte disturbances report changes in energy, mood, and affect—which can change religious experience. In severe cases, metabolic and toxic encephalopathies caused by electrolyte changes or medication totally disrupt cognitive processes with disorientation and hallucinations.

At the level of the cell, people present with a variety of psychopathological symptoms caused by the fact that a cell type has turned malignant and has invaded the central nervous system. Naturally such cell changes influence tissue, organ, nervous system, personal, and social levels as well.

At the level of tissue, organs, and organ systems, we may note a disease process affecting, for example, the adrenal glands, which subsequently disturbs mood and influences the central nervous system—and religious experience. Clearly many disease processes affecting the nervous system also affect religious experience.

On the two-person level, we may encounter people who reject religion because of an extremely negative experience with another member of their religious community or because of a bond with a nonreligious person who models atheism. On the triadic level, disruptions of faith can occur as people become involved in triangles. Certainly many family disturbances disrupt religious experience.

At other systems levels, we examine the cultural and subcultural aspects of religious experience. For example, some charismatic sects practice dissociative experiences including hallucinatory trances as part of their liturgical expression. Some members' behavior may exceed group norms, and other members may then bring the individual to the emergency room, having correctly diagnosed a psychotic state in which behavior foreign to the group has been exhibited. The psychiatrist in such an instance is greatly aided by gathering collateral history from group members and understanding the cultural norm for the group.

On the family level, we can examine the influence of the religious tradition on the family. It may help stabilize family life, may have little influence, or may cause conflict. Likewise, the absence of religious experience within a family may diminish cohesiveness. Strong religious faith may prevent participation in traditional family life, as in the case of Roman Catholic priests and nuns. We need to see how individuals interact with family tradition and whether their response is phase appropriate. For example, adolescent rebellion against religious values or adolescent asceticism may not be pathological unless prolonged and disruptive to the individual or family. An individual may have changed religions, and this for many reasons: marriage, availability of a denomination in a new location, more supportive atmosphere in a different church, theology more compatible with the individual's world view, reaction against parent's religion, need to assert individuality in relation to family of origin. The effects of such a change on the family level and the restabilization required by individual and family may be important issues for the individual.

On the personal level, we need to inquire into the meaning of the experience for the individual: Have the person's thoughts or feelings about religious experience changed? Has behavior associated with the experience changed? There are also intrapsychic feedback loops. For example, have psychological stressors brought on a mood disturbance, or has a primary organic mood disturbance brought on the psychosocial stressors? Also, combinations of such factors typically feed into negative feedback loops and aggravate problems at several levels. Common depression can start as a primary neurobiological illness which creates a negative mindset with resulting cognitive distortions (Beck, Rush et al. 1979), including overgeneralizations, the screening out of positive affect, and such behavioral changes as withdrawal. This process can lead to further demoralization due to lack of mastery, worsening of mood, worsening of cognitive view, and even further worsening of behavior. Thus a negative feedback is created that affects mood, behavior, and cognition. Depression also influences social interactions and the central nervous system. The defect can start at any level, but if it reaches sufficient severity, it can affect neighboring levels, and a spiraling negative feedback loop can be set up. However, this interrelationship also means that intervention at other levels may be possible—and may be necessary to break negative feedback loops. For example, cognitive therapy without medication has been effective in treating mild to moderate depression, even in the presence of such biological symptoms as sleep and appetite disturbance. On the other hand, it does not always work. Medication may be necessary. Medication may improve both symptoms and cognition in one individual and yet fail in another, making psychotherapy a necessary adjunct. The systems of thinking, feeling, and behavior interact, which accounts for the success of behavior therapy in treating some emotional disorders, the success of cognitive therapy in some, and of medication management in others.

Many different models have been created to conceptualize personality. Traditional psychoanalytic concepts of ego, id, superego, and defense mechanisms have their clinical relevance. Self psychology as founded by Heinz Kohut has particular relevance to the examination of how people experience themselves as religious beings. Internal-object-relations theory can aid in evaluating how a person conceptualizes God. Psychodynamic concepts of transference and attachment to people and objects is relevant to the evaluation of religious experience.

In our practices we may encounter someone who has difficulty establishing relationships based on trust, obedience, and commitment, which one author describes as the building blocks of faith (Droege 1972). These issues will be played out in the therapeutic relationship. The client may confront these same impediments in establishing a prayer relationship with God. This person may, however, participate fully in other aspects of church life, even agreeing cognitively with the church dogma. In psychotherapy, a person's relationship to God and the impediments to developing it could feasibly be addressed with transference interpretations or by addressing the cognitive distortions involved. This could potentially free the person to develop a fuller, more satisfying relationship with God. In addition, if the patient viewed God as a real entity in his or her life, the transference interpretations could be made of the patient-God relationship even if the therapist were an atheist or of a different religious group. This would be similar to interpretations of relationships based on information reported in therapy but involving people the therapist does not know.

Therapists may encounter patients with inconsistent views of God deriving from conflictual internal object relations. These can also become the focus of therapy as attempts are made to integrate the objects, and hence integrate the image of God.

Just as therapists should not view all religion as pathological, they should not view it all as healthy. A situation like that in the Jim Jones community is a prime example. In such a situation, a therapist may be ethically compelled to intervene to prevent harm. Much depends on the therapist's ability to understand comprehensively the content and meaning of the religious experience. Religion cannot be viewed automatically as the opiate of the people unless one is willing to admit that opium can be put to both good and bad use, depending on the individual and the circumstances involved.

Merely knowing a person's denominational label is misleading, since within a denomination there can be extreme variation in religious experience. One may encounter Roman Catholics whose religious liturgy is charismatic or conducted in Latin. Some mainline Protestant parishes are very supportive of a person seeking psychotherapy, and others of the same denomination may be antagonistic. Just as few therapists adhere rigidly to one model of psychotherapy, so few clergy adhere rigidly to all the official dogma of their denominations. Ministers' personalities may play a big role in the theologies they espouse. Furthermore, the congregation is not the only medium in which religion is developed. Many people watch a variety of nationally broadcast television programs whose message may influence them more than local congregational life. One may also note a cross-fertilization of theologies within individuals as a result. This can lead to inconsistencies in personal theology and anxiety over the resulting conflict.

It is important to assess how integrated the religious experience is within the personality. An example is an antisocial personality in which one aspect of the person may be very active and constructive in community religious activities, while the other unintegrated part of the personality is overtly criminal.

Clergy, psychiatrists, and others counseling people with religious issues should realize that not everyone who presents complaining of a religious issue has a primary religious problem. The issue may have arisen in the context of another illness which should be addressed as a primary problem. To counsel the individual as if the issue were real and to ignore the underlying disorder could be detrimental. We encounter people with major depression with guilt over having committed an unpardonable sin when no such sin has been committed or who develop guilt over an actual act that is followed by a secondary depression. At times the religious aspects of guilt may need to be dealt with in therapy. A clergyperson may be the best therapist for certain basically theological conditions that influence the religious self and internal object relations reflective of religious issues. Close collaboration and mutual referral between the two professions can greatly benefit the people the professions serve.

Case Presentation

The following case examines the evaluation and treatment of a patient who presents with a common complaint. Many people who experience psychiatric difficulties consult clergy. For those who complain of disrupted faith, perhaps we should have at our disposal a differential diagnosis of this inherently psychospiritual crisis. Such an experience is for many people as traumatic as the loss of a significant other.

Applying a standard DSM-III diagnostic approach, we must be careful not to confuse diagnostic levels. Syndrome categories are listed on Axis I such as major depression, panic disorder, or schizophrenia. These serve to provide a diagnosis to aid in the establishing of treatment and formulating prognoses. Axis II categorizes personality factors in a very rough way. Axis III reminds us that we must evaluate physical conditions, and Axis IV is for the evaluation of psychosocial stresses. Axis V indicates the highest level of functioning over the past year. This paradigm allows us to think in terms of the biopsychosocial model (Engel 1980). However, in the religious realm, this systems classification is too coarse to provide the fine tuning necessary to deal with the issues. I would like to take a case in which the presenting complaint was disruption of faith and analyze it from a systems perspective.

Mrs. N, a forty-five-year-old married woman of Methodist background, presented initially with complaints of fatigue, lethargy, low energy and motivation, and poor self-esteem. She additionally complained that she could not sleep well: she often took two hours to fall asleep, awoke frequently through the night, and woke up two hours earlier than usual. She reported a pervasive lack of interest in activities that had once been pleasurable to her. She could not give an exact time of onset, but reported she had not been "happy" for a number of years. She reported that her libido had been low. Eventually even participating in group activities gave her no pleasure, and she began to isolate herself at home.

Her minister, noticing her absence from church activities, referred her to the psychiatrist. She had attended church regularly and was an active member of a ladies' prayer group. Her minister had never known her to express doubts about her faith. He attempted to discuss her doubts, to listen empathically to her fears, and to clarify issues for her. Several visits resulted in little relief. She complained that her husband was irritating her and stated she was contemplating divorce. She even mentioned occasional thoughts of suicide but felt that she would not act on them. She cried frequently during sessions with her pastor, sometimes for no apparent reason. When there was no clear reason for her crying she searched for reasons, blaming her husband, her parish, eventually her minister, and God for causing her suffering through their insensitivity to her needs. Her pastor referred her to a local psychiatrist, who evaluated her using the biopsychosocial approach.

Initially a symptom profile was obtained to clarify the Axis I syndrome diagnosis. The symptoms clearly indicated Mrs. N suffered from a major depression. No history of mania, psychotic symptoms, panic attacks, agoraphobia, other phobias, or psychosis was obtained, and she had no history of depression.

Mrs. N. was given an Axis I diagnosis of major depression, single episode, without psychotic symptoms. In view of the duration of her illness, a secondary diagnosis of a dysthymic disorder was made as indicative of chronic low-grade depression occurring for at least several years prior to the onset of her major depression.

The evaluation of her personality profile on Axis II was temporarily deferred in view of the present system profile and pending further data.

In evaluating medical conditions on Axis III, the psychiatrist learned that Mrs. N.'s only medical illness was hypertension treated with propranolol for several years. She had routinely visited her internist to have her blood pressure rechecked and medications renewed, but she failed to mention to him that she was feeling depressed. When the psychiatrist asked why, she replied that she felt her internist most likely would not care or would be unable to help. She felt that she would have to make it on her own. A physical examination revealed her blood pressure was well controlled and routine lab tests revealed no abnormalities of her thyroid function, blood count or chemistries, B_{12}, or urinalysis. Pelvic examination was normal. Pap smear was negative, and routine screening mammogram was normal. She did complain of a change in her menstrual patterns and hot flashes. The internist diagnosed only hypertension and possible onset of menopause. He agreed in consultation with the psychiatrist to discontinue propranolol and to treat her with a different antihypertensive agent without central nervous system side effects. The internist agreed with the psychiatrist that propranolol could have contributed to her depressive syndrome. During a washout period with no propranolol she noted that her energy level lifted slightly and that her spontaneous crying episodes ceased. Her overall mood, however, did not lift. She was subsequently started on an antidepressant medication, nortriptyline, and reported a slight increase in energy over three weeks with a fluctuating improvement in her sleep pattern, energy, and motivation. Her enjoyment of life returned briefly at times. An antidepressant blood level revealed a level of 40 with a normal range of 50–150. A slight increase in the dosage of her antidepressant relieved her symptoms more consistently and her activity level increased. Thoughts of suicide faded away, but she continued to demonstrate a negative mindset and low self-esteem.

Further psychological workup revealed that her level of functioning in the past year, as evaluated on Axis V, was only fair. However, her level of functioning five years ago had been good. The psychiatrist determined that cognitive therapy to correct cognitive distortions was indicated. She proved receptive to this and began to feel again more in control of her thoughts. It was explained to her that her thoughts, feelings, and behaviors all influence each other and that improvement in one area could benefit another. She was told that medication would improve her emotional tone and activity level, which would in turn help stabilize the mood-regulating center of her central nervous system, basically acting much as a temporary cast does on an injured leg. It was explained that medication would be used for six to twelve months and, depending on her progress, could be tapered off gradually and finally discontinued. Since she had had no prior episodes of depression, her prognosis for recovery was good and medication was likely to be temporary.

She was encouraged to return to previous activities, such as church, and to focus on her sense of mastery and pleasure as she did so. She began to participate in some activities and to attend services but had particular difficulty reintegrating into her ladies' prayer group.

To evaluate Axes II and III, a more detailed psychosocial history was obtained. The patient's family of origin consisted of her mother, father, and one older sister, who had often ignored her. Her older sister had apparently been more attractive and outgoing and was clearly her father's favorite. She recalled times when she had finally gotten her father's attention, only to have her sister steal him from her. Mrs. N.'s father had been a busy traveling salesman, frequently away from home; she had been emotionally distant from him. She described her mother as having a pervasively negative, judgmental attitude, demanding excessively good behavior of the child. Her mother picked her friends and clung to her. She was unwilling to allow Mrs. N. much leeway in making her own life decisions as her mother both viewed her as incompetent and expected her to act mature. Mrs. N. was generally unhappy at home. She left at age seventeen and married at age twenty. She had a son six years later.

As an adult she had little contact with her sister, who continued to snub her. Her parents' health began to fail, necessitating daily visits to help them with their basic care. Her father became cranky and demanding, and her mother griped when she arrived later than she had promised. Mrs. N.'s sister lived out of state. On her infrequent visits home the father cheered up and complained less. Her sister criticized her and continually asked her why she had not done more to make her parents more comfortable. Mrs. N. began to resent taking the brunt of all the complaints.

Around the time Mrs. N.'s parents were failing in health and their demands became greater, her husband's career as an executive for a large firm became more demanding as he attempted to climb the corporate ladder. His job frequently took him away from home and drained his energy. Feeling drained, he became more demanding on his wife for attention and sex, but did not act genuinely concerned for her feelings. She began to withdraw. As she did this he became more demanding, feeling that she was rejecting him. He began an affair and withdrew even further emotionally, leaving her feeling more isolated.

During this period her son made plans to leave for college. She felt desperate at the thought of losing him. She disliked his girlfriend because she encouraged him to attend a school out of state.

The patient had previously attended a church prayer group of six to ten women who met under the direction of a woman about the patient's age. This group had been one of Mrs. N.'s major supports, and as her mood dropped, she attempted on several occasions to discuss her concerns over her loss of faith with the group. The group leader attempted to persuade her to have more faith, witnessing to her about the marvelous relationship she herself had with God. Mrs. N. found little relief in this. She felt incompetent at believing. The other ladies in the group did not intervene on her behalf and colluded with the leader by not offering examples of their own struggles with faith. Mrs. N. began to believe that this depression was what God wanted for her and that He was punishing her for sins she was unaware of but must have committed. She was told repeatedly by the leader of the group that "all things work out well for those who love the Lord." Since the patient felt that "everything was going badly" she assumed that she must not love God. She assumed that God hated her and that she would be damned, so might as well stop the suffering by ending it all. The patient's background did not include hellfire-and-brimstone theology but did include belief in the need for a personal salvation by a personal Savior. This was part of the theology of the ladies' prayer group. Interestingly, however, this was not a prominent aspect of her church's preaching, as her minister preached universal salvation.

Intervention Options

The psychiatrist outlined the following possible levels of intervention. Under organic causes he noted a partial contribution by propranolol. It was felt that the hypertension had perhaps been triggered or exacerbated by the recent stresses. No disturbances at the level of subatomic particles or atoms were observed. The disturbance occurred at levels from the molecular and cellular to the tissue and central nervous system. The plan to control this situation was to stop propranolol and start a different hypertensive, which resulted in cessation of her affective lability. The psychiatrist further hypothesized that the end point had been an organic disturbance in her central nervous system secondary to the multiple biopsychosocial stressors. Biological treatment was effectively prescribed. The organic factors had begun to pervade the person level, as well as the two-person, family, and community subculture relationships for this woman. On the personal level, the psychiatrist noted disturbances in cognition, affect, and behavior. Also, disturbances in Mrs. N.'s experience of her self and in internal object relations were noted, as these were being played out again in her present relationships. Mrs. N. exhibited a significantly negative mindset, and cognitive therapy was applied to correct her faulty cognitions. The patient was encouraged to resume previous activities, and support in doing this was elicited from her friends, family, and pastor.

The severe marital stress, the illnesses of her parents, and the impending move of her son were felt to be issues for psychotherapy. The psychiatrist noted the disturbed relationship with her husband and involved him in her psychotherapy in a supportive way, initially as a preparation to exploring the crisis in their relationship. The pattern in the patient's relationships to her father, husband, pastor, internist, and therapist all were addressed eventually within transference interpretations in order to increase the patient's awareness of her expectations concerning how men would treat her.

The triangled relationship involving the patient's sister and father was addressed as it was learned that she actually was developing similar feelings towards the woman who led her prayer group and toward God. This triadic level of interpretation was made, and the patient began to see that God need not be a distant male image inclined to accept women more perfect than herself. She was informed that some of her faith experience was mood dependent (as are certain personality traits), and that her faith in God likely would be strengthened as her mood improved. The pain of the triangled relationship between her, her husband, and his girlfriend was addressed.

Mrs. N.'s anger towards and withdrawal from her church group was addressed with a group level of interpretation. Her mother's tendency to cling to Mrs. N. while also demanding that she grow up was correlated with the behavior of the woman in the group who told her to be more mature and strong in the faith, and thus kept her in an immature, child role. Her self-image as inadequate, unlovable, and incapable of mature relationships was dealt with in individual psychotherapy. Her internal object relations were explored, particularly her reenactment of clinging behavior with her son as he was about to leave for college and the anger directed toward his girlfriend in this triangle. These issues were interpreted and clarified on multiple levels.

On the family level, it was decided to help the patient arrange to get care for her parents. Her parents' demands that Mrs. N. care for them were addressed, and the patient became able to enjoy the relationship with her parents more after home health care was obtained. Mrs. N. was encouraged to become more assertive in her relationship with her sister and to see her more realistically as a fallible human being. This perception enabled her to stand up to her sister and demand that she help in the care of their parents. She found that she was actually able to feel close to her sister after this.

On a community and subculture level, the psychiatrist met with her minister to discuss her situation (with Mrs. N.'s consent). It was recommended that the pastor attend the women's prayer group to provide theological assessment and subsequent consultation. They decided it would be most fruitful for the minister to provide role modeling by discussing his own faith difficulties to lessen the tension that had built up in the group concerning perfection of faith. In therapy, she addressed her anger over these demands for perfection and began to realize that the group members were also acting unconsciously. She became more tolerant of the group and more able to ask the members to tolerate her doubts.

The initial crisis interventions with medication and cognitive therapies to improve her mood and diminish psychosocial stresses helped reestablish her social interactions at church, improved her self-esteem, diminished her symptoms of depression, and offered her hope and enjoyment in life again. Unfortunately, the marital difficulties had become severe and required marital therapy. The patient had become strong enough to engage in the rigors of marital therapy to reestablish trust and commitment to the relationship for both parties. She began to see herself as a more lovable being and to see God as continually present within rather than as distant. She ceased to fear God and began to trust that He would not reject her. She became even more secure in this belief as trust, fidelity, and communication were reestablished in her marriage and as she worked through her anger appropriately. She no longer was intimidated by threats of damnation but participated in her religious experiences more out of genuine love, joy, and celebration. Her mood stabilized quickly—and within the cost limitations of her insurance policy and other financial means.

Comments

Dialogues between psychiatry and religion have in the past addressed psychopathology of religion in terms of extreme psychopathology (often of a schizophrenic or obsessive-compulsive nature) or on the basis of pure character pathology. It is my experience in the private practice of psychiatry that depression and panic disorders are the most common maladies affecting faith. These are, however, given short shrift in the literature. It is here that the psychiatrist and minister most often collaborate. Faith and various levels of religious experience can be distorted and even lost during the course of an affective illness. It is common to encounter patients suffering from panic disorder who, due to their fear of having panic attacks in group situations, cease attending church for years on end. These people thus lose their ability to experience faith corporately. This loss is often painful for those who had enjoyed church as a major source of psychosocial support.

Psychiatry has focused too often on the pathological aspects of religious experience. This is in many ways equivalent to addressing sexual experience merely from the perspective of the bizarre, atypical, and perverse. Clearly the more common sexual maladies involve those of loss of function, as in impotence or inhibition of sexual desire. To fail to intervene in altered religious experience using a full systems perspective (as one would in a situation of inhibition of sexual desire or impotence) does the client a disservice. It is my experience that the loss of a once relatively sound faith experience is more common in psychiatric practice than the more bizarre examples of distorted faith. Also, it needs to be recognized that some ministers are aware of this loss of faith in their members who have entered treatment. Some misread this to mean that patients have lost faith as a result of therapy, when in reality emotional illness itself can be the causative agent and the loss may go uncorrected unless dealt with in therapy. It would have been an error merely to counsel this woman on issues of loss of faith without delving into the other systems involved. Likewise, it would have been inadequate to involve this woman in psychotherapy without addressing the other aspects of her life that this model allowed her psychiatrist to address. Not only was the patient's faith restored, but some of her neurotic doubts—which previously had lingered in the background and partially disrupted her faith experience—were relieved, allowing her to deepen her faith.

Contrary to the popular notion that an analysis of relationship difficulties diminishes a person's need for a creator or for a relationship with one's Creator-God, the opposite seems in this author's experience more often to be the case. In evaluating a person's religious experience we may see a pathological alteration in religious beliefs. In the example presented here we see Mrs. N.'s ongoing fear of her own lovability to God and concern about the distance and relationship between herself and God. These issues, however, did not interfere totally with her faith experience. Only when her psychological state changed did faith become untenable for her. What we see here is both an interplay between longstanding traits and a change into a temporary state. This illustration shows the constant flow and interaction of multiple systems issues over time.

It is interesting how patients' religious experiences often are restored with the administration of psychotropic agents to relieve the dread of panic or the anhedonia of depression that leaves one feeling incapable of experiencing joy. An important concept here is that of the mood-dependency of religious experience. When the affective nature of this experience is altered, the person may experience a disruption of relationship with God and with his or her religious community. Just as marital relationships can be destroyed through the course of depression, so a relationship with God and the church can be affected adversely. Perhaps all relationships have a mood-dependent quality.

Clearly, we are all vulnerable beings, and it is perhaps frightening for us to think that even our religious experience can be altered by a biological or sociological change or disruption of our affective tone. Any church worker is aware that changes in church program will make it more difficult for some in the congregation to maintain their affective tone, causing complaints to surface. Perhaps in the hustle and bustle of today's society the affective tone associated with religion is sought only within the framework of corporate worship. Christians are often told they should experience the peace of Christ. Perhaps this admonition gives an unconscious message that a relationship with God must occur in a prayerful, meditative setting and so cannot be generalized into the present rapid pace of life. Thus, people are taught that the faith experience revolves around a very narrow affective tone and that God cannot be present during other heightened, positive or negative affective states such as anger, or even extreme joy.

Whereas some denominations seem to preach that a narrow emotional tone in a subdued range is an indicator of a true faith experience, other denominations tend to feel that highly emotional, ecstatic states are more desirable. It is possible that people can become obsessively addicted to either the affective or cognitive components, and at times the behavioral components, of their religious experience. Perhaps this addictive or obsessive-compulsive quality needs to be recognized and diagnosed in some people. Perhaps a goal of therapy can be to broaden people's definition of the affective range over which they define their faith experience. Defining only limited prayerful moments as religious may indicate too great a reliance on the affective component in religious experience. Interpretations along these lines can perhaps widen a person's perspective to define religious experience more broadly and as occurring over multiple systems levels, so that the whole experience is not seen as somewhat isolated and frail.

Theological Implications for Christianity

As culture has entered the "Age of Narcissism" there has been an increasing focus on a personal God and a personal salvation. The present study shows that a multitude of factors enters into the cognitive, emotional, and behavioral matrix of faith. It is instructive psychologically that any faith in God is accompanied by considerable doubt. If we continue to see faith as an achievement rather than as an endowment, then faith in a loving God and personal salvation must be accompanied by an equally strong dread of a hateful God and damnation.

We should perhaps consider that anything that alienates our fellow humans from the love of God (including a theology of fear) may indeed by offensive to God. Love and support for those who struggle with their religious experience (which includes us all) would certainly better support faith than threats of damnation. Moral behavior taught on the basis of empathy for one's fellow humans, rather than to save one's soul, could lead to deeper compassion and greater genuineness in all of us.

Using this model I must conclude that faith is truly a gift that can be fostered in a proper milieu or fail to thrive if any of a number of possible systems breaks down. We will never know why one person was given the opportunity to develop faith, while another was destined to be raised in an environment not conducive to it. But given that this is so, we must be careful not to kick each other when we are down with threats of damnation. As members of the human race we bear an ethical imperative to demonstrate empathy and understanding, not rejection, neglect, and intimidation towards our fellow human beings. Many churches declare that salvation is dependent upon the acceptance of a given belief system. The biopsychosocial model, however, shows that faith is multiply determined.

I am convinced that a theology of fear as preached in certain churches and households can contribute to psychopathology. Such a theology can lead to tremendous disturbances in religious experience and away from religious concerns. Those who preach this theology bear some moral responsibility for such a negative outcome.

I advocate further study and understanding of the biopsychosocial components of faith and religious experience and that we strive towards greater empathy with others in their faith struggles by making a place for tolerance of doubt in our religious discussions.

Paul Tillich (1948) wrote that we are in eternity now and that eternity is not something that begins in the future. Perhaps we should strive to purge our theologies of conditions upon this eternity. To do so would require us to stop claiming that salvation is faith-dependent. In fact, I suspect that discussing doubts and fears openly in our churches would be more deepening of our faith than any attempts to strive for perfect faith. We should explore those dynamics at play in ourselves, as individuals and corporately, that make us think that we have a greater or lesser claim to salvation than our fellow human beings.

References

American Psychiatric Association. 1980. *Diagnostic and Statistical Manual of Mental Disorders*, third edition. Washington, DC

———. 1987. *Diagnostic and Statistical Manual of Mental Disorders*, third edition-revised. Washington, DC.

Barnhouse, R. T. 1986. "How to Evaluate Religious Ideation." In *Psychiatry and Religion: Overlapping Concerns*, ed. L. Robinson. Washington, DC: American Psychiatric Press.

Beck, A. T., A. J. Rush, B. Shaw, and G. Emergy. 1979. *Cognitive Therapy of Depression*. New York: Guilford Press.

Berger, P., and K. Brodie, eds. 1986. *American Handbook of Psychiatry, Vol. 8: Biological Psychiatry*, ed. S. Arieti. New York: Basic Books.

Blumer, D. 1977. "Treatment of Patients with Seizure Disorders Referred Because of Psychiatric Complications." *Maclean Hospital Journal* (June): 53–73.

Droege, T. A. 1972. "A Developmental View of Faith." *Religion and Health* 11, 4: 313–28.

Engel, G. 1980. "The Clinical Application of the Biopsychosocial Model." *American Journal of Psychiatry* 137: 535–44.

Engel, G. L. 1977. "The Need for a New Medical Model: A Challenge for Biomedicine." *Science* 196: 129.

Gill, M. 1982. *Analysis of Transference, Vol. 1: Theory and Technique*. New York: International Universities Press.

Knall, P. 1985. "Current Theoretic Concepts in Psychosomatic Medicine." In *Comprehensive Textbook in Psychiatry*, Fourth Edition, ed. H. I. Kaplan and B. J. Sadock. Baltimore: Williams and Wilkins.

McFarlane, W. R., C. C. Beels, and S. Rosenheck. 1983. "New Developments in the Family Treatment of Psychotic Disorders." In *Psychiatric Update: Volume 2*. Washington, DC: American Psychiatric Press.

Matteson, A. and S. Kim. 1985. "Psychological Factors Affecting Physical Conditions (Psychosomatic Disorders)." In *Comprehensive Textbook in Psychiatry*, Fourth Edition, ed. H. I. Kaplan and B. J. Sadock. Baltimore: Williams and Wilkins.

Miller, J. G. and J. L. Miller. 1985. "General Living Systems Theory." In *Comprehensive Textbook of Psychiatry*, Fourth Edition, ed. H. I. Kaplan and B. J. Sadock. Baltimore: Williams and Wilkins.

Nicholas, M. 1977. *The Theory and Practice of Group Psychotherapy,* Third Edition. New York, Basic Books.

Nichols, M. 1984. *Family Therapy Concepts and Methods.* New York: Gardner Press.

Ogden, T. H. 1983. "The Concept of Internal Object Relations." *International Journal of Psychoanalysis* 64: 226.

Poznanski, E. 1985. "Depression in Children and Adolescents: An Overview." *Psych. Annals* 15, 6: 365–67.

Robinson, L. 1986. *Psychiatry and Religion: Overlapping Concerns.* Washington, DC: American Psychiatric Press.

Schwaber, E. A. 1985. *The Transference in Psychotherapy: Clinical Management.* New York: International Universities Press.

Tillich, P. 1948. *The Shaking of the Foundations.* New York: Scribner's.

Van Dooren, H. 1987. "The Significance of Religion in Clinical Practice." Annual Meeting of the American Psychiatric Association, Chicago, IL, May.

von Bertalanffy, L. 1968. *General Systems Theory.* New York: George Braziller.

Yalom, L. 1985. *The Theory and Practice of Group Psychotherapy,* third edition. New York: Basic Books.

CHAPTER TEN

RELIGIOUS AND CREATIVE STATES OF ILLUMINATION: A PERSPECTIVE FROM PSYCHIATRY

Philip Woollcott, Jr., M.D.
Prakash Desai, M.D.

Neither psychiatry nor religion has come to terms with the nature of mystic experiences. Use of the term *mystical* tends to imply either regressive psychopathology, an otherworldly state of religious bliss, or just plain mystification. Consequently, the study of mystic experiences has been pushed to the periphery of both psychiatry and religion. Scientific inquiry into the nature of reality has largely shunned these purely subjective experiences. In the religious sphere, Western orthodoxy has found incorporation of mystic experiences either unacceptable or at best a problematic enterprise. In Eastern cultures, such as India, both the clinical and the folk tradition regard mystic experiences as exceptional achievements, and mystics themselves as objects of veneration.

In this paper we attempt to bridge the chasm between religion and science in the study of mystic experience. We take as given the fact that some persons have such experiences, a reality that must be understood. We recognize at the outset that the major problem confronting discussion of the subject is the absence of a language in which to speak about these issues. As the mystic Suso stated, "Then did he hear things which no tongue can express" (Laski 1961, 367).

From the standpoint of science, the study of mystic states is related to a central problem of psychology—the enigma of consciousness itself and its various forms (John 1976). Our usual scientific methods of data gathering, analysis, and verifiability have not been to much avail in the area of those very aspects of consciousness that are most related to our humanity. We have as yet no scientific explanation for the qualities of subjective experience. Yet dreams and hypnosis have been investigated extensively. Mystic states await a formulation that will lend itself to further study. The pursuit of such a formulation is the purpose of our paper. Our approach will be phenomenological, with an orientation that attempts to integrate psychodynamic, physiological, and cultural features.

The subject of mystic experiences contains such a hodgepodge, such a variety of phenomena (James [1902]1958), that some sort of preliminary theoretical frame must be imposed on the data just to get started. Otherwise, the results depend upon which part of the elephant one has grasped. From the standpoint of scientific psychology, mystic and religious illumination represent a particular form of a larger spectrum of "discrete" states of consciousness (Tart 1977), each of which has its own specific characteristics. These states range from deep-sleep imagery to full-waking consciousness, including daydreaming, nocturnal dreams, reverie and other relaxation states, sensory-deprivation states, hypnagogic and hypnopompic states, inspirational creativity, psychedelic states, meditative states, states of rapture and religious ecstasy, states of dissociation, fugue states, and psychotic states, particularly hallucinatory states. Only the last three are clearly pathological (Fromm 1977).

Definition and Etymology

For the purpose of this paper, mystic states are viewed as sudden, time-limited altered states of consciousness (ASC) associated mainly with a subjective experience of the interrelatedness of all things. Mysticism is a pivotal element in religious experience, although not limited to religion. The word *mysticism* derives from the Greek, referring to those "who cover their eyes and lips" (*Webster's New International Dictionary* 1971). By closing off the senses, the mystic becomes disconnected from the anchoring effects of objects, thoughts, and perceptions. The mystic ASC is characterized by sudden onset, diffuse affect, a profound sense of unity or harmonious interconnectedness, and clarity of perception, especially the experience of light. When part of religious conversion or illumination, the cognitive content or "message" usually links the particular predicament of the individual to the broader social context, including, in the religious person, the Deity.

Psychology of Religious Experience

In a series of publications Philip Woollcott reported an analysis of the psychology of religious experience utilizing data from two sources (1962, 1969). The first comprised reports of patients, clergy, and other religious volunteers. The "research tool" used was an in-depth, relatively open-ended interview in which the subject was encouraged to describe any religious or mystic experiences beginning in childhood, emphasizing adolescence, and continuing to the present. The interview lasted ninety minutes to two hours and in approximately twenty cases was supplemented by a full battery of psychological tests administered by an experienced clinical psychologist (Pruyser 1968). The second source of data comprised published autobiographical accounts of religious figures, notably Augustine, Martin Luther, and Ignatius of Loyola (Woollcott 1966, 1963, 1969).

From these studies a number of psychological features stand out, which may be briefly summarized as follows:

1. *Religious conversion must be understood not as an event but as a three-phased process:* a preliminary phase, usually characterized by intense inner conflict approaching despair; the "illumination" proper, representing an altered state of consciousness associated with a subjective experience of interconnectedness which includes a vision or message; and a subsequent phase in which major shifts in values and meaning may occur, as well as character change and increased energy and resolve.

2. *Moral and psychological conflict resolution is a prominent part of religious conversion.* In the case of creative individuals, there may be a correspondence between the problem solving of the subject and existing social or religious problems (e.g., Martin Luther). As Bion has noted, the mystic may often become the creator for the social group that authenticates the mystic (1977), the mystic vision thus serving not only as a solution to the mystic's inner conflict but as a solution or new path for the existing culture or religious group to which the mystic belongs.

3. *The role of self-restraint and limitation of sensual activity is a central feature of mystic experience.* Disciplining of appetites and desires is the *sine qua non* of the mystic way and the first step in the achievement of *samadhi* in the traditional Yoga tradition (Eliade 1975). This is equally true of the monastic mystics of the West, but such discipline has been largely forgotten in contemporary or "popular" meditation training in the West, which often begins with the postures.

4. *The crux of significant religious experience is often the mystic component, and new religions are given birth in the experience of mystic enlightenment of their creator.* The test of "authenticity" of mystic illumination is the enduring effect on the personality of an expression of a deep identification with all others and the world, as experienced in some form of "creative" action, usually in the social sphere.

5. *Experiences of religious illumination are often associated with the formation of adaptive "transitional phenomena" or "illusions" (holy objects, myth, rituals) that bridge the chasm between the mystic's inner vision of*

unity and interconnectedness and existing religious and social beliefs. In other terms, the rituals and beliefs of the religious tradition are revitalized and challenged by the mystic vision. Modifications in existing religious beliefs or rituals brought about by the mystic vision may in time become codified themselves, to be eventually again "disrupted" by a subsequent mystic vision. Thus, the development of religious belief seems to follow a developmental model of homeostasis followed by disruption, followed by a new, more evolved homeostasis. Such a model has been described as a basic organismic evolutionary process which can be identified in child development (Kegan 1985). A similar pattern has also been observed in the evolution of social systems and ideas (Kuhn 1962).

6. *Normal and pathological narcissism are central to the religious struggle, and aggrandizement is the main psychological hazard of religious illumination or conversion.* This risk has been recognized and described by the monastic traditions (Merton 1967) and in the Hindu tradition (Saradananda 1978) in the East. Various pathological outcomes of mystic experiences are described in a subsequent section.

7. *The psychological essence of "mature" or "creative" religious illumination is not regression or need gratification but integration of dissociated elements into conscious experience.* Divisiveness, scapegoating, and fanatic belief are indications of a miscarriage of the mystic illumination. A "healthy" or creative result is an integration involving not only the inner life of the mystic but also a perception of a common ground in ideas, things, and persons previously considered disparate, if not contradictory. The true mystic, in short, sees harmonious interconnection not previously recognized by others.

8. *The more creative mystics seem to have a relationship as an essential ingredient.* This relationship has a "sublimating" effect, channeling the "mad" excesses of the mystic's experience and behavior, e.g., Sri Ramakrishna. Suicidal depression, hallucinations, and confusion are frequently associated with the mystic "breakthrough" experience, even in cases of the great saints and religious figures.

9. *The phenomenology of the mystic illumination for the religious subject and for the creative writer, scientist, or artist is largely indistinguishable.* Often religious language is the only one available to express the intense affects and psychological alterations of the illumination experience. The individual's language, culture, and values strongly influence mystic expressions, their content and interpretation.

Review of Literature

The classic description remains William James's *The Varieties of Religious Experience* ([1902]1958). James described a progressive obliteration of space, time, and the sense of self to the point of dissolution, a transient enlargement of the perceptual field, a sense of union with the universe, together with a sense of revelation by means of a direct perception associated with depths of truth and lucidity beyond ordinary experience. The world appears new and luminous. James emphasized that the language of music and poetry was better suited to communicate such ineffable experiences. James, who had such experiences, saw them as a return from the solitude of individuation to a merger with the all.

Freud's most explicit statements about mystic experience are mainly in two publications: the first chapter of *Civilization and Its Discontents* and one of the metapsychology papers, *On Narcissism*. Freud came to discuss the "oceanic feeling" as a result of his correspondence with Romain Rolland.

In commenting on such an experience, Freud made several observations. In the first place, he recognized the reality of such a subjective state and allowed that in a particular situation, namely that of being in love, the loss of ego boundaries was normal and natural. "There is only one state— admittedly an unusual state, but not one that can be stigmatized as pathological. . . . At the height of being in love, the boundary between ego and object threatens to melt away. Against all the evidence of his senses, a man who is in love declares that 'I' and 'you' are one and is prepared to behave as if it were a fact" (1930, 21:65).

Freud then went on to provide a theoretically consistent interpretation of such ego states. He stated, "our present ego feeling is, therefore, only a shrunken residue of a much more inclusive—indeed, an all-embracing—feeling which corresponded to a more intimate bond between the ego and the world about it. If we may assume that there are many people in whose mental life this primary ego feeling has persisted to a greater or less degree, it would exist in them side by side with the narrower and more sharply demarcated ego feeling of maturity, like a kind of counterpoint to it. In that case the ideational contents appropriate to it would be precisely those of limitlessness and of an oneness with the universe—the same ideas with which my friend elucidated the 'oceanic feeling'" (1930, 21:68).

Freud was careful not to attribute pathology to the erasure of "every trace of sexual interest" in the anchorite or mystic meditator by emphasizing that "he [the anchorite] may have turned away his interest from human beings entirely and yet may have sublimated it to a heightened interest in the divine, in nature, or in the animal kingdom, without his libido having undergone introversion to his phantasies or retrogression to his ego" (1914, 14:80).

Federn (1952) conceived of an early split in the ego between the body ego, which follows the development of the self and object relations, and the "cosmic ego," which begins with the primary awareness of unity in the infant and remains in the unconscious throughout life. Despite theoretical difficulties related to primary narcissism and autoeroticism, Federn's view is closer to the thesis in this paper. Freud also viewed the oceanic feeling as remaining with the individual throughout life (1930).

Hartmann and Lowenstein (1960) described "automatization" of certain ego functions as a part of psychic structure—i.e., those parts of the personality that "have a slow rate of change" (Rapaport 1951). Gill and Brenman (1959), in their studies of hypnosis, coined the term *deautomatization* to account for the undoing of certain ego structures and functions. Deikman utilized this concept of deautomatization to explain phenomena associated with mysticism (1963, 1966). By having subjects meditate on a vase for thirty minutes daily over a period of several months, Deikman was able to reproduce a number of the phenomena described by mystics: a quality of intense realness, unusual sensations, a sense of unity, ineffability, and transsensate phenomena. He thought that the liberated energy experienced as light during the mystic experience may be the core sensory experience of mysticism.

The emergence of modern psychoanalytic ego psychology, especially Kris's concept of regression in the service of the ego (1952), has led to a series of writings in which mystic states, as well as states of creative illumination, are examined in a less reductionistic way.

Bach (1977) defines state of consciousness as an organized notion that emphasizes the primacy of subjective experience, ranging from more or less nonconscious to highly conscious, with a particular emphasis on the vicissitudes of self-awareness. There is in states of consciousness a dimension of subjective awareness that has its roots in diurnal variation.

From a quite different perspective, E. R. John, in a recent review, defined *mind* (under which rubric he subsumed such phenomena as consciousness, subjective experience, the self-concept, and self-awareness) as an "emergent property of sufficiently complex and appropriately organized matter." However, John pointed out that reality is not our experience of reality. What dimension or aspect of this cooperative interaction of processes "might produce the rich, diverse qualities of this abstraction from reality (consciousness)" is unknown (1976, 45).

As these two latter viewpoints indicate, consciousness itself is not readily defined, and the particular definition depends on the orientation of the definer. At least four different orientations are relevant to this discussion: (1) physiology, (2) psychology, (3) physics, and (4) philosophy.

A detailed discussion of the varied components of consciousness as well as misconceptions concerning it are beyond the purpose of this study.[1,2]

Tart (1977) has elaborated further on a typology of "discrete states of consciousness," defined on the basis of biological and physiological givens on the one hand and by learning and acculturation on the other. He described a multidimensional space to map various discrete states of consciousness. Each dimension represented one of these components as a "hardware" or "software" variable in the "map."

Developmental Approaches

Margaret Little has proposed that a "primary unity" between infant and mother forms the basis of all subsequent relationships and very likely of the deeply moving experiences of nature, art, and religion as well (1981). Burrow (1964) termed this initial bond "primary identification" and attributed to it much the same significance as Little. What we know about this period of life is inferred from the observations of infants and, to a certain extent, from work with adult patients. This initial structure of the infantile mental life may be termed the "pristine ego," which we define as a primordial, largely neurobiologically determined structure of the mind, which exists from birth as a primary awareness, a state of consciousness in which there are as yet no distinctions. Our "essence," to the extent that we can become aware of it, is not yet an "I" but a unity of "I" and "other."

The study of human development has been conceived by Piaget less as a steady, unremitting process than as a series of homeostatic balances (Kegan's "evolutionary truce," 1985) interspersed with transitional disruptions, leading to a new homeostatic balance at a higher level of development. This cyclicity continues throughout life. In early life most of the changes are characterized by physical predominance; in later life, by mental predominance. Each stage of homeostatic balance is characterized by a particular composition of self and object that defines our perception of the world and the meaning and value we give things (Piaget 1932). Generally, development moves from embeddedness to individuation, from fusion with the world to relationships, from egocentricity to sociality in an increasingly broad sense.

There is in Kegan's work a tension between self-preservation and self-transformation throughout development. It is our thesis that mystic states represent the evolving manifestations of an innate psychobiological (neurophysiological) propensity for unity, for affiliation with our fellowman and with the natural world. True mystic states represent a relatively rare form of unitary consciousness associated with a breakthrough or disruption of homeostatic balance. In addition to mystic states of unity, experiences of awe, rapture, the numinous, creative insight, and the so-called "eureka experience" refer to related states of unitary consciousness that tend to be dissociated from our ordinary "objective" consciousness.

Neurophysiological Approaches

Recent studies (Galin 1978; Tucker 1984) indicate that people have the capability for at least two major modes of consciousness: a logical, sequential, analytic mode, which is processed primarily, but not exclusively, in the left hemisphere of the brain; and an intuitive, holistic mode that develops primarily in the right hemisphere. It would appear that mystic disciplines attempt to enhance "intuitive" knowing associated with the right hemisphere integrated with enhanced clarity and "one pointedness," which may represent left-brain activity. Mystic disciplines and meditation thus may promote integration and rebalancing of left and right hemispheric functions (Deikman 1966). The sudden appearance of mystic states suggests a phenomenon in the brain similar to what has been described as "kindling" (Racine, Burnam et al. 1973).

According to Goleman (1976), meditation delinks the limbic neurophysiological arousal patterns through attitudinal modification (similar to biofeedback). However, he contends that meditators are characterized not only by limbic inhibition but by greater specific cortical alertness. The experience of the self and the state of consciousness vary with each "deepening" level of meditation, with advanced meditators reporting obliteration of all perception and, finally, a state where there is neither perception nor sense of self. The latter is experienced as a unity with the all or cosmos.

D'Aquili (1886) has described an "aesthetic-religious continuum," one pole of which is represented by the aesthetic sense and the opposite pole by what he terms the epistemic mystic state of absolute unitary being (AUB).

When in the state of AUB, which would appear to correspond to the true mystic state, people lose all sense of discrete being; the difference between self and other is obliterated; there is no sense of passing time. Such experiences are often described by religious individuals as a perfect union with God—the *unio mystica* of the Christian tradition. This is a rare state, according to d'Aquili, and possesses a sense of transcendent wholeness without temporal or spatial division.

According to d'Aquili, these rare AUB states are attained through the "absolute" functioning of the "holistic operator," the neurological substrate which is probably the function of the parietal lobe on the nondominant hemisphere. However, d'Aquili makes the interesting proposal that during AUB there is not only maximum discharge from the holistic operator and other neural structures on the nondominant side, generating a sense of absolute wholeness, but also a simultaneous maximal firing of structures on the left or dominant hemisphere. Therefore, the experience of absolute unitary being is not a sense of merger or undifferentiated wholeness only, but also, and paradoxically, a state of intensive clarity of consciousness and perception, since both hemispheric systems are maximally firing.

D'Aquili proposes that whenever the sense of wholeness exceeds the sense of discrete elements, there is an affective discharge via the right brain–limbic connections. This tilting of the balance toward an increased perception of wholeness, depending on its intensity, can be experienced as beauty, numinosity (religious awe), religious exaltation, or finally, AUB.

Fischer, in his study of yogic *samadhi* (attainment of inner light), presents a cartography of various states of consciousness. (See figure 10.1.) Fischer's conception that ecstatic mystical rapture and yogic *samadhi* may arrive at a similar endpoint through quite different paths—tropotrophic or ergotrophic—is a useful one. Fischer's diagram (1975) represents one of the few attempts to integrate psychological, physiological, and "religious" categories.

Julian Davidson (1976) emphasized shifts between physiological states of tropotrophic and ergotrophic stimulation as inducing altered states of consciousness, including mystic states of unity (*samadhi*). However, he felt that the specific determining factors belong with set and setting (as with LSD research) rather than physiological phenomena.

Phenomenology

Suddenly, with a roar like that of a waterfall, I felt a stream of liquid light entering my mind, I felt the point of consciousness that was myself growing wider surrounded by waves of light. (Gopi Krishna 1974, 2)

Mystic states come suddenly, are generally dissociated, and cannot be predicted, although certain disciplines may increase the probability of their occurrence. Mystic states are temporary phenomena, rarely lasting for longer than a few hours. Then they fade away, leaving vestiges of emotion, perception, and thought which in some cases may be experienced as having extraordinary and enduring meaning. There may be associated creative insights, enhanced energy and resolve, and a sense of inner peace.

One may feel inspired to express the vision accompanying the mystic experience in some form, but the vision itself is ineffable. The very nature of mystic experiences tends to exclude them from the "real" world, its strivings and practical demands.

The phenomenon of mysticism is more than a feeling. It has a cognitive component that has persisted through the ages. If one examines the accounts of mystics, one perceives a common thread that runs through culturally and historically diverse documents: a deep identification with all beings, so deep and immutable that once envisioned, its repudiation seems to divide the self against itself. In some cases, an experience in youth is "reviewed" and reassimilated at subsequent stages of life, even into old age (Syz 1981). In the mystic illumination the subject feels convinced of this unity with others and the world.

Because of the power and at times blissful nature of mystic states, people have attempted throughout history to cultivate them. The meth-

Figure 10.1: Varieties of Conscious States

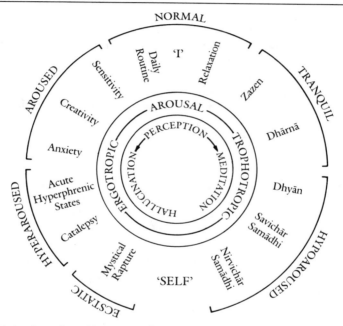

Varieties of conscious states are mapped on a perception-hallucination continuum of increasing ergotropic or hyperarousal (left half) and a perception-meditation continuum of increasing trophotropic or hypoarousal (right half).

Note that a labeling in terms of psychopathology has been omitted from this map. Hence it is perfectly normal to be hyperphrenic and ultimately ecstatic in response to increasing levels of ergotropic hyperarousal. The creative rapture of a St. Teresa, however, will envelop the cognitive repertoire of the whole perception-hallucination continuum. The radiating center of this repertoire may be the ecstatic state characterized by a very high sensory-to-motor ratio, and an erotic euphoria or orgasmic intensity. Visualize Bernini's rendition of St. Teresa's ecstasy (Peterson 1970). An analogous very-high-sensory-to-motor ratio is also characteristic for the most hypoaroused state: nirvichār samādhi; recall the picture of Ramakrishna in samādhi (Lemaitre 1963); his smile very closely resembles an euphoric-orgasmic mystical smile. A subsequent publication should separately cartograph states of consciousness during sleep, certain composite (drug-induced) states and those states of consciousness which can be assigned to the realm of psychopathology.

SOURCE: Fischer 1975:234.

odology of this cultivation varies but inevitably involves creating an ASC, often through a combination of regulation of breath and control of thought, or deprivation or regulation of the senses.

Mystic states, including religious and creative illumination, are related psychologically to other "breakthrough" experiences such as trances, faith healing, hypnotic phenomena, and, on a pathological level, to multiple personality. In all of these there is a sudden breakthrough of previously dissociated or unconscious aspects of experience into consciousness, resulting in a broader, more integrated and in some cases a novel or new field of perception and thought.

The after-effects of mystic and creative illumination often include a sense of rejuvenation and newfound energy, liberation from prior conflict and depression, a profound sense of joy, and a sense of having "another life," or a "new world" (Laski 1961). In religious subjects, a feeling of closer contact with the Deity, with other people, and with the nonhuman universe as well is frequently described (Searles 1960). In this respect, this state is not unlike the feelings described by those in love.

A sense of new knowledge in the form of a message or vision is often described—a message that resolves or transcends previous painful contradictions or personal struggles by linking the conflicts of the subject with broader social values:

> The necessity to find ever-new solutions for the contradictions in his existence, to find even higher forms of unity with nature, his fellowmen, and himself, is the source of all psychic forces which motivate man, of all his passions, affects and anxieties. (Fromm 1955, 25)

A sense of greater coherence and expansion of the self is common. At times this results in a grandiose or megalomanic identification with the Deity. This indeed was the outcome of one of Saint Ignatius's earlier "partial" conversions, prior to his famous experience at Cardoner. Ignatius reported, following this prior ecstatic experience, an elated sense of "vainglory" which did not last and which was followed by a depression. Following his enlightenment at Cardoner, his vision sustained him through long hardship. This second illumination, although more creative and productive, was accompanied by a pronounced humility (Woollcott 1969).

The aftereffects of the "higher" forms of mystic illumination tend to be creative, adaptive, socially valuable—not grandiose, divisive, or schismatic. However, the effects of religious illumination may be radical and controversial vis-à-vis existing social values. What is especially noteworthy in the aftereffects of the higher mystic illumination is the attitude of dedication and commitment, rather than strident or polemic efforts.

A feeling of renewed physical health and vigor without anxious or hypomanic drivenness is commonly described. This "healing" effect of mystic illumination is in need of much further study. The psychoanalyst Nathaniel Ross has stressed the importance of "an objective and dispassionate study of whether religious or mystic claims to have improved or enriched human relationships is valid" (Ross 1975).

Creative writers have stressed the importance of the dissociated component of creative illumination. The more disconnected, the more forceful the "vision," the more it is "surrendered" to, the more likely it is to be "true poetry" (George Eliot, in Laski 1961, 306). This ability to "turn off" the thoughts and reactions that usually filter and organize what is perceived, to be open, and to "surrender" to the illumination is found in both religious and creative people who seem to have had intense and life-changing experiences of illumination.

Archaic types of mystic illumination may be distinguished from more "creative," developmentally evolved forms of mystic consciousness along three axes: (1) degree of clarity of perception, (2) degree of integration versus projection, and (3) level of moral or ethical development as reflected in relationships. Generally, regressed merger states are characterized by a lack of clarity and relatively primitive moral and psychological development. For example, fanaticism may be associated with pseudo-religious ecstasy, a high level of perceptual clarity, but with marked projection, often of paranoid proportions, and highly disturbed ethical development—self-righteousness, omnipotent grandiosity associated with amoral or immoral destructive hatred of the "scapegoat" (i.e., merger or unity at expense of projection). More creative mystic or unity states are associated with a paradoxical combination of intense clarity of perception (enhanced ability to make distinctions), profound sense of integration or interconnectedness (absence of projection), and highly developed moral behavior often associated with principles reflecting broader social concerns and repudiation of narrow, culture-bound prejudices. (See tables 10.1 and 10.2.)

Methodological Considerations

The problem with the scientific study of mystic states is primarily methodological. We must first raise the question of whether subjective experience, especially the ineffable, nonobjectifiable subjective states that characterize mystic and religious experience, can be scientifically studied at all.

Let us examine first the question of whether *empathy* might be used as a scientific tool for studying subjective experience generally. Then we will consider the more specific problems associated with mystic states. The

Table 10.1   A Developmental Psychology of Mystic States

	Dionysian Frenzy	Erotized Mystic States	Mystic Illumination
Developmental Level	Preoedipal, "paranoid position"	Oedipal, "depressive position"	Postoedipal, Creative
Self	Grandiose, narcissistic	Triumphant Guilty	"True" self, identified with transcendent values
Object Relation	Idealized or devalued	Ambivalence God and Devil	Object constancy Concern for all others
Affect	Manic omnipotence Persecutory anxieties	Ecstasy Erotization Guilt	Serenity Joy
Defenses	Splitting Projective identification	Repression Reaction formation	Sublimation
Group	Fanatic religious cult	Charismatic	Religious commitment Care of others Moral code

phenomena of empathy suggest that individuals are far more contiguous than our usual "objective" perception would indicate. In his original description of empathy, Waelder (1960) described the scientific merit of empathy as an approach to human subjectivity. More recently, Basch (1983) described empathy "as the highest transformation of affective communication . . . a form of cognition, value-free and open to scientific evaluation." Margulies (1984) has also emphasized the legitimacy and importance of subjective experience as scientific data, and of empathy as a scientific instrument.

When it comes to mystic states of consciousness, however, their apparent discontinuity from everyday objective consciousness raises serious problems for the use of the "empathic" method to study states of consciousness for which one has no memory traces. How can we empathize with someone who is devoting a life to the mystic way when we have never been on that road, much less had a mystical experience? There are limitations of empathy and objectification of mystic states, and therefore, of the scientific study of religious experience and mysticism.

Despite their baffling obscurities, Freud believed dreams to be the royal road to the unconscious mind and proceeded to examine them rationally by the exploration of his own dreams and those of his patients, using the method of free association (Freud [1900] 1961). Stahl (1975) has suggested that Freud's method of dream analysis may serve as a model for studying mystic experience. In such an approach, the problem of the empathic limitation might be partially overcome by having the scientific student of mysticism personally undergo training in the mystic way and then examine personal experiences as rationally as possible, comparing them to those of colleagues undergoing the same experiential learning experience. Notable autobiographical accounts of such a disciplined self-examination of a personal transformational experience have been reported by the psychiatrist Hans Syz (1981) and more recently by the Indian psychiatrist Ravi Kapur (1985).

A Psychological Theory of Mystic States: Trigant Burrow's Cotention

Although avowedly nonmystical, the "phyloanalytic" approach to human behavior developed by the former psychoanalyst Trigant Burrow and his associates (1964, 1984) contains striking similarities to some of the more recent developments in meditation research and the consciousness disciplines that have attempted an integration of Eastern practices, such as Yoga and Zen, into the frame of empirical psychological study and research (Walsh 1980; Gellhorn and Kelly 1972; Tart 1975; Shapiro and Walsh 1985; Green and Green 1977).

In his concept of the "organism as a whole," Burrow denotes a total action pattern ("cotention") that is a primary physiological given. Burrow views the so-called normal world of symbols and objects as an aspect of secondary distortion and social conditioning through language and family life. This prevailing social conditioning results, he believes, in a partitive, egocentric behavior pattern ("ditension") responsible for much of our interpersonal and social strife. According to Burrow, man's "egogenic" strivings represent a deviation, a "decentering" from the primary mode of human phylic solidarity with fellow humans. Burrow utilized group techniques to diagnose and correct the excessive emphasis of each member's "I-persona" (similar to narcissism) as expressed in the "ditentive mode."

His description of "cotention"—a time-limited state of organic continuity with others and the world associated with a decrease in egocentric striving—is similar to a mystic state. Burrow spent many hours engaged in solitary self-reflection in order to try to understand tensions and reaction patterns, as he called them, which seemed to be experienced in the cephalic region of the head during the usual ditentive state. It was during this process of self-reflection that he became aware of a different subjective reaction of wholeness and calm which he termed "cotention" to distinguish it from the more partitive, striving, ego-related ditensive attitude so prevalent in the behavior of himself and the other colleagues in his research group.

Table 10.2   Altered States of Consciousness

Category	Neoplatonic Trance (Mystic Consciousness)	Dionysian Frenzy
Ego functions	Regression and reintegration (regression in service of ego) Integrative, unifying Basic ego functions intact, even enhanced Higher-level ego defenses only	Clearly regressed Divisive, disorganizing Repressed ego state gains ascendancy Primitive ego defenses: splitting, omnipotence and devaluation, denial, projective identification
After effects	Associated with "rebirth" and new personality structure	Return to same personality structure
Object relations	Bad objects integrated Synthesis of internal and external object representation (wholeness) Integration of good and bad objects	Bad objects projected Primitive, part objects predominate, often fantastically distorted Dichotomy between good and bad, self and object representations. We and They sharply differentiated.
Self system	Cohesive sense of self Identity integration Humility, sense of "we-ness" I–Thou	Primitive identification or fusion with grandiose self-object Identity diffusion or submission to group identity Omnipotent, narcissistic, magical, manic sense of power I–It
Instinctual Vicissitudes	No special object of drives Aggression and sexual instincts sublimated	Fusion of sex and aggression Aggression and sexual instincts released
Perception	Open Clarity increased Heuristic vision Deautomatization Hallucinations rare	Constricted Intense but confused, dissociated Ecstatic vision Less deautomatization Hallucinations possible
Cognition	Universal symbolism Clear Intuitive, penetrating insights	Esoteric symbolism Confused Magical insight

Affective component	Calm	Excitement
	Bliss	Ecstatic frenzy
	Peace "which passeth all understanding"	Intense excitement, restlessness
	Neutrality, paradoxical detachment and commitment, desirelessness	"Manic" quality, hysteroid, frenetic
	Compassion	No compassion
	Nonerotic, noetic, heuristic passion	Erotic
	Agape	Eros
	Stable, unified	Unstable, spreading, contagious
	Nonambivalent	Ambivalent
	No anxiety	Great anxiety, if not ritualized
Social implications	Sense of being like others	Sense of specialness and superiority
	Humanizing	Dehumanizing
	Maximal integration of both individualness and groupness	Mob, cult, group instrument of collective forces
	Intellectual functions still intact	Intellectual functions suspended
	Rarely drug induced	Often drug induced
	No ritualization	Ritualization
	Crosses cultural and historical lines	Bears stamp of particular culture or subculture
	Complex	Simplistic
	Inclusive	Exclusive
	No scapegoating	Scapegoating
	Cotensive (Burrow)	Ditensive (Burrow)
Group implication	Task-work group (Bion)	Basic assumption group phenomenon
	Union based on shared vision and task	Union based on dogma
Value orientation	Ethical	Moralistic
	Individual and social responsibility	Group responsibility only
	Humility	Omnipotence
	Creative	Noncreative
	Humanizing	Dehumanizing
	Truth	Idolatry
	Sense of sacred	Sense of magical

Burrow's view that the cotentive reaction pattern had a biological basis in the brain provided a link to the physical, comparable to Yoga. Another "mystic" feature of Burrow's thought is his insistence that there is another deeper, more basic approach to reality that does not involve the symbol. Thus, Burrow's cotention, like mysticism, becomes another, more direct way of knowing. The experience of cotention involved distinct physiological features (e.g., steadying of eye movements, decreased respiration) as well as mental features (sense of calm and social affinity). These were so qualitatively distinct from the usual ditentive mode of "normality" that Burrow felt a fundamental, organic aspect of the species must be involved, one which had a neurophysiological basis (Burrow 1984). In contrast to the symbolic, partitive ditentive knowing associated with symbol and language, Burrow speculated that cotention must represent a fundamental holistic mode of the species or, as he preferred to say, of the phylum. Hans Syz has suggested that Burrow's choice of the broader term *phylum* may reflect an unconscious preference for a more cosmic term than *species* (Syz 1981).

Essentially, Burrow came to believe that psychoanalysis, in treating individual neuroses, was dealing with secondary symptoms of a more basic, organismic dissociation or displacement—the "social neurosis" endemic to humans. This organic decentering, he proposed, is too entrenched and too fundamental to the functioning of the organism to respond to the "mental or symbolic plan of enquiry" of traditional psychoanalysis or psychotherapy. He wrote that these ditentive deviations are universal and, like the proverbial mote, present in treater as well as patient, in investigator as well as research subject. Therefore, the usual techniques of psychoanalysis or psychotherapy cannot resolve them, for they cannot be objectified in the patient. The cure, he proposed, requires a group format in which the therapist and group member are equally subject to confrontation and interpretation. This method of social analysis he called *phyloanalysis*.

In terms of specific techniques developed from his researches to produce the desired cotention, he encouraged the subject to sit or lie down in an attitude of repose and to become increasingly sensitive and aware of the position of the eyes when in their "relaxed" state, i.e., when not engaged in "symbolic or projective attention." With the eyelids closed, the eyes are focused as steadily as possible on a point a few yards away directly in front at the center of the field of vision. An effort is made to exclude the usual flow of thoughts and distractions. These techniques were arrived at utilizing physiological correlates (e.g., slowing and deepening respiration) to promote and enhance the generally latent "cotentive" mode.

Burrow noted that these efforts to center on a more harmonious induce the desired cotention, he encouraged the subject to sit or lie down tegration included the respiratory, vasomotor and circulatory, and cerebral activity. His descriptions are similar to the claims of the mystics that their discipline affects the basic physical and metabolic functions of breath, circulation, digestion, and hormonal activity as well as the mind. Parenthetically, it was from similar observations of yogis that the idea of biofeedback developed (Green and Green 1977).

In summary, Burrow proposed that the problems of human beings are basically socioneurotic problems; i.e., individual neurotic difficulties are *derivative* of a primary specieswide defect in sociality. Burrow hypothesized that this social defect is due to our unique symbolizing and language facility, which has deflected the innate biological sociality of humans into an excessively self-referent attitude or mode. Burrow claimed to be able to detect and clarify this self-referent, acquisitive, competitive mode by examination of human interaction in small groups. He called this mode of behavior "ditention." He related the ditentive mode to what he called the "I-persona"—the competitive, self-centered motivations of humanity as a whole.

After years of research and, we would add, mounting frustration and discouragement regarding the resistance to change associated with the ditentive attitude in his experimental groups, Burrow reported he was able to detect evidence of a more fundamental, latent cooperative mode in himself and others. He termed this cooperative mode "cotention" and published studies in which he reported differences between cotention and ditention with electroencephalographic and other neurophysiological measurements. He proposed that the cotensive mode was derived from the primary identification between infant and mother. He sometimes called cotention the "preconscious mode." Although some scientists and therapists (for example, the family therapist, Nathan Ackerman) were attracted to these ideas, Burrow's main advocates at the time were creative writers and artists (D. H. Lawrence, among others) (Burrow 1964).

Burrow went against prevailing individualistic trends in Western thought and was repudiated by most of his fellow psychoanalysts. He emphatically disavowed mystic, teleological, or religious elements and persistently sought physiological correlations and scientific support for his findings. Nevertheless, his view of an innate communal solidarity of the phylum, as well as the somewhat contemplative techniques he used to discover the cotensive mode, has mystical, if not religious overtones. Furthermore, the dualistic nature of his theory, with the struggle to overcome ditention (bad) and enhance cotention (good) may reflect his own repudiated Christian background (his mother was a Southern grand dame and a devout Roman Catholic) (Syz 1981).

A Case Example: Sri Ramakrishna

The life and experiences of the Indian saint Sri Ramakrishna afford us an opportunity to understand the nature of mystic experiences. Set in a religious context, Sri Ramakrishna's experiences were varied and spontaneous, as well as induced, and they had a profound impact on his life as well as that of his culture. The knowledge about his early childhood and even later adulthood come to us from hagiographic accounts of his disciples (e.g., Saradananda [1911–16] 1978), where fact and legend have merged. This very fact reveals not only the Indian attitude toward history but also a tradition in which myth making about heroes has been second nature. A religious man and especially a mystic lends himself to the forces of culture, thus legitimizing his role as a pathfinder.

Ramakrishna was born in 1836 in a village near Calcutta in the province of Bengal. Biographers tell us, from anecdotes and memories of contemporaries, that his parents themselves had visions relating to Ramakrishna's birth. As a child, he was known to be unruly, mischievous, and given to impersonating women. In one incident he was reported to have entered a strictly regulated women's quarter dressed as a woman and gone unrecognized. He especially enjoyed devotional singing and was reported to be lost in the rapture of the rhythm. His father's sister was known to have been possessed by the spirit of a goddess, and Ramakrishna later recalled that it would have been splendid if the spirit had possessed him. At least on one occasion, the story goes, while participating in worship, Ramakrishna became so engrossed that he lost consciousness. Later accounts of such behaviors characterized them as trance states, but his father was worried that the young boy suffered from "fits," and his mother was concerned that he had come under the influence of an "evil eye."

After his father's death from chronic dyspepsia and dysentery when the boy was about seven, Ramakrishna became restless and pensive and was known to wander alone at the cremation grounds. He frequented the pilgrim-house where the wandering monks lodged to become familiar with them, but the mother feared that he might be tempted by the monks to go away with them. In the following months, Ramakrishna remained preoccupied and had episodes of loss of consciousness and of his sense of self and time. Some years later he came under the protection of his eldest brother, who had migrated to Calcutta to make a living as a teacher and priest and who was also known to have premonitions about the future. It is said that he predicted the event of his wife's death accurately. Ramakrishna became a temple priest at the age of nineteen. Soon after that his brother died.

Following his brother's death, Ramakrishna's behavior became strange, his mind agitated. He spent hours in worship of Kali, the mother goddess of Bengal, and in meditations. He felt despairing and desperate and contemplated suicide. He later described his state of mind:

> Just as a man wrings a towel forcibly to squeeze out all the water from it, I felt as if somebody caught hold of my heart and mind and was wringing them likewise. . . . I was in great agony. I thought there was no use in living such a life. My eyes suddenly fell upon the sword that was then in Mother's [Kali's] temple. I made up my mind to put an end to my life in that very moment." (Saradananda [1911–16] 1978, 162)

Instantly, he had a vision that he described as follows:

> It was as if the houses, doors, temple, and all other things vanished altogether; as if there was nothing everywhere! And what I saw was a boundless infinite Conscious Sea of light! . . . a continuous succession of Effulgent Waves coming forward, raging and storming . . . and lost all sense of consciousness." (Saradananda [1911–16] 1978, 163)

His behaviors, especially his tendency to fall into a state of unresponsiveness and sometimes unconsciousness, led those around him to suspect insanity. Doctors were consulted and various medications given (Saradananda [1911–16] 1978, 164, 165, 175). His mother thought that he was possessed by a ghost and brought him to an exorcist (Saradananda [1911–16] 1978, 202).

During the years that followed, Ramakrishna came in contact with a series of individuals: sponsors, intellectual and religious leaders of the community and, most important, both mentors and disciples. Having received the patronage of a wealthy sponsor, he returned to the Kali temple in Calcutta and met with the curious, the devout, and the skeptic alike. It was here that his first mystic experience occurred, but there was no end to his travails. He continued to be rapt in worship and meditation, caring not for his physical well-being, and was known to frequently pass into altered states of consciousness. His family's concern for the health of his mind was unabated, and they arranged his marriage, hoping that would alleviate whatever was ailing him. However, Ramakrishna was not to be deterred from his path of seeking divine vision.

A holy woman entered into Ramakrishna's life, taught him specific devotional practices, and arranged for a conference of scholars and pundits to pass judgment on his religious authenticity. A model existed, particularly in the history of Bengal, of a saint whose emotional frenzy and ecstasy was a matter of folklore. The assembled group conferred a similar status on Ramakrishna. In a sense, at this point, he was invested by the community with holiness.

The next twelve years Ramakrishna spent in intense religious practices from every known tradition, including Islam and Christianity. The intellectuals who spearheaded reform movements within Hinduism, incorporating Western influences, came to regard Ramakrishna as a major contributor to the resurrection of Hindu ideals. Finally, in the disciples—especially Swami Vivekananda, whose arrival had been accompanied by another divine vision—Ramakrishna's spiritual leadership in India was consolidated. The bonds that developed between him and his disciples, particularly Swami Vivekananda, brought organization and stability to the life of Sri Ramakrishna, elevating his message to the status of a movement in India.

The hallmarks of Ramakrishna's mystic experiences are in concordance with our understanding of such experiences. Spontaneous or induced, the experiences had in common a profound affective tone. There was a perception of interconnectedness of all things, so that the boundaries between subject and object were obliterated and the predominant cognitive aspect was of a religious nature.

It must also be emphasized that the period prior to his ascension to sainthood was one of intense psychological turmoil, often mistaken by those around him as possession or insanity. (June McDaniel [1987] has extensively treated the subject of madness and ecstatic states in relation to culture and religion.) But when the community reinterpreted his experiences and set Ramakrishna into the prevailing religious tradition, his experience was legitimized. Also, the succession of mentors and disciples was an important grounding. In his incorporation of deities of other religions, Ramakrishna restored to his followers a sense of mastery over the Western missionaries and a pride in their native traditions during a time of onrushing Western modernity in India.

Mysticism and Creativity

Many scientists emphasize the role of a mystical perspective in their own scientific breakthroughs. Much of Newton's theoretical system developed from a mystical experience (Bion 1977). Such developments occur in agnostic as well as religious persons. The mystic vision appears to be a central stimulus for religion, but once religion becomes institutionalized, mysticism may have little to do with religious practice and may be held in suspicion by the religious hierarchy. It seems important, therefore, to examine mystic states in their own right, independent of any theological or teleological assumptions. For example, poets and writers have described the instantaneous nature of inspiration in which the entire conception or idea or story is grasped, which may then require months of working out through rational, empirical means (Ghiselin 1963).

Nathaniel Ross states that regressive unions that infiltrate the more

objective, reality oriented ego perspectives may even be required for optimal function (1975). Rose describes how in creative inspiration, the
boundaries of our separateness and identity "are repeatedly dissolved and
recreated as we dip back and re-emerge from looser and earlier arrangements of reality." He has described case material of pathological, normal,
and creative fusion (1972). A different view is expressed by Singer (1977)
who views this open, flexible outlook as part of an adult personality style
rather than a regression.

Greenacre wrote that some gifted children describe ecstatic states of a
"peculiarly exalted type." They combine a prominent mystical and religious flavor with collective and cosmic themes. Such gifted children describe a haunting and compelling sense of boundlessness and a general
sense of power and awareness that reach beyond the limits of the self. In
some ways, such experiences of gifted children may represent precocious
experiences of unitary consciousness. Although Greenacre described this
material within the context of classical psychoanalytic theory, she nevertheless noted that creative ability that appears in this form may be "beyond
the scope of psychoanalytic research" (1958).

It has been proposed that religious practices and their mystic coloring
may derive affective overtones from their association with important early
relationships, essentially serving as "transitional" objects or phenomena
(Winnicott 1953). Greeley (1975), following Eliade (1964), sees mystic
experience as a return to a powerful primordial myth of paradise, common
not only to primitives but to all humans. Some of the profound affective
experience associated with mysticism reflects a vision of reality distinct
from "objective" experience which yet has a particular clarity and meaning
of its own. We would consider the transitional experiences described by
Pruyser (1984) in regard to imagination and childhood and Csikszentmihalyi's (1975) concept of play and "flow" to be developmental forerunners of mature mystic and creative experiences. (See, for example,
DeNicolas's *Powers of Imagining* [1962], a study of Saint Ignatius of Loyola.) The capacity for creative imagery is also highly correlated with hyp-
notizability (Hilgard 1986).

The Eureka Experience

The so-called eureka experience generally associated with a creative breakthrough may be considered a secular variant of mystic illumination. The
word *eureka* derives from the Greek, meaning simply, "I've found it." The
paradigm for the eureka experience was Archemedes who, after long study
and concentration, suddenly discovered in a flash how to determine the
alloy in the king's crown. What we wish to emphasize by this term is the
human capacity to become rapt—to develop a total psychological absorp-

tion in the object. This process involves a period of disciplined concentration and screening out of distractions, followed by a sudden breakthrough of insight in which some hitherto unknown experience or previously unorganized concept suddenly becomes manifest. The eureka experience has an emotional component of exhilaration, even ecstasy, and is a variant of mystic experience.

Without the capacity for becoming rapt (carried away) by the particular subject, conflict, or problem, there can be no subsequent eureka experience. The relationship of such processes to the unconscious, and the breakthrough of previously repressed or unintegrated contents of the mind into consciousness, as well as the ego capacity to "let go" without becoming disorganized (Rose 1972), have been described in the psychoanalytic literature as a psychological means of switching from a more motivation-powered and problem-solving behavior to a process in which one becomes so totally absorbed in the object of study that one "loses oneself," enabling the individual to "see" new relationships and connections not previously recognized.

The "high" associated with the eureka experience is complex. Like mystic experience generally, it probably includes a neurophysiological discharge mechanism, which is given a particular character by aspects of the object-relations history of the individual.

The eureka experience, like mystic states, is frequently associated with the presence of another person—a guide, a mentor. If such a guide or mentor is not present, there is usually a highly cathected object representation, such as God. The unusual work and discipline involved in the preparatory stage of such experiences should be emphasized, as well as the subsequent working through of the insight.

The eureka experience often involves resolution of internal conflict, particularly around narcissistic phenomena. In such cases a change and alteration in the *self* follows the experience (Kohut 1971, 1977). After the eureka experience, there is a new knowledge *and* there may be new sense of self as well. Despite the unique subjectivity of the eureka experience, its most significant and meaningful forms invariably involve a highly developed social context. Finally, the eureka experience is almost always experienced as healing, as therapeutic. In this respect it is similar to descriptions of the "aha" experience associated with insight in psychotherapy.

Mysticism: A Darker Side?

Expressions of the mystic and of the fanatic or cult member seem at times dangerously similar. Both are fearlessly sure of themselves. Fanatic zeal and moral passion or commitment are not easily distinguished. As noted previously, such observations suggest different levels of mysticism or unitary consciousness. In table 10.1, different levels of development are linked to archaic and higher mystic states. It also seems useful to compare various affective-cognitive expressions of unitary consciousness with an assessment of the object relations in any given case. Existing theory has no place for higher forms of unitary consciousness, such as true mystic states or, for that matter, creative illumination. The differentiation of such "higher" states from pathological states is as yet not well understood, and the distinctions in the tables 10.1 and 10.2 must be considered tentative. In addition to the developmental model in table 10.2, a phenomenological examination of "higher" and "lower" mystic states is found in table 10.2.

Even the most esteemed mystics may at times explain the world's problems with simple formulas and do so with sublime freedom from self-doubt: all evil apparently lies outside the explanatory system. One cannot help but wonder whether this treatment of the darker side constitutes a form of "pathological mysticism" that distorts rather than augments reality. It would seem that it does and that the mystic vision is "subject to many diseases" (Buber 1970). The presence of projection and a hated scapegoat signifies the presence of such diseases (Cohn 1970).

Cult members and fanatics generally seem to regress to and remain fixed at the level of archaic merger states, whether ecstatic or traumatic. Such states are characterized by loss of and withdrawal from the object and a deadening of human sensibilities. The element of human cooperativity is missing. There is destruction of the necessary kinship with others which alone can authenticate and complete the self. What then happens to the solitary mountaintop mystics in the best of the Indian tradition? Even here one finds an intense, devoted relationship to a guru, and if not an actual person, then the memory of such a person, or the image of a God made real and personally meaningful.

In the case of severe narcissistic injuries, on the other hand, the primary other failed the developing self, so that the self may turn for fulfillment, not to the ideal other or the image of that ideal, but to a compensatory grandiose self-image fused with an idealized object. In this case there is no true recognition of an "other," except in the service of the grandiose self. Such individuals may gravitate to religious cults and pathological "mystic" expressions. In such cult members or leaders, other people have no meaning other than as an extension of the narcissistic needs of the self (or group). Consequently, persons or groups outside the cult easily become targets of hate or violence—even persons previously loved. There is an "addictive" clinging to the cult and its beliefs, which embody the grandiose ideal-self–ideal-object merger. In "healthy" or higher forms of mysticism, the capacity for distinction (for "one-pointedness") and for clarity of perception parallels the development of unity. It is a paradoxical state.

In pathological forms of cultic belief, there is a similarity to the picture seen clinically in compulsive addictions. There is intense craving in proportion to the absence of any meaningful relationship and commitments. This "emptiness" of the addicted or "cultic" personality presents a severe obstacle to treatment. Whereas writings and poetry of the great mystics, even the most solitary ones, overflow with devotion, there is neither true devotion or commitment in the fanatic cult member.

In some ways the fanatic expresses in such group behavior a caricature of the universal psychosis of social humanity. According to the mystic commentators, this is a disease that all people share: disavowal of the organismic unity with our fellow human beings.

Discussion

> Our greatest blessings come to us by way of madness.
> Plato, *Phaedrus* 244A

The phenomena of mystic and creative illumination suggest that there exist quite different states of awareness, dissociated from our ordinary consciousness, which appear suddenly, as if a threshold of some kind had been reached, bringing with them for a limited period of time an altogether different cognitive and perceptual state. From a clinical standpoint we are familiar with pathological or traumatic experiences, memories, and affects, which may be repressed or split off from our usual conscious awareness— possibly to appear later directly or in the disguised symbolic form of symptoms. Thus, the mechanism of dissociation is familiar to us as a primitive defense mechanism and a form of psychopathology. Indeed, we have every reason to believe that there exist quite commonly such pathological forms of religious and mystic experience. The religious traditions in both the West and the East have warned us of "false prophets" and of the narcissistic pathologies to which the spiritual life in its mystic form is susceptible (Merton, 1967).

Saint Ignatius himself was remarkably candid about the "vainglory" and suicidal depression that followed his earlier state of rapture prior to his final conversion at Cardoner, which resulted in a major personality change and the eventual founding of the Jesuit order. What is the difference between these two states in Ignatius? Phenomenologically, they seem much the same if one examines only the experience of the ecstasy itself (Woollcott 1969). The preliminary and subsequent phases are, however, very different. There are many records of experiences of religious and creative illumination in the lives of our greatest poets and saints, including hallucinations, trances, delusions, and loss of boundaries of the self. In fact the very creative power of the vision may be related in the mind of creative individuals with its foreignness, its otherworldliness, its intrusive disruption of their normal consciousness (Laski 1961).

Hallucinations and delusions are common in the dissociative syndrome of multiple personality, leading frequently to a misdiagnosis of schizophrenia. The dissociative experience itself, especially at the time of the "breakthrough" of dissociated material, seems to be associated with the temporary appearance of disturbances in thought and consciousness, which in clinical experience is generally related to psychosis but in the case of dissociation may express a more temporary disorder. The situation is similar to the psychedelic experience. If the set and setting are supportive, a nonpsychotic, even "transcendent" and ecstatic, transformation of perception and cognition may occur. If the situation is nonsupportive, severe anxiety or even psychosis may result.

If we lay aside our clinical bias that mystic states are a form of regressive psychopathology, we confront an interesting observation, which may be expressed in the form of a question. Why would the expression of human creativity and religious genius be connected with a dissociation of experience? Why are mystic states dissociated? Is there something about the content of experiences of mystic illumination that could explain why they so rarely enter our conscious experience, and then only for a short while?

Mystic experiences, including religious and creative illumination, are related psychologically to other dissociative phenomena, such as shamanistic trance, faith healing, hypnotic phenomena, and, on a pathological level, multiple personality. The breakthrough of previously dissociated aspects of experience into consciousness, resulting in a broader, more integrated field of perception, seems to represent a common psychological mechanism that may be associated with integration, healing, and increased well-being, but which may also result in pathological outcomes. The presence or absence of a supportive environment is an important factor in outcome. This suggests a deep psychological link between mystic states and a deeper level of as yet poorly understood social forces in the personality. Bion has proposed the existence of a "proto-mental state" preceding self-object separation and language acquisition, which may be the source of "basic assumption" group behavior (Bion 1977). This protopathological mental state may also contain deeply repressed or dissociated archaic social tendencies.

Burrow suggested that the "objective" mode associated with self-object differentiation may be essentially incompatible with the initial infant-mother "dual unity," which must be repressed. Mystic and creative illumination may represent more evolved developments of this largely repressed unitary consciousness. I say "more evolved" because we do not know what the infant experiences. The infant's brain and neurophysiology is far different from that of the adult. Although mystic states have been described in children and are fairly common in adolescence, they reach their full state only in adulthood.

Since the mystic vision of identification with all other beings seems much the same in different cultures and periods of history, this experience may spring from our innate neurophysiology. It is as if the mystic illumination represented a social ethic embedded in our brain and mind, apparently contradicting our biological strivings for instinctual gratification.

Our thesis is that mystic states represent a breakthrough that links the developmental line of largely dissociated experiences of unitary consciousness with the developmental line of the self and object relations which we experience in our ordinary "objective" consciousness. Mystic states as well as other related states (religious awe, eureka experiences, numinous experiences) disrupt the homeostasis of the self and its "objects," creating a risk of regressive and especially narcissistic solutions, but also the possibility of a more advanced level of development of the self and its relationships. Creative forms of mystic enlightenment involve a more integrated view of the world and a broader sense of relationships, including social ethics and values.

Paradoxical Integration

There appears to be an inherent conflict between the yearning for fusion associated with the largely dissociated experience of unitary consciousness and the strivings for individuality. Mystics at their best seem to achieve an integration between polar opposites. The advanced yogi may seek *samadhi* or "oneness with God." This union is associated paradoxically with a separation of and control over the demands of the instinctual drives of sexuality and aggression, as well as functions of the body not ordinarily under the control of the will (e.g., respiration, eye movement). In other terms, the yogi's achievement of the unity of *samadhi* is associated paradoxically with a high degree of "field independence" through control of the breath and concentration.

Thus, on close scrutiny, the achievement of mystic states seems to be associated with certain paradoxical developments of an equally high degree of perceptual clarity, "one-pointed" attention and concentration, motor control, affective modulation, ethical discrimination, and independence in relationship to the environment, which are generally associated with a high level of ego strength and maturity of object relations. Thus, efforts to explain mystic states as regression to infantile states do not correspond to clinical observation.

Summary

We may summarize our hypothesis of a developmental line of unitary consciousness as follows. We begin life in a state of union with the environment. Consciousness itself springs from this unity or *is* this unity. Without the response of the consciousness of another, neither consciousness nor life could proceed further. Thus, in its fundamental nature, consciousness is *interactive*. ("The very Being of man . . . is the deepest communion" [Bakhtin 1961].) We have no direct knowledge of what the infant actually experiences of this primary identification or consciousness. What we have done is to adultomorphize about it on the basis of what we observe in children, in the mystic, or in regressed patients. There seems to be a consensus among developmental psychologists, however, of the role of a firm establishment of this "primary unity" between infant and mother for subsequent development (Little 1981; Mahler, Pine, et al. 1975). Even from its earliest origins, this primary bond is characterized by a synchronous rhythmical connectedness between two quite different organisms. "Those fortunate individuals who, in early infancy, have been able to enjoy and internalize the emotional experiences of a rhythmical adaptive interaction of the mouth differentiated from the breast are receptive to later experiences such as human sexual love and aesthetic and religious experiences" (Tustin 1981).

Cognitive and perceptual development create awareness of disunity—of separation between the self and the environment—and the basic unitary experience of interconnectedness of the child is lost. Throughout the separation-individuation phase (Mahler, Pine, et al. 1975) and, indeed, through life, the individual struggles to differentiate his or her unique humanity from the surrounding human and nonhuman environment (Searles 1960).

In our unconscious, however, remain traces of our original sense of oceanic continuity and connectedness with the universe, which in our development we have dissociated and put behind us. We are ambivalent toward this primary state of unity; we fear becoming immersed again in its limitless chaos yet long to recapture its blissful interconnectedness. We have referred in previous studies to this basic human ambivalence as the "fusion-individuation conflict" (Woollcott 1981). The fusion-individuation conflict is only resolved by means of a continuation throughout life of various direct or symbolic forms of merger experiences between the developing self and the dissociated experience of unitary consciousness and its derivatives.

In this conception, the unitary model of consciousness evolves in a parallel developmental series with, and in proportion to, the developing structures of the self and object relations, and of the brain itself. Connections between the developing self and object relationships, the evolving line of development of unitary consciousness, and the neurophysiological structures of the brain are manifested by complex affective-cognitive states such as awe, wonder, the numinous, states of creative insight, eureka experiences, and mystic states. The fact that such experiences occur only temporarily in brief "quanta," as well as their cognitive and space-time distinctions, reflects the discontinuity or dissociation which exists between the development of the self of everyday reality and the development of unitary consciousness. Finally, the meaning of the unitary states and their "cognitive" component of a deep fraternal bond among people which occurs during mystic experience is unknown.

In conclusion, there are two paradoxically related experiences that are the focus of our study of mysticism. One is the solitary individual's experience of a sense of interconnectedness of all things. The other is the primacy of relationality in human experience. The true mystic unity is a primal dynamic connection, a uniting. A so-called mystic experience that leads away from relationships with others and the world, or one that divides relationships between the all good and the all bad, between the holy and the evil, is a false or pathological mysticism. True mysticism is characterized by an identification with all beings. This is the radical mystic experience of the poet John Donne, expressed in "No man is an island": How do people who have never had a mystic experience appreciate the poet's creation? People may not understand the poet's mystic experience per se, but they can "empathize" with the poet's insight or vision. The poetic vision stirs something deep inside all of us, an essential affinity with others and the world.

This paradoxical connection between mystic illumination and relationality and love is eloquently expressed by the blind poet Jacques Lusseyren, who lost his eyesight through an accident at the age of seven and a half. He later wrote (in "The Blind in Society"):

> Barely ten days after the accident that blinded me, I made the basic discovery . . . I could not see the light of the world anymore. Yet the light was still there. . . . I found it *in myself* and what a miracle!—it was intact. This "in myself," however, where was that? In my head, in my heart, in my imagination? . . . I felt how it wanted to spread out over the world. . . . The source of light is not in the outer world. We believed that it is

only because of a common delusion. The light dwells where life also dwells: within ourselves. . . . The second great discovery came almost immediately afterwards. There was only one way to see the inner light, and that was to love. (Erikson 1981, 330)

Notes

1. Julian Janes (1976) describes consciousness as follows: "We have said that consciousness is an operation rather than a thing, a repository, or a function. It operates by way of analogy, by way of constructing an analogue space with an analogue 'I' that can observe that space and move metaphorically in it. It operates on any reactivity, excerpts relevant aspects, narratizes and conciliates them together in a metaphorical space where such meanings can be manipulated like things in space. Conscious mind is a spatial analogue of the world and mental acts are analogues of bodily acts. Consciousness operates only on objectively observable things" (65–66).

2. Ludwig (1966) defined altered states of consciousness as any mental state induced by various physiological, psychological or pharmacological maneuvers or agents which can be recognized subjectively by the individual himself (or herself) or by an objective observer of the individual as representing a sufficient deviation in subjective experience or psychological functioning from certain general norms for that individual during alert, waking consciousness. This sufficient deviation may be represented by a greater preoccupation than usual with internal sensations or mental processes, changes in the formal characteristics of thought, and impairment of reality testing to various degrees.

References

Bach, S. 1977. "On the Narcissistic State of Consciousness." *International Journal of Psychoanalysis* 58:209–322.

Bakhtin, M. M. 1961. *Problems of Dostoevsky's Poetics.* Minneapolis: University of Minnesota Press.

Basch, M. F. 1983. "Affect and the Analyst." *Psychoanalysis Inquiry* 3:691–703.

Bion, W. 1977. "The Mystic and the Group." In *Seven Servants,* 62–71. New York: Jason Aronson.

Buber, M. 1970. *I and Thou,* trans. Walter Kaufman. New York: Scribner's.

Burrow, T. 1937. "The Organism as a Whole and Its Phyloanalytic Implications." *Australian Journal of Psychological Philosophy* (December).

———. 1964. *Preconscious Foundations of Human Experience,* ed. W. E. Galt. New York: Basic Books.

———. 1984. *Toward Social Sanity and Human Survival, Selections from His Writings,* ed. A. S. Galt. New York: Horizon Press.

Cohn, N. 1970. *The Pursuit of the Millennium,* revised edition. New York: International Universities Press.

Csikszentmihalyi, M. 1975. *Beyond Boredom and Anxiety: The Experiences of Play in Work and Games.* San Francisco: Jossey Bass.

d'Aquili, G. E. 1986. "Myth, Ritual and the Archetypal Hypothesis." *Zygon* 21 2(June): 141–60.

Davidson, J. 1976. "The Psychology of Meditative and Mystic States of Consciousness." *Perspect. Biol. Med.* (Spring): 235, 345.

Deikman, A. J. 1963. "Experimental Meditation." *Journal of Nervous and Mental Disease* 136:329–43.

———. 1966. "Deautomatization and the Mystical Experience." *Psychiatry* 29:324–38.

DeNicolas, A. T. 1962. *Powers of Imagining, Ignatius of Loyola: A Philosophical Hermaneutic of Imaging Through the Collected Works of Ignatius de Loyola,* translation. Albany: State University of New York Press.

Eliade, M. 1953. *The Yearning for Paradise in Primitive Tradition: Diogenes.* Chicago: University of Chicago Press.

———. 1964. *Shamanism: Archaic Technics of Fantasy.* New York: Pantheon.

———. 1975. *Patanjali and Yoga.* New York: Schocken.

Erikson, E. H. 1981. "The Galilean Sayings and the Sense of 'I.'" *Yale Review* 70:321–62.

Federn, P. 1952. *Ego Psychology and the Psychoses,* ed. Eduardo Weiss. New York: Basic Books.

Fischer, R. 1971. "A Cartography of the Ecstatic and Meditative States." *Science* 174 (November 26):897–903.

———. 1975. "Transformations of Consciousness: A Cartography." *Confinia psychiat.* 18:221–44.

Freud, S. 1914. *On Narcissism,* Standard Edition, Volume 14.

———. 1930. *Civilization and Its Discontents,* Standard Edition, Volume 21.

———. 1961. *The Interpretation of Dreams,* Standard Edition, Volume 5 (1900). London: Hogarth Press.

Fromm, Erik. 1955. *The Sane Society.* New York: Rinehart.

Fromm, Erika. 1977. "Altered States of Consciousness and Hypnosis: A Discussion." *Int. J. Clin. Exp. Hypn.* 25:325–34.

Galin, D. 1978. "Implications for Psychiatry of Left and Right Cerebral Specialization. A Neurophysical Context for Unconscious Processes." *Arch. Gen. Psychiatry* 31(October):572–83.

Gellhorn, E. and W. F. Kelly. 1972. "Mystical States of Consciousness: Neurophysiological and Clinical Aspects." *Journal of Nervous and Mental Disease* 154:6.

Ghiselin, B. 1963. *The Creative Process.* New York: New American Library.

Gill, M. and W. Brenman. 1959. *Hypnosis and Related States: Psychoanalytic Studies in Regression.* New York: International Universities Press.

Goleman, D. 1976. "Meditation and Consciousness: An Asian Approach to Mental Health." *American Journal of Psychotherapy* 30:40–54.

Gopi Krishna. 1974. *Higher Consciousness: The Evolutionary Thrust of Kundalini.* Bombay: D.B. Taraporevala Sons and Co.

Greeley, A. M. 1975. *The Sociology of the Paranormal.* Beverly Hills, CA: Sage.

Green, E. and A. Green. 1977. *Beyond Biofeedback.* New York: Dell.

Greenacre, P. 1958. "The Family Romance of the Artist." *Psychoanalytic Study of the Child* 13:9–35.

Grinberg, L., D. Sor, Tabakcle, and E. Granchedin. 1977. *Introduction to the Works of Bion.* New York: Jason Aronson.

Hartmann, H., E. Kris and R. M. Lowenstein. 1960. "Comments on the Formation of Psychic Structure." *Psychoanalytic Study of the Child* 2:11–38.

Hilgard, E. R. 1986. *Divided Consciousness, Multiple Controls in Human Thought and Action.* New York: Wiley.

James, W. 1958. *The Varieties of Religious Experience* (1902). New York: New American Library.

Janes, J. 1976. *The Origin of Consciousness in the Breakdown of the Bicameral Mind.* Boston: Houghton Mifflin.

John, E. R. 1976. "A Model of Consciousness." In *Consciousness and Self-Regulation: Advances in Research,* Volume 1, ed. Gary E. Schwartz and David Shapiro, 1–50. New York: Plenum Press.

Kapur, R. 1985. Personal Communication.

Kegan, R. 1985. *The Evolving Self: Problem and Process in Human Development.* Cambridge: Harvard University Press.

Kohut, H. 1971. *The Analysis of the Self.* New York: International Universities Press.

———. 1977. *The Restoration of the Self.* New York: International Universities Press.

Kohlberg, L. and C. Powers. 1983. "Moral Development, Religious Thinking and the Question of a Seventh Stage." *Zygon,* 16, 3(September): 203–59.

Kris, E. 1952. *Psychoanalytic Explorations in Art.* New York: International Universities Press.

Kuhn, T. S. 1962. "The Structure of Scientific Revolutions." In *International Encyclopedia of Unified Science,* Volume 2, Number 2. Chicago: University of Chicago Press.

Laski, M. 1961 *Ecstasy: A Study of Some Secular and Religious Experiences.* Bloomington: Indiana University Press.

Little, M. 1981. *Transference Neurosis and Transference Psychosis: Toward Basic Unity,* 110–25. New York: Jason Aronson.

Ludwig, A. 1966. "Altered States of Consciousness." *Arch. Gen. Psychiatry* 15:225–34.

Mahler, M., F. Pine, and A. Bergman. 1975. *The Psychological Birth of the Human Infant.* New York: Basic Books.

Margulies, A. 1984. "Toward Empathy." *American Journal of Psychiatry* 141:1025–33.

McDaniel, J. 1987. "Madness and Ecstasy." Ph.D. dissertation. Chicago: University of Chicago Press.

Merton, Thomas. 1967. *Mystics and Zen Masters.* New York: Farrar, Straus, and Giroux.

Piaget, J. 1932. *The Language and Thought of the Child.* London: Routledge and Kegan Paul.

Plato. 1961. "Phaedrus" 244A, in *Ecstasy,* by M. Laski.

Pruyser, P. 1968. Personal Communication.

———. 1984. *The Play of the Imagination.* New York: International Universities Press.

Racine, R. J., W. M. Burnham, J. G. Gratner, et al. 1973. "Rates of Mood and Seizure Development in Rats Subjected to Electrical Brain Stimulation: Strain and Interstimulus Interval Effects," *Electroencephalogr. Clin. Neurophysiol.* 38:1.

Rapaport, D. 1951. *Organization and Pathology of Thought.* New York: Columbia University Press.

Rose, G. 1972. "Fusion States." *Tactics and Techniques in Psychoanalytic Therapy,* ed. P. Giovacchini, 170–88. New York: Science House.

Ross, N. 1975. "Affect as Cognition: With Observations on the Meanings of Mystic States." *Rev. Psychoanal.* 2:79.

Saradananda. 1978. *Sri Ramakrishna, The Great Master* (1911–16), 2 volumes, trans. Swami Jagadananda. Madras, India: Sri Ramakrishna Math.

Schachtel, E. G. 1958. *Metamorphosis: On the Development of Affect, Perception, Attention, and Memory.* New York: Basic Books.

Searles, H. 1960. *The Nonhuman Environment in Normal Development and in Schizophrenia.* New York: International Universities Press.

Shapiro, D. and R. Walsh, eds. 1985. *The Science of Meditation: Research, Theory and Practice.* New York: Aldine.

Singer, J. L. 1977. "Ongoing Thought: The Normative Baseline of Altered States of Consciousness." In *Alternative States of Consciousness,* ed. N. E. Zinberg. New York: Free Press.

Stahl, F. 1975. *Exploring Mysticism.* Berkeley: University of California Press.

Syz, H. C. 1981. *Of Being and Meaning,* trans. Bjorn Merker. New York: Philosophical Library.

Tart, C., ed. 1969. *Altered States of Consciousness.* New York: Wiley.

———. 1972. "States of Consciousness and States of Specific Sciences." *Science,* 176:1203–10.

———. 1975. *States of Consciousness.* New York: Dutton.

———. 1977. "Putting the Pieces Together: A Conceptual Framework for Understanding Discrete States of Consciousness." In *Alternate States of Consciousness: Multiple Perspectives on the Study of Consciousness,* ed. N. E. Zinberg. New York: Free Press.

Tucker, N. 1984. "Brain Hemisphericity, Mysticism and Personal Wholeness." *Zygon* 19:89–91.

Tustin, F. 1981. *Autistic States in Children.* London: Routledge and Kegan Paul.

Waelder, R. 1960. *Basic Theory of Psychoanalysis.* New York: International Universities Press.

Walsh, R. 1980. "The Consciousness Disciplines and the Behavioral Sciences: Questions of Comparison and Assessment." *American Journal of Psychiatry* 137:663–73.

Winnicott, D. 1953. "Transitional Objects and Transitional Phenomena." *International Journal of Psychoanalysis* 34:2.

———, ed. 1965. "Ego Distortion in Terms of True and False Self." In *The Maturational Processes and the Facilitating Environment: Studies in the Theory of Emotional Development,* 140–152. New York: International Universities Press.

Witkin, H. A., R. B. Dyk, H. F. Patterson, D. R. Goodenough, and S. A. Kemp. 1962. *Psychological Differentiation.* New York: Wiley.

Woollcott, P. 1962. "The Psychiatric Patient's Religion." *Journal of Religion and Health.* 1 (July 4):337–49.

———. 1963. "Erikson's Luther: A Psychiatrist's View." *Journal of the Scientific Study of Religion* 2:243–48.

———. 1966. "Creativity and Religious Experience in St. Augustine." *Journal of the Scientific Study of Religion* 5:273–83.

———. 1969. "Pathological Processes in Religion." In *Clinical Psychiatry and Religion,* ed. E. Mansell Pattison. Boston: Little, Brown.

———. 1981. "Addiction: Clinical and Theoretical Considerations." *Ann. Psychoanal.* 9:189–203.

CHAPTER ELEVEN

THE CONGREGATION AS A HEALING RESOURCE

Herbert Anderson, Ph.D.

Religious communities have always had an obligation to be agencies of healing. The sacred writings of every major religious tradition are replete with references to divine intervention on behalf of the sick and suffering. Religious communities demonstrate this concern of God for people who are ill or troubled through acts of mercy and service, through clear and prophetic preaching on behalf of the helpless, and through the development of human solidarity in community. The practice of psychiatry has a similar mandate to work for healing even though it has not felt obligated as a discipline to explore the healing potential of religious belief and practice. The intent of this essay is to examine the circumstances under which religious community life and the practice of psychiatry might be considered allies for the sake of mental health and healing.

The impetus for exploring the relationship between psychiatric practice and religious community life has come from many quarters. Both perspectives recognize that psychiatry and religion share a common commitment to the emotional and spiritual well-being of humankind. This common cause is enhanced by the growing consensus in both religion and psychiatry that human nature is inescapably communal. A wholistic approach to the treatment of psychological distress that takes seriously religious belief and practice is the logical consequence of a biopsychosocial perspective on human nature. For that reason, I propose that it is not only appropriate but even necessary to regard every social context, including one's religious community, as a potential source of both illness and health.

In this essay, the term *religious community* will be used to refer to an assembly of people whose beliefs about God combine with a common identity, a shared history, regular worship, and common values in order to effect personal and social transformation. Something like a local community or congregation is a vital expression of and support to religious life in both Jewish and Christian traditions. Through services of worship and gatherings for fellowship, individuals are drawn out of their isolation and differences into communities of friendship and support. Through programs of education, knowledge of a religious tradition and its meaning for contemporary life is transmitted in ways that also promote community solidarity and responsible discipleship in the world. Through their networks of care, religious congregations attend to the needy in their midst by providing a hospitable and healing environment.

Although a religious community or congregation has characteristics that are common to other human social systems, it is also shaped by values and practices that are unique to its own beliefs and identity. Images of the religious congregation as a "caring community," "therapeutic community," or "nurturing community" suggest more emphasis on health than such images as "prophetic community," "servant community," or "base Christian community," in which the primary emphasis is on social change for the sake of justice. Although the emphasis varies with the governing values, most religious communities seek to balance the needs of the individual and concern for the larger human community.

In this essay I will argue that both the means and the end of healing have a social dimension. Mental health occurs in community for the sake of community. "By the crowd we have been broken, by the crowd we must be healed." Restoration to emotional well-being invariably happens in some corporate context *so that* the restored individual might participate more effectively in his or her communities of significance. That participation is in turn enhanced by the ways in which a congregation is a potential resource for mental health by being a healing and sustaining community. A religious congregation is therefore a place of sending *and* a place of healing.

Throughout human history religious communities have been organized very differently in order to respond to different needs. For that reason, one must be cautious in making general statements about the relationship between religious congregations and mental health. Despite the limitations imposed by this particularity, some of the following general questions need to be asked in order to determine whether and under what circumstances a religious community might be a resource in the promotion of mental health.

1. Should churches and temples provide mental health resources to meet a variety of special individual needs, *or* should the focus be on creating a wholesome community that is itself the therapeutic resource?

2. If it is a therapeutic resource, what are the unique features of a religious community that are likely to contribute to emotional well-being?
3. If religious communities were to take seriously emotional well-being as a significant agenda for their ministry, how would that affect what congregations do?

It is my conviction that the religious community has the potential to be a natural ally in preventive mental health because it is involved in the ordinary physical, developmental, and spiritual struggles of daily life. Because of its accessibility to people in life-cycle crises from birth to death, a religious congregation has an unprecedented opportunity to exercise positive influence on the growth and health of persons in its orbit. At the same time, however important such emphasis on prevention might be for the enhancement of human wholeness, it is necessary to remember that a religious community is not another health provider. The primary role for religion in relation to health is to promote it rather than provide it. A religious community needs to serve the values of health without losing its soul or its uniqueness or without becoming another health center.

Religious Communities and the Community Mental Health Movement

Although there is a much longer history to the relationship between religious communities and mental health, we begin this exploration with the emergence of the community mental health movement in the United States in the middle of the twentieth century. It was a time of great expectation for religious congregations as well as for psychiatry. Religious congregations, it was said, were one of the local social systems that had unprecedented opportunities to contribute to the preventive dimensions of mental health. It was also expected that religious congregations would be one context of care for the mentally ill that would enable them to remain connected to their primary environments.

In order to equip congregations to function as effective therapeutic resources, there was a widespread effort during those years to acquaint parish clergy and other religious professionals with the range of mental health issues. Clergy were often referred to as the first line of defense in mental health. Moreover, it was assumed that clergy would have a significant role in mental health centers as one link to the available and appropriate resources of the community that had been mobilized for prevention, diagnosis, treatment, and rehabilitation of the mentally ill. Given this emphasis, it is not surprising that a substantial portion of the literature on religion and mental health written at this time (circa 1955–1970) focused on the interaction between clergy and "other" mental health professionals (Maves 1952; Hofmann 1960; McCann 1962; Clinebell 1965, 1970; Pattison 1969).

The involvement of religious congregations in the community mental health movement was thought to be necessary and desirable in both prevention and treatment. Without the support of churches and synagogues, it was said, the mental health "revolution" would be slower and less effective. Religion also added to the movement an emphasis on values and meaning that included an awareness of transcendence in human life. Moreover, the capacity of the church to involve itself in every aspect of community life provided a desirable model for the development of certain aspects of community mental health centers. Whether in fact it can be said that religious communities were such a model, it was expected that a comprehensive mental health center would take initiative in response to human need. Such initiative, long held as the sacred trust of religious leaders of congregations, was regarded as an expression of the mission of community mental health centers to bring the mentally ill within the therapeutic orbit of the centers through consultative, educational, and preventive efforts.

The community mental health movement had something to contribute to religious communities as well. Churches and temples needed the mental health "revolution" in order to remain true to their mission and relevant to the needs of individuals in a psychologically oriented age. Howard Clinebell predicted that if religious groups and leaders did not respond to the opportunities this new movement afforded, then mental health centers would become the *de facto* churches by meeting the growth needs of individuals in a psychologically oriented age. Although there were some efforts to promote the maintenance of human community for the sake of individual well-being, most notably *The Church and Mental Health* (1952) edited by Paul Maves, it was assumed from the beginning of the community mental health movement that a religious congregation would seize the moment by allowing mental health to become the leavening concern that permeated all of its life and ministry with individuals.

The mental health of individuals was clearly the focus of *Mental Health through Christian Community*, written by Howard Clinebell in 1965. The book was intended to be a practical guidebook for maximizing the mental health ministry of a congregation. Every activity of a religious congregation, he suggested, should seek to enable people to love themselves, others, and God more fully in order to live more creatively. For Clinebell, the concern for mental health is at the very center of the mission and purpose of religious communities. It deals with that which in Christian ethics is regarded as the most precious part of God's creation—personality. Everything in the life of a religious congregation, from worship to education, preaching, and pastoral counseling, should be measured according to its capacity to exercise positive influence on the growth and health of persons. For Clinebell, the restoration of persons to wholeness and the promotion of life in all its fullness were the ultimate aims for all programs of a religious congregation.

There are four presuppositions (Clinebell calls them facts) that undergird this close connection between religious communities and mental health: (1) Spiritual health and mental health are inseparably related because no understanding of mental health is complete if it ignores spiritual health. (2) Mental health deals with that which is of central importance to churches and temples, namely, the wholeness and fulfillment of people. (3) The concern of religious communities for the mental health of all people is a particular manifestation of a larger commitment to human well-being in the face of widespread suffering. (4) Religious communities have a unique contribution to make to the mental health movement by bringing an emphasis on values and meaning and on relatedness to the Spirit that permeates all of existence (Clinebell 1965). These presuppositions appear again in the introduction to a volume Clinebell edited in 1970 entitled *Community Mental Health: The Role of Church and Temple*. This second volume is explicitly linked to the "community mental health movement," which Clinebell regarded as the most exciting new concept in psychiatry since Freud.

The growth of an individual within a community is the theme that dominated most of the early literature on the relationship between religion and mental health. It was consistent with the aim of the community mental movement, which sought to provide for the total mental health needs of individuals within a particular geographic area. Although some attention was given to modifying the structures of a society that precipitated emotional crises, the growth and health of individuals was generally thought to be primary. Even when there was an emphasis on the health of the community, it was for the sake of individual well-being. The balance between the individual and the community that is the ideal for the life of religious congregations and for mental health was tilted in favor of the individual.

This overemphasis on personal emotional health as the aim of the ministry of a congregation is today regarded by many religiously oriented people as potentially self-serving and certainly secondary to a concern for social justice. They believe that the mental health of individuals is achieved more effectively by changing the social structures that diminish well-being and dissipate the human spirit. From that perspective, it is not enough to suggest that concern for the mental health of individuals is the only or even primary focus of the mission and purpose of a religious congregation. It is necessary to build human communities marked by justice and love. Such religious communities are in turn committed to seek the health of individuals in order that they might serve more effectively or exercise their religious vocation more courageously or simply be engaged in the world for the sake of peace and justice.

In 1963, R. A. Lambourne, M.D., an English physician and clergy-man, developed in *Community, Church and Healing* a perspective parallel to and yet very different from the religious dimensions of the community mental health movement in the United States. Lambourne suggested that through the ordinary deeds of changing a wet bed, cooking a meal, dispensing medicine, or making intercessory prayer, the local religious community becomes a therapeutic community and an occasion of grace. His emphasis on the community as a healing force emerged out of the "growing recognition in medicine that the social pathology of disease makes every aspect of community life relevant to the prevention and treatment of disease in the individual" (1963, 12). Sickness is never simply a private, individual matter. It is public or communal in its origins and in its consequences. Not only is the one who works for healing a representative of the community; so also is the sick one. Everyone shares in each other's flesh and sin and sickness. Because personality is corporate, healing acts need to be public acts within the community that are public signs of the rule of God in human life.

What is particularly significant about Lambourne's approach is his emphasis on the communal nature of human nature. In this, it differs considerably from the individualism of Clinebell. It has consequences for the healing arts as well as our understanding of sickness. From Lambourne's perspective, a community is judged by how it responds to the sick ones in its midst and by the ways in which people identify themselves with the predicaments of others. "We come then to the paradoxical fact that the local church, in so far as it is a fellowship of love, becomes so by being what it is in acts of love to the sick and troubled amongst them. . . . (F)ullness of life is a life of self-committal to others from the depth of one's being to the depth of another's being, and . . . this involves suffering love" (1963, 118–19). Whole people are those who are joined to the suffering of others. There can be no full health without sharing the burdens of sickness in a community of care.

The consequences of this perspective for religious communities are worth noting. Human wholeness can never be separated from community. From the Christian perspective, to belong to community means loving one another and having all things, including sickness, in common. Lambourne differs from Clinebell and others who were influenced by the community mental health movement not only in his strong sacramental and mystical emphasis on community life; he shifts the focus away from health as the end of religious life to healing as an act of identification with those who suffer. The mark of a religious community that embodies the love of God is its capacity to embrace the suffering of its own members and the sufferings of its neighborhood. The religious congregation is a fellowship of love and a community of sufferers who visit the sick, offer a cup of cold water to the thirsty, and help one another carry their heavy loads. Its mission is to be a sign of God's love by welcoming into its midst the sick and the troubled. Such a community, I submit, would be a rich resource for psychiatry.

What Lambourne pictures in mystical language as the sacramental Body of Christ bound to one another as a community of sufferers, E. Mansel Pattison, M.D., presents in a systemic mode in *Pastor and Parish: A Systems Approach* (1977). Both Lambourne and Pattison emphasize the health of the community. Pattison is quite specific on this point. The congregation can and should be the kind of social system that produces a whole, holy person. "It is precisely the wholesome system that will be therapeutic and corrective to its membership. . . . Therapy may not be the *goal* of the system, but it can be a result. While not denying this, I hold that the primary function of the minister is pastoral care of the social system of the church to the end that the church system can provide the necessary basis for *being*" (1977, 12). The function of the religious leader is to "direct the whole body" to the end that the parts mesh with one another and exercise mutual care.

The shift in focus from the earlier literature on the congregation and mental health is slight but significant. The emphasis moves away from the individual toward the health of the community in order that it might be a healing resource. "The church as living system is effective when it is proclaiming, symbolizing, moralizing, and fostering morality, teaching and facilitating growth, sustaining itself and its members, providing help and healing in time of stress and crisis" (Pattison 1977, 47). The religious congregation that attends to its health as a system may become, for example, a halfway place to which emotionally fragile individuals might be referred for support and safe social interaction. The mission of the religious congregation is its own well-being in order that it might be a healing place.

The convergence of a systemic perspective on human nature and the biblical view of corporate personality that Lambourne espouses leads to the conclusion that neither mental illness nor emotional healing can be understood or effected apart from community. The religious congregation is one communal context in which to explore the biopsychosocial unity of the person. At minimum this would mean for clinical practice that no case history is complete that does not record some understanding of an individual's thoughts and feelings about his or her place and purpose in the world. It could also lead to a greater emphasis on the religious community as a locus for change and healing.

Inevitably, there is an individual focus to therapeutic practice in the interest of human wholeness. Particular persons experience emotional pain that is particular to their own life history. The movement toward mental health depends on providing resources that will enhance each individual's growth. The religious community may be one such mental health provider, but that is not its unique function. It is a community of care and a healing fellowship. Its purpose is to be a place of hospitality and love and justice in which the stranger is welcomed, the lonely are embraced, and the alienated find refuge. To have this healing effect, religious community life must not be seen as essentially in the service of mental and/or spiritual health. Mental health is most likely to be realized as a by-product of relating in depth to God, self, and others.

The Character of a Religious Community

The religious community is a human system and as such has characteristics common to all human systems. The identity of a human system is determined by invisible boundaries that mark out its membership but do not close off interaction within the system or between the particular community and its environment. The interdependence of parts and the specialization of functions within a system are enhanced when the boundaries are clear but permeable. A community that is open to people and ideas from outside its membership is most likely to be a place of continued growth. For a human system to function effectively, it also needs to be clear about what is expected of its membership. Generally, those expectations are expressed in rules and myths that govern the behavior of members.

The clarity with which communication occurs and decisions are made within a human system depends on the absence of covert rules or rigid roles or hidden alliances or ambiguous messages. A human system that has movable loyalties that are also visibly dependable and shared responsibilities that are openly negotiated will foster the development of trustworthy and secure relationships in which autonomy and self-esteem flourish. Values like fairness and justice and honesty also enhance trust within a human system and increase the possibility that the uniqueness of individuals or parts of the whole will be respected.

Within every human system, there needs to be a balance between the whole and its parts. Communities function best when a delicate reciprocity is sustained between being together and being separate, between individuation and participation. When a human system does not attend to the individual needs and concerns of its members, the whole community suffers. If, however, there is insufficient commitment to the system as a whole and too much resulting individualism, the human system ceases to be the kind of context in which parts prosper and individuals grow.

All these features of a human system are interrelated. The wholesomeness and the effectiveness of any human community are enhanced by their presence. Therefore these features are essential for a religious community as well. What is important for us to explore in this essay is whether there are characteristics unique to religious community life that would make it a particularly valuable resource for psychiatry in the interest of enhancing emotional well-being. Although it is foolhardy to assume easy agreement on the nature of the religious community as a human system, there are at least four religious values that seem unique to religious community life: unconditional love, self-giving service, forgiveness, and hope. I suggest these values as illustrative but not exhaustive of the qualities that might uniquely characterize religious community life and that would, if embodied, make it a positive resource for the promotion of mental health.

Unconditional Love

A religious community is an open and inclusive system in which people are welcomed without conditions and cared for without strings attached. It is a place that is obligated by its own ideals to show hospitality to strangers and where the alienated, lonely, and disenfranchised find a place to belong. In order to be an inclusive community, it honors difference and lives through the conflicts that emerge because of that diversity. How people relate to one another matters, not only because it enhances well-being, but also because it is intended to express the gracious and unconditional love of God.

For those who wonder whether they are lovable, the religious community may be a place of affirmation and acceptance. For those who have struggled to overcome a personal history of conditioned acceptance, it is a free space in which to discover one's unique lovableness. One of the great paradoxes of life is that a community is most likely to become a place of safety when it no longer attempts to heal or convert or fix or change. Persons are accepted as they are. Within such an accepting community, it is more likely that a person could discard the defenses, masks, and disguises that impede spiritual and psychological health (Williams 1968; Tillich 1952).

Self-Giving Service

Every human system has determined the values and procedures it regards as necessary to maintain its existence. The natural and necessary disposition of a system to seek to maintain itself (sometimes even at the expense of its membership) is in contrast with the self-giving emphasis of religious community life. A religious community needs to maintain its life in order to give that life away. This necessarily conservative nature of a human system is always in danger of becoming self-serving only for the sake of survival.

A religious community is always extending itself to larger and larger human communities. For that reason, a religious community is always on the edge of survival. In fact, survival is not the religious norm: service and sacrifice are. Therefore, from a religious point of view, health even of the community as a whole can never be an end in itself. It is always for the sake of service. A religious community becomes one context in which people who are preoccupied with themselves or obsessed by their own needs are invited to look beyond their own horizons to larger and larger communities of human need (Minear 1959).

Forgiveness

A religious community is a place to practice living with imperfection because it is a forgiving community. It is a place where acceptance is unconditional and where a person is not condemned for failures. Forgiveness may well be *the* religious ideal that most clearly distinguishes a religious community from other human systems. A community that centers its life around forgiveness is likely to discourage secret-keeping and personal deception and to encourage candid conversation and vulnerability, all of which in turn promote the development of congruence and personal integrity (Patton 1985).

Hope

Hope is central to religious life in and out of community. It is a characteristic of a religious congregation insofar as that community stands against despair and debilitating powerlessness and stands for the possibility of something new happening that will contradict what binds us to the past. From a religious perspective, hope is realistic. It is neither naive nor innocently optimistic. It seeks to include hopelessness and despair as a part of hope.

With hope there is also courage to be future oriented. A religious community embodies that hope by being open to the future and realistic about living with what is possible in the present. Moreover, there can be no immediate solution to present dilemmas that does not take into account the need to live into a future that is simultaneously open and contingent. Because hope is at the center of religious existence, it is a characteristic of religious community (Moltmann 1976).

Meeting the Goals

Several comments are in order on this excursus into characteristics of the religious community. The first is obvious. Most religious congregations fail to embody fully and consistently the values they espouse. Nonetheless they regularly challenge themselves to achieve the highest possible standards of human interaction. While the gap between the real and the ideal is serious, it is the presence of the ideal that ensures communal self-criticism in the interest of wholeness. Because it frequently fails to achieve its ideals, a religious community needs to be a forgiving community as well as a community of the forgiven.

Second, the increase in individualism and consequent privatization in American society makes it more and more imperative that we find ways to attend to the formation and maintenance of significant human communities. It is self-evident that every human being is unique. The process of individuation is necessary to actualize as fully as possible each individual's autonomy and destiny. And yet we are inescapably social creatures who need one another, not only to survive, not only for companionship, but for meaning in life. Social relations are not merely secondary phenomena of human existence but rather are primary components of the biopsychosocial organism.

In order for a religious congregation to maximize its potential as a healing and sustaining human community, some shift is necessary in the practice of ministry. Leaders need to give greater attention to the community as a whole—and to develop a style of leadership marked by differentiation from the community (Friedman 1985). Insights from the human sciences need to be applied to communal as well as individual wholeness. Leaders should see the nurture of congregations as every bit as important as the healing or guiding of individuals. To undergird these efforts, it will be necessary to establish a normative vision of the religious community, an ideal against which to measure our outcomes, and a set of expectations by which those outside of religious communities (including psychiatrists) might determine the therapeutic usefulness of such a human system.

The Healing Ministry of Religious Communities

A religious community cannot ignore its obligation to be an agency of healing. It is *an* inevitable agenda for every church and synagogue, even if it is not *the* agenda. The concern of God for human well-being is made concrete within religious congregations through their compassionate efforts on behalf of the physically impaired and the emotionally distressed. That commitment to healing and health is not, however, an end in itself.

The promotion and maintenance of health is always propaedeutic to vocation. The religious community promotes health in order to increase service. Making community participation a goal of healing has the effect of guarding against the privatization of health.

This ministry of healing belongs to the whole. If one follows a systemic perspective, as this essay does, then every context, including one's religious community, is a potential source for both illness and health. Because of the biopsychosocial nature of human nature, all psychological healing must have some connection with community life. If we have been broken in social contexts, it follows that healing needs to be communal as well. And the religious community is itself a potential healing source.

If healing is from the whole as well as from within the individual, then the health of the community *is* significant. When it fulfills its best ideals, a religious community provides an experience of unconditional acceptance that renews basic trust; it fosters attitudes of sacrifice and service that encourage people to transcend preoccupation with themselves; it provides a world view by which individuals might interpret their experience and a set of ethical guidelines beyond rules that help people decide how to act. According to its best ideals, a religious congregation is a compassionate community that takes into its life human pain and suffering *and* takes initiative to eliminate those structures and situations in life that diminish self-esteem and drain the human spirit.

This shift in focus from individual health as the primary agenda of a religious community to the congregation as a healing resource has consequences for congregational activities on behalf of mental health. The remainder of this essay will explore those ways by which religious communities might be engaged for the sake of emotional well-being. Because the congregation is a holding environment, a believing community, and a supportive context, *prevention* is likely to remain one dimension of its ministry through and to its people. To be the kind of environment that fosters human growth and sustains people in ordinary and extraordinary crises, a religious community will need to attend to its communal character.

Some religious communities may have the resources to provide direct mental health services. Others may be located in environments that mandate providing therapeutic care to the poor or the dispossessed. However, a congregation that provides physical space for a health-care clinic or simply organizes direct therapeutic service is more likely to attend to individual mental health needs than to community well-being. A religious community that serves the values of health through therapeutic *intervention* should take care to retain its uniquely religious perspective.

The third type of congregational activity on behalf of mental health is more like *maintenance* than either prevention or intervention. The early literature on religion and community mental health identified the religious community as a context that could assist in the process of reentry for the institutionalized mentally ill. Ex-patients do need an atmosphere of receptivity and acceptance to help them renew old friendships, recover old social patterns, and return to places of work and play. Because of the effects of deinstitutionalization, the task facing our society today is to find sociocultural milieus to assist in maintaining the chronically mentally ill. The religious community knows itself to be a fellowship of love most clearly through its ministry with the sick and troubled. Because suffering and pain are not regarded as alien to the religious community, it may be uniquely suited to provide one context of care for the chronically mentally ill.

Prevention

A religious community is, by its nature, a resource for preventive mental health. Because of its concern for just societies and humane institutions, it is committed to the elimination of conditions that produce emotional illness and to the promotion of conditions that foster mental health. Because of its wholistic approach to human life, a religious congregation is attentive to the physical and psychosocial needs of people as well as their spiritual longings.

Through its teaching and preaching, a religious congregation seeks to develop beliefs and attitudes that provide a positive framework for interpreting experience and determining behavior. Through its rituals, a religious community continues to point to the transcendent dimensions of everyday existence. It promotes an attitude toward being human that celebrates life and engenders self-esteem. It engages people in lively discourse on critical personal, social, and political issues of the day in the context of a shared ideology. At a time when many traditional values are in flux, it is reassuring to have a community of shared beliefs to which one might repair for critical reflection and support.

A religious community is also a natural resource in the interest of preventive mental health because it is able to respond to ordinary and extraordinary crises in individual and family life. There is an intimacy about life in a religious community that makes it possible for people to be known and cared for when they are vulnerable. Religious rituals support people through significant transitions from birth to death. A religious congregation welcomes the young into a hospitable, nurturing environment. Those who are sick, dying, or grieving are sustained by compassion and concrete actions. In the early stages of a crisis, a modest amount of emotional support and guidance may be enough to help an individual or a family through a difficult situation (Friedman 1985; Anderson 1984).

Although it is no longer the case that the majority of individuals in emotional or mental distress turn first to a clergyperson for assistance, religious professionals and religious communities still have the kind of access to people that makes preventive intervention possible. Even without making mental health a central part of its mission, a religious community may avert a serious emotional crisis by its ordinary ways of caring for persons.

A religious community is also a natural mental-health resource because it is a bridge between the individual and society. Sometimes it is primarily intent on creating a safe haven that shelters people from the pain inflicted in and by society. Such a religious community is likely to place individual mental health at the center of its mission. From that perspective, religious life is considered a personal and private matter more than a public one. Others may regard working for peace and justice in the public world as the core of religious life and essential for human wholeness.

Religious communities are compelled to work in the public arena to withstand those social, political, and economic forces that threaten human dignity. From that perspective, individual emotional needs are set aside for the sake of a bigger cause and a greater need in the larger society. Religious communities have throughout history struggled to find a balance between the personal good and the social good. Individuals are likely to select a religious community that corresponds with their preference in this private/public dialectic. However a religious community achieves a balance between personal good and social good, the tension will remain. A healing ministry is inevitably a social ministry.

Although in one sense prevention is like breathing for a religious community, there are specific programs that enhance even further its preventive ministry. The following illustrations suggest the variety of ways that congregations have organized their ministry to promote mental health.

- The Community of Christ the Servant established a "health cabinet" in order to mobilize the unrealized potential of the congregation for becoming a healing community. The cabinet's task was to be a catalyst in the community so that the membership might see more clearly how helpful they could be to one another in preventing illness. The cabinet was made up of health professionals and others from the congregation committed to health and healing. While the cabinet was not involved in the diagnosis and treatment of individuals, its purpose was to promote healthy behavior and to ensure strong support for individuals who were not well. The intent was to make the healing ministry inclusive of every aspect of the congregational life and mission (Lundin 1977).

- Sinai Temple developed a variety of special groups that attend to the particular needs of the elderly and the disabled. This achievement illustrates very well the opportunities of a religious community to provide supportive contexts for a wide range of human needs. This congregation emphasized a ministry to the elderly because it was located in a popular retirement area. Its programs included "friendly visitors" who regularly saw home-bound people and could thus often detect changes in physical and mental condition that even the elderly person was not aware of; a "senior friendship center" that provided activities three days a week; a "widowed persons service" that provided a support group for newly widowed men and women; and an advocacy group for the disabled that was able to change the town building code regarding public access.
- The Stephen Series is one of many training programs that have been developed in the last couple of decades to enlarge the pool of persons within religious communities who can care responsibly for those who are sick and troubled. Sometimes these training programs are aimed at special populations—for example parents of teenagers, children of divorcing parents, the hospitalized, or adult children of alcoholics. People are trained to staff a telephone crisis service or a rape hotline or to be a listening friend for someone recently released from psychiatric hospitalization. Such training programs have extremely wide potential for extending care to people facing a wide range of problems and thus helping to prevent more serious illness (Haugk 1984; Stone 1983).
- Education is a significant activity in most religious communities. Through education, beliefs are shared and evaluated, and ethical norms are articulated and passed on to subsequent generations. Although some religious communities limit their educational efforts to theological or biblical matters, many others offer courses on problems in living designed to enhance physical and emotional well-being. Topics such as AIDS, teenage suicide, child abuse, dying and grieving, and changing roles for women and men in society are frequently a part of religious-education programs. Groups for support as well as education are organized for parents with young children, single parents, widows and widowers, or adult children of alcoholics. Congregations also sponsor more extensive workshops on such topics as family life, communication in marriage, and self-esteem and the human person, utilizing the resources of the health sciences as well as the religious tradition. Although there is no guarantee that such educational efforts will forestall serious illness, the religious community is still a significant context for helping people learn more effective ways of handling problems in daily living.

Intervention

The emphasis on prevention as one form of a congregational ministry is a logical extension of the religious commitment to physical and emotional well-being. It is a continuation of the community's care of its membership in the everyday crises of life. By embodying its highest ideals, a religious community becomes a holding environment in which its values and relationships help people endure problems of living and grow because of them.

The role of religious communities in providing direct therapeutic intervention is less self-evident. The primary purpose of the church and the temple regarding health is to promote care. From a religious perspective, care, not health, is a basic human right. Care is essential to the dignity of every human being as a creation of God. The religious congregation advocates the care of all sick or troubled persons as a concrete expression of God's care. If religious communities are engaged in providing care consistent with this self-understanding, they are most likely to respond to the needs of the poor, powerless, or alienated.

Although the interventive role of religious communities is less clear than their preventive role, there are three ways by which they have become involved in direct therapeutic intervention: (1) through the development of specialized ministries of chaplaincy and pastoral psychotherapy; (2) by founding wholistic health-care clinics or supporting a 'parish nurse program in the local religious community; and (3) in the growing recognition that the religious congregation is in a strategic position to intervene where there is physical or sexual abuse or substance abuse.

SPECIALIZED MINISTRIES

The development of the clinical ministries of chaplaincy and pastoral psychotherapy grew out of efforts around the turn of the century to apply psychological principles to the practice of religion. This early interest in linking the psychology of religion with the traditional religious practice of *seelsorge* moved in several directions. Nonetheless the work of people like Elwood Worcester, Richard Cabot, Russell Dicks, Flanders Dunbar, Anton Boison, John Sutherland Bonnell, and Seward Hiltner had at least one concern in common: increasing competence among clergy in pastoral care in order to enhance human growth toward maturity (Holifield 1983; Stokes 1985). The rise of the therapeutic professions had not diminished the pastoral responsibilities of religious communities, but it did elevate the standards of care by which they would be judged.

The Association for Clinical Pastoral Education and the American Association of Pastoral Counselors are the two organizations that have been responsible for developing and certifying competence in clinical ministry.

Both the chaplain and the pastoral counselor have a liminal role between religion and health. A chaplain is understood to function in the place of a local congregation to provide pastoral care for those whose life crisis has necessitated institutionalization. The chaplain helps the patient transcend the moment of pain or illness by being a symbolic link to the patient's religious community and history. The specialized ministry of pastoral counseling in a community often began in the unused back office of a local congregation. Many pastoral counselors are still located in a religious facility and depend on referrals from pastors and rabbis for some of their client load. There is some possibility that the development of pastoral psychotherapy, with its emphasis on the individual therapeutic relationship, may have unwittingly contributed to shifting the focus away from the religious congregation as a healing resource.

The secularization of society and the professionalization of specialized clinical ministries over the last fifty years has meant that chaplains and pastoral counselors are thought of less and less as an extension of local religious communities and more and more as part of the health-delivery system. Nonetheless, the clinical minister of counseling or care is considered a representative leader of a religious community. What pastoral counselors and chaplains do is inevitably an interventive action on behalf of communities of religious practice. More attention should probably be paid to maintaining an organic connection between specialized ministries and religious communities so that the clinical ministries retain their essential communal character and the transcending power of their source.

CLINICS

The development of a health-care clinic in a religious facility is one way for a congregation to engage directly in a healing ministry. Proponents of such clinics believe that the location makes a difference in the healing process because the context symbolizes the presence of God as the ultimate source of healing and because recipients have more confidence that their treatment will be compassionate and personal. The idea of wholistic health-care clinics in religious facilities was developed by Granger Westberg in the early 1970s. The intent was to acquire, construct, equip, and operate a church-based health-care facility whose team of pastors, physicians, psychologists, and others would together focus on all aspects of an individual's health needs (Westberg 1979; Tubesing 1979).

The Trinity Health Care Clinic of Minneapolis is an example of such a clinic. Its declared purpose is to provide a more personalized style of caring for the sake of health. Its staff includes two physicians, two psychologists, a nurse, a lab assistant, an administrative assistant, and a part-time bookkeeper. The stated purpose of this ministry of healing is the discovery, restoration, and maintenance of wholeness in an individual that can take place under the authorship of God and within the context of a fellowship. On the basis of information provided in an extensive health inventory of the physical, emotional, and spiritual aspects of the patient's life, the treatment team and the patient together arrive at a plan for attaining and maintaining health. This emphasis on the patient as a full partner of the team is supported by the belief that responsibility for one's own health is a sign of the dignity that God has given all persons (Droege 1982).

A health-care clinic in a religious facility is a sophisticated and ambitious program of intervention on behalf of individual health. There are not many religious congregations, however, that have the size, money, talent, and vision to provide the facilities and support the staff necessary for such an operation. Because of their cost, whole-person health-care clinics have tended to be established in communities that already have adequate medical resources. Such clinics are not usually established to serve people who long for healing or who are barely surviving the rigors of living or who are alienated from centers for healing. If, however, a health-care clinic in a religious facility were dedicated to providing preventive education, medical care, and therapeutic interventions more easily for those who are unwilling or unable to utilize medical and mental health centers, it would perform a ministry consistent with the ideal of self-giving service that is one of the marks of a religious community. Unfortunately, the cost of such a venture is generally prohibitive.

The recent development of the parish nurse program offers a less costly alternative and one that may indeed serve the purpose of religious communities to work toward ensuring health care for all humankind. Health care has become so technical and impersonal that the poor and uneducated are afraid to seek help even when it is free. The parish nurse program offers wholistic health care by responding to the physical, spiritual, economic, and emotional needs of the person. One such program in the economically deprived area of Cabrini-Green, a public housing project in Chicago, is a collaboration of 3C's Medical Center and six parishes, each of which has at least one nurse.

The intent of the parish nurse program is to reach out to people through health education and counseling, advocacy and systems referrals, physical assessment, and crisis intervention in order to connect people with the needed health resources. The advantage of this program is that it is not a costly operation requiring extensive investment in facilities. And it is a particularly useful ministry of advocacy for those who are overwhelmed by problems of living and who do not know where to go for help or whether to trust the help that is available. It is an appropriate intervention of a religious community in support of its conviction that care is a basic human right.

PASTORAL INITIATIVE

Initiative has long been regarded as a sacred privilege for pastoral ministry. Pastors and other religious professionals have historically been allowed and sometimes encouraged to intervene on behalf of the spiritual well-being of congregation members. There are today three specific human situations in which pastoral initiative in intervention would be useful and even necessary in protecting the powerless or minimizing suffering.

Because of the access to people in families, leaders of religious communities are likely to have early knowledge of sexual, physical, or emotional abuse of children or violence toward spouses. The obligation to report knowledge about child abuse has raised serious questions about clergy confidentiality. It has, on the other hand, prompted serious reconsideration about methods of intervention that will nonetheless honor the sacred trust of pastoral initiative. Religious communities are also now being used as one resource in developing a strategy of intervention where there is alcoholism in the family. Interventions of this kind differ from the more casual pastoral initiatives because they require careful planning and competent, responsible execution. Such interventions are able, however, to build upon community members' care for one another and trust in pastoral initiative that no other helping professional enjoys (Pellauer, Chester et al. 1987).

Maintenance

Any community of God's people is a broken community living in a broken world. Injury, fear, anxiety, stress, abuse, pollution, the possibility of nuclear annihilation, racism and sexism, and the never-ending stream of emotional casualties all point to this brokenness. Because of the tenacity of evil in the world and the pervasiveness of ill-health, healing in this life is never complete. And yet, paradoxically, wholeness is possible in the midst of pain, sickness, and suffering. We experience that peace in the midst of a community of sufferers as a gift that comes from God through the compassion and care of others.

Because health is never fully possible, the ministry of healing is an ongoing necessity for religious congregations. That ministry remains valid and meaningful even when no significant contribution is made to the cure of individual sickness or situational distress. We care for the chronically ill, offer companionship to the dying, and console those who grieve losses and injustices in life, even when we cannot change what is wrong. Healing is what we do, not what we expect. A religious community receives human pain and enters into human brokenness out of compassion for those who suffer and as a sign that God is present even when health is absent. The emphasis on the congregation as a healing community rather than a health center is also a reminder that finally health is a gift from God.

There is today a growing population of the chronically mentally ill who are neither institutionalized nor adequately cared for by the limited resources of community-based programs of treatment. The National Institute of Mental Health estimates that 2.4 million Americans should be classified mentally ill and that approximately 1.5 million of them now live in the community. In a study paper prepared for distribution by the Evangelical Lutheran Church in America entitled *Chronic Mental Illness: A Congregational Challenge,* it is estimated that up to 80 percent of chronically mentally ill people depend for their survival on the daily care of family members or friends or are struggling alone to exist day to day. Some of these people need to be institutionalized. Others are quite able to function independently within a supportive setting. Still others need ongoing, dependable, and structured supervision.

The chronically mentally ill have a diminished capacity for coping with ordinary problems of living and yet are often likely to reject the very resources they need to survive. In order to salvage a small amount of self-esteem, they disregard in anger the treatment they need. They ignore treatment in order to avoid the label of mental illness. This population of mentally ill may never have been institutionalized, but adequate maintenance programs for them have not emerged. There is an enormous need for local supportive contexts to help to maintain the chronically mentally ill.

As the Lutheran study paper clearly points out, this population presents a serious challenge to religious congregations and a unique opportunity for cooperation between religion and psychiatry on behalf of the marginalized mentally ill. Because of its capacity to "hold" in its midst people who are sick and suffering, the religious community is an appropriate context to assist psychiatry in the maintenance of the chronically mentally ill, particularly those without family or friends. In consultation and cooperation with mental-health professionals, a religious community could become a surrogate family or provisional support system that would keep in touch with chronically mentally ill persons between crises.

Both consumers and providers of mental-health services for the chronically mentally ill would benefit from the active involvement of religious communities on both the national and local level. Religious communities could lend their support to citizens' groups such as the Alliance for Mental Illness in advocating on behalf of the needs of the chronically mentally ill. Those who care for the chronically mentally ill also need support. The emotional strain that mental illness creates for families and friends is often overlooked in efforts to offer care to the one who is ill. Those who have refused treatment in order to avoid the label of mental illness might be more willing to participate in a maintenance program located in a religious facility.

It is true, as several essays in the volume have pointed out, that religious communities have not always been exemplary in their response to mental illness. The mentally ill have been regarded as possessing evil spirits, or being witches, or at least heretics. Sometimes the illness itself is in reality a response to negative or destructive religious beliefs and practices. And some religious congregations become uneasy when people who are mentally ill are too visible, out of justifiable fear that their unpredictability will become disruptive. If, however, a religious community embodies its highest ideals, it will be a place that holds people in pain; that loves the chronically cranky without needing to be loved in return; and that does not overlook the need to care for those who are mentally ill even though cure is not possible.

Conclusion

We began this essay by asking whether and under what circumstances a religious community might be regarded as a resource for psychiatry. It is a difficult question to answer, partly because of the diversity of religious communities and partly because of the complexity of issues related to health and healing. Religious communities and the discipline of psychiatry share a commitment to human well-being insofar as that is possible. Both are compelled by compassion to care for those who suffer emotional pain and disease. And both are intent on helping people live more effectively in their communities. In order to accomplish that task, both religion and psychiatry mediate between the individual and society.

The possibility of concrete cooperation between psychiatry and religious communities hinges on several factors. It depends on a shift in the focus of ministry away from the individual toward the community as a whole. The primary purpose of ministry from this perspective would be to nurture the congregation to become a more wholesome community of justice and unconditional love. The religious community has the potential to be a unique place in which to bring isolated and alienated people back into a circle of belonging in which acceptance, recognition, mutual purpose, love for one another, genuine forgiveness, and the worship of God work together to mitigate isolation and foster wholeness (Marty and Vaux, 1982). It is difficult to argue on behalf of the religious community as a healing resource until there is a commitment to maximize its potential as a community of care. Such a change in emphasis is most likely to occur if there is a parallel rediscovery of the communal identity of human nature, which is at the center of the Judeo-Christian tradition. In a similar way, the recognition by psychiatry that the religious congregation is a legitimate healing resource is most likely to happen as psychiatry adopts a more systemic perspective on the genesis and resolution of mental illness.

References

Anderson, Herbert. 1984. *The Family and Pastoral Care*. Philadelphia: Fortress Press.

Clinebell, Howard J. 1965. *Mental Health Through Christian Community*, Nashville, TN: Abingdon Press.

————, ed. 1970. *Community Mental Health: The Role of Church and Temple*. Nashville, TN: Abingdon Press.

Droege, Thomas A. 1982. *Ministry to the Whole Person: Eight Models of Ministry in Lutheran Congregations*. Valparaiso, IN: Valparaiso University.

Friedman, Edwin H. 1985. *Generation to Generation: Family Process in Church and Synagogue*. New York: Guilford Press.

Haugk, Kenneth. 1984. *Christian Caregiving: A Way of Life*. Minneapolis: Augsburg Publishing House.

Hofmann, Hans, ed. 1960. *The Ministry and Mental Health*. New York: Association Press.

Holifield, E. Brooks. 1983. *A History of Pastoral Care in America: From Salvation to Self-realization*. Nashville, TN: Abingdon Press.

Lambourne, R. A. 1963. *Community, Church and Healing*. London: Darton, Longman and Todd.

Lapsley, James N. 1972. *Salvation and Health*. Philadelphia: Westminister Press.

Lundin, Jack W. 1977. *A Church for an Open Future*. Philadelphia: Fortress Press.

Marty, Martin E. and Kenneth L. Vaux, eds. 1982. *Health/Medicine and the Faith Traditions*. Philadelphia: Fortress Press.

Maves, Paul, ed. 1952. *The Church and Mental Health*. New York: Scribner's.

McCann, Richard V. 1962. *The Church and Mental Health*. New York: Scribner's.

Minear, Paul S. 1959. *Horizons of Christian Community*. St. Louis: Bethany Press.

Moltmann, Jürgen. 1976. *The Theology of Hope*. New York: Harper and Row.

Pattison, E. Mansell. 1969. *Clinical Psychiatry and Religion*. Boston: Little, Brown.

————. 1977. *Pastor and Parish: A Systems Approach*. Philadelphia: Fortress Press.

Patton, John. 1985. *Is Human Forgiveness Possible? A Pastoral Care Perspective*. Nashville, TN: Abingdon Press.

Pellauer, Mary, Barbara Chester, and Jane Boyajian. 1987. *Sexual Assault and Abuse: A Handbook for Clergy and Religious Professionals*. San Francisco: Harper and Row.

Siirala, Arne. 1964. *The Voice of Illness*. Philadelphia: Fortress Press.

Stokes, Allison. 1985. *Ministry After Freud*. New York: Pilgrim Press.

Stone, Howard. 1983. *The Caring Church: A Guide for Lay Pastoral Care*. San Francisco: Harper and Row.

Tillich, Paul. 1952. *The Courage to Be*. New Haven: Yale University Press.

Tubesing, Donald. 1979. *Wholistic Health*. New York: Human Sciences Press.

Veroff, Joseph, et al. 1981. *Mental Health in America: Patterns of Help-Seeking from 1957–1976*. New York: Basic Books.

Westberg, Granger, ed. 1979. *Theological Roots of Wholistic Health Care.* Hinsdale, IL: Wholistic Health Centers.

Whitlock, Glenn E. 1973. *Preventive Psychology and the Church.* Philadelphia: Westminister Press.

Williams, Daniel Day. 1968. *The Spirit and the Forms of Love.* New York: Harper and Row.

CHAPTER TWELVE

BETWEEN BROKEN BRAINS AND

OPPRESSIVE BELIEFS: TROUBLED MINDS

James B. Ashbrook, Ph.D.

In 1937 a psychiatrist and a Protestant minister took steps to establish a religio-psychiatric clinic in New York City. Fifty years later that interdisciplinary collaboration between psychiatrist Smiley Blanton and minister Norman Vincent Peale reflects a widespread phenomenon in the delivery of mental-health resources to people with troubled minds (Carr, Hinkle, et al. 1981). Their efforts, significant in their own right, also represent a variety of associations and alliances between members of the two professions.

In exploring the implications of a public philosophy for psychiatry, the issues of "the role of religion in human life" and of appropriate models of "the relationship between religion and mental health" have their most concrete focus in the interface between the practice of psychiatry and the practice of pastoral counseling and pastoral psychotherapy. The concern for broken brains seems to fall within the province of psychiatry (Andreasen 1984; Sachs 1986). The concern for oppressive beliefs seems to belong to the province of religion (Bonino 1975; Cone 1970; Gutièrrez 1973; Moltmann 1983; Ruether 1983). Between the two provinces lies the ambiguous and ubiquitous realm of troubled minds.

What does it mean for people to be in pain—physically, psychologically, socioculturally, spiritually? How are people helped to deal with pain that never remains confined to only one dimension of this multidimensional creature we know as *Homo sapiens*? How do specialists in the respective fields of medicine and ministry understand what they are each about distinctively and what they are both about collaboratively? How, in short, do the practices of psychiatry and pastoral counseling influence one another?

An answer to this interdisciplinary relationship includes knowledge of historical developments as well as information about current activity. First,

I sketch an historical overview. Then, I report conversations between psychiatrists and pastoral counselors about their collaboration. Finally, I suggest issues in that public space of shared responsibility in the field of mental health.

Historical Overview

One striking characterization of the twentieth century has been what Philip Rieff called "the triumph of the therapeutic" (Rieff 1966). Not immodestly, Freud linked his discovery of the unconscious with the Copernican and Darwinian revolutions (Freud 1917). Each revolution successively dethroned humanity—first from the center of the universe, then from lordship over the other animals, and finally from mastery in its own household, the mind. Despite spectacular advances in science, human pain found powerful expression in psychic suffering.

Not everyone believed in the primacy of psychic reality. But the alleviation of personal suffering became increasingly important for those who resisted "true belief" in specialized disciplines, particularly reductionistic medicine or imperialistic theology. Some physicians shifted from organic medicine to dynamic psychiatry. In retrospect, we might identify that trend as a demedicalizing of physicians who chose to work with troubled minds more than organic symptoms. Similarly, some ministers shifted from theological orthodoxy to clinical pastoral care (Holifield 1983); we might identify that trend as a detheologizing of clergy (Strunk 1985; Thornton 1970).

Individual ministers sought out individual psychiatrists who exhibited an openness to working relationships. James Ewing, executive director of the American Association of Pastoral Counselors, conducted personal interviews with many of the pioneers in the field of pastoral care and counseling. Invariably, he came upon such a pairing of professionals. To his discerning eye, an unconscious complementarity was evident. "Scratch a psychiatrist," he reports, "and you find a hidden minister. Scratch a minister, and you find a hidden physician." Each completed the other's unconscious longing (Ewing 1987).

Whether that dynamic interpretation is accurate, a description of the interfacing of practitioners through the middle part of this century is informative (Committee on Psychiatry and Religion 1960, 1968). They are part of that phenomenon that has been identified as "the fifth profession" (Henry, Sims et al. 1971). Apart from ministry, the four core professional groups active in the mental-health field have included psychoanalysis, psychiatry, clinical psychology, and social work. An analysis of the public and private lives of those practitioners showed a "similarity of work style and of viewpoint" (Henry, Sims et al. 1973). Psychiatrists and psychoanalysts did not practice physical medicine, psychologists did little empirical research, and social workers did not utilize knowledge of public welfare and community organization (Henry, Sims, et al. 1971, 180). And, I would add, pastoral therapists did not engage in normative ministerial practices. In short, their separate career backgrounds held little relevance to their final involvement in the practice of psychotherapy.

The conclusion of the study of 4,000 mental-health professionals demonstrated that "the life ways of psychotherapists constitute a homogeneous and integrated system of belief and behavior that most often begins in family-situated early religio-cultural experiences and that progresses selectively toward a common concept of a psychodynamic paradigm for the explanation of all behaviors" (Henry, Sims, et al. 1973, x). Quite simply, "To be a psychotherapist is to live in a unidimensional world defined in terms of psychodynamic language" (Henry, Sims et al. 1973, 217). More than formal education and training, members of the fifth profession, including pastoral therapists, share a life-style, a belief, an ideology. Their understanding emphasizes "the individual explanation and the individual context" (Henry, Sims et al. 1973, 231). The times, however, are bringing an "awareness of broadened social and community involvement in both the development and alteration of mental distress. . . . The need for altered systems of prevention and care. . . . The need for personnel both more broadly located in the social system and more flexible in their beliefs, convictions, and professional skills" (Henry, Sims et al. 1973, 232). The common bias requires more differentiated concerns.

For our purposes, I reluctantly bracket out the presence and importance of clinical psychologists and social workers. Empirical methodology and social structures are not inconsequential in contributing to our knowledge of human beings. Further, practitioners in each of these professions have influenced both psychiatry and ministry in basic understanding as well as practical functioning (Siskind and Lindemann 1981). An adequate mapping of mental health concerns includes these two core professional groups. They play substantive roles in "the evolution of psychotherapy" (Zeig 1987). In the public sphere of mental health professions I locate them in the middle of a continuum, with medicine and theology on the opposite ends. But more of that refinement later.

Between the 1920s and the 1960s, psychiatrists and clergy moved toward the public space of alleviating the suffering of troubled minds (Klausner 1964a, 1964b). Developments can be summarized as follows.

Clergy looked to psychiatrists for more mastery and proficiency in their methods of helping. Traditional theology and conventional ministerial practice simply missed concrete human beings, especially in their pain. "Love" was not enough. "Belief" was not enough. "The Church" was not enough. Theological instruction and moral imperatives failed to meet the needs of more and more people. Theology proved inadequate in ministering to troubled minds because it was too rationalistic in its formulations and too repressive in its applications.

Stressed by the burden of multiple roles and restive under institutional constraint, many clergy turned to the empirical "know-how" of dynamic psychiatry for answers. New techniques, based upon depth psychology, would result in greater effectiveness in ministry, or so went the hope. Clinical pastoral training, exposure to what Anton Boisen called "living human documents" (Boisen 1936; 1960), led the way from parish-based ministry to institutions that serviced specialized needs: mental disorder, criminal behavior, physical disease. From parish ministry to institutional chaplaincy to specialized pastoral psychotherapy (Lee 1980; Wise 1987), clergy sought the instrumental competence and prestige of psychiatry.

In parallel fashion, psychiatrists looked to clergy for more meaningful practice and a sense of the mystery of healing. Traditional practitioners had time to help only a small percentage of mentally ill people. The suffering that pervaded the wider community called for attention. And clergy provided a bridge, perhaps the most accessible bridge, to that ongoing reality.

The role of consultation, support for other professionals within their own spheres of responsibility, also became a challenging opportunity for many psychiatrists. Neither the physical mechanisms of human functioning nor the dynamic understandings of human coping satisfied the more religious longings of many psychiatrists. They found more shared values with some clergy than with many physicians. In truth, the practice of psychiatry failed to contain the larger interests of individual practitioners.

Some psychiatrists experienced "uncertainty about the efficacy of techniques" and grew restive under narrow instrumental relationships with both patients and colleagues (Klausner 1964b, 21). Clergy represented a way to get at the mystery of human life, and through some kind of working relationship with the clergy, the psychiatrist would, he hoped, become more effective. From restrictive institutional settings and isolated private practice, psychiatrists sought the more humanized caring and companionship associated with the clergy.

The emerging relationship of clergy and psychiatrists, as part of the practice of psychotherapy, reduced the strain each carried as a result of deviating from the mold of the "ideal" minister and the "ideal" physician, respectively (Klausner 1964a, 104–106; 1964b, 17–18). Pastoral counselors rejected magical religion. They sought to move beyond infantile neurosis by concentrating on transferential dynamics. Psychiatrists, in turn, abandoned mechanized medicine. They probed the intrapsychic and interpersonal realms of human suffering. While the psychotherapeutic role was less radical for psychiatrists than for clergy, the working relationship reflected the psychiatrists' search for more integrative values.

Through the years both psychiatrists, as specialists within medicine, and pastoral counselors, as specialists within ministry, have been viewed by colleagues with ambivalence. The focus of their work—psychic reality—has been questioned as fanciful. It represented something deviant from the main task of their separate professions. Their expertise elicited apprehension about what they saw that their colleagues did not see, namely, unconscious pathological derivatives in normal behavior. Their clientele consisted of individuals whose difficulties did not respond to conventional approaches.

On the way to the present, however, unexpected changes have occurred. The previous movement toward convergence, as each practitioner exhibited a variation from the dominant reference group, is no longer as evident. Psychotherapy still can be used to describe a shared activity in the public space of working with troubled minds, but there are forces at work to distinguish psychiatrists and pastoral therapists more sharply. Each is turning back toward its generic group.

In psychiatric practice, the phenomenon is most clear in what is termed "the new psychiatry" (Maxmen 1985). *New* refers to a remedicalizing of psychiatry, a rejection of classical orthodox psychodynamic explanations of human suffering. In short, its hallmarks consist of medication and a narrower focus on symptoms in contrast to meaning and symbolic expressions.

The phenomenon of reidentifying with one's generic profession is also apparent in pastoral therapy. Clergy struggle to articulate what is distinctively "pastoral" about their therapeutic work (Borchert and Lester 1985; Browning 1983; Capps 1979, 1981, 1984; Clinebell 1984; Gerkin 1984; Oates 1978, 1981; Patton 1983; Wimberly 1982, see Note 1). I speak of it as a retheologizing of pastoral counseling and psychotherapy. It comes with a rejection of the idolization of dynamic explanation. It includes a recovery of the language of faith and communities of belief (Ashbrook 1982). In short, in contrast to emphasis on simplistic psychic forces and privatized existence, its hallmarks consist of dynamic religious understanding and basic communal belonging (Karl and Ashbrook 1984).

There are significant variations in this historical overview. Most psychiatrists and ministers did not participate in developing working relationships, much less engage in working alliances.

Based on an analysis of what task needs doing and what practitioner should do it, one investigator (Klausner 1964a, 154–74) identified at least five prototypes of practitioners: the reductionists who simply subsumed all problems under the rubric of either psychiatry or religion; the dualists who rejected role differentiation and perceived themselves as adequate to handle every difficulty; the specialists who took a more limited view of their jurisdiction and granted legitimacy to other professionals; the self-sufficient innovators in each specialty who utilized the techniques of other groups but with differing goals; and the rebels who competed with other practitioners.

But the main directions remain. A significant number of psychiatrists and ministers cultivated working relationships in the service of people with troubled minds (Robinson 1986). Within the last decade or so, powerful forces have uncoupled some of that interdisciplinary cooperation. Something of the flavor of the current ambiguity can be discerned in the issues of whether psychiatrists and clergy are allies or rivals (Tiedeman 1982), strangers or partners (Barnhouse 1981). Beyond the metaphysical issue of whether religion is an illusion (Freud [1927] 1957) lies the pragmatic issue of the interface between the practice of psychiatrists and the practice of specialized pastoral therapists.

What is the character of working relationships between psychiatrists and pastoral therapists? Is there any evidence of professional working alliances? Does interdisciplinary association move beyond supportive contact to mutually collaborative endeavor?

Since I could not speak for psychiatrists and chose not to speak for pastoral therapists, I invited twelve pastoral psychotherapists to identify and interview a psychiatric colleague with whom he or she worked.[2] An interview schedule asked for feedback from the psychiatrists about the working interface of the two specialties. Results came from practitioners in New York, New Jersey, Maryland, the District of Columbia, Virginia, Georgia, Kentucky, Indiana, Illinois, Texas, and California. I have drawn my impressions from the taped sessions.

Thematic Issues

The responses, of course, were shaped by the questions raised. The focus of the interview was how psychiatrists viewed the practice of pastoral psychotherapy.[3] Specific questions included:

- Why do you bother with contact with those who practice pastoral psychotherapy, i.e., what interest do you have in them and what they do?
- What kinds of contact do you have and would like to have with such specialists?
- What do you need or want to know about the practice of pastoral psychotherapy?

- What questions and concerns do you have about the practice of pastoral psychotherapy?
- What part do your personal religious convictions contribute to your associating with pastoral psychotherapists?
- What do you need or want to know from pastoral psychotherapists about the practice of psychiatry?
- Are there other issues about the practice of pastoral psychotherapy that are of interest and concern to you?

Responses immediately uncovered the inadequacy of these probes, especially when they were followed in a mechanical, step-by-step manner. In the first place, the psychiatrists being interviewed were already involved in a collaborative enterprise with a pastoral counselor or psychotherapist. Thus, to ask what they knew or needed to know was redundant and in some cases a cause for irritation. At the same time, a few of the respondents knew little about pastoral counseling as a specialized ministry. For instance, they were unaware that it has its own professional organization and certification process (American Association of Pastoral Counselors 1986–87). Many used the occasion to voice appreciation of the working relationship, an exchange that had remained primarily implicit through the years. One or two waxed eloquent about life, its meaning, and its complications. One blanched at the very prospect of being interviewed. Another grumbled about it but went along until the issue of his personal religious convictions came up; to that he declared, "To hell with this, I don't want to do it." A few were indifferent to what pastoral therapists thought about the practice of psychiatry. Some cared little about the practice of pastoral psychotherapy beyond the satisfying working relationship that already existed.

Rather than report responses according to the questions, therefore, I have grouped them thematically. While I do not claim the issues raised represent psychiatrists in general, I did find a converging consensus from these practitioners who already have located themselves at the interface between the two specialties. They undoubtedly represent a minority of psychiatrists and so represent those most favorable to, and most informed about, the specialized ministry in counseling and psychotherapy. Psychiatrists in general are probably less interested and even less knowledgeable.

Regional emphases ought to be noted. Respondents from Maryland, the District of Columbia, Virginia, Georgia, and Kentucky tended to express more personal religious interest than those elsewhere. At the same time, respondents in New York and Illinois, as well as elsewhere, reported that individually significant help from clergy specialists had contributed to their own growth as persons and professionals. Overall, the individual working relationships tended to start serendipitously or as the result of initiative by the clergyperson in search of professional consultation. While the psychiatrists were receptive to contact, in no instance had they initiated it.

What, then, were the themes of their responses?

Proper Care for Patients

First, they uniformly expressed concern for the proper care of people in pain. This was viewed as a shared goal even as they acknowledged the complementarity of the respective roles of psychiatry and ministry. Some took the narrower view of the new psychiatry, which specifies biological symptoms; others recognized the broader view of problems in living; all wondered about issues of meaning. But a pragmatic concern to alleviate individual suffering pervaded the conversations.

As part of that concern, two subissues emerged, one associated with each specialty. From the psychiatric side were voiced apprehension and even dismay concerning the escalating role of the family physician in diagnosing and treating mental illness. HMOs and profit-motivated medical care reduce the contribution of the psychiatric specialist. Psychiatrists worry about inaccurate diagnoses, overmedication, improper treatment, and loss of a patient constituency. On the religious side all expressed uncertainty about assessing and practicing the religious and ethical dimensions of proper care. Ironically, current conditions of treatment often exclude the expertise of both the psychiatrist and the pastoral counselor.

Professional Competence

Second, and inextricably tied in with the theme of proper care, was a universal concern about the professional competence of the pastoral therapist. All the relationships reflected respect for the psychotherapeutic competence of the pastoral specialist. Yet almost all the respondents voiced concern that pastoral therapists should not only maintain but "guard and enhance" therapeutic expertise.

Proper training represented the clearest means to that end. Since all the interviewers were involved extensively in the specialty of pastoral counseling, their psychiatric respondents used those training programs as models for what contributes to competence in the practice of pastoral psychotherapy. The components were clear: clinical and didactic training in recognizing and assessing psychotic symptomatology; intensive and varied supervised clinical practice; didactic training in theories of personality, psychopathology, and treatment modalities; personal therapy; and interdisciplinary collaboration in patient care—all over a period of several years and after generic education in theology and ministry.

The certification procedures of the American Association of Pastoral Counselors—and parallel professional organizations expressive of specialized ministries—seemed of secondary importance. Perhaps that reflected lack of information as much as anything else. I suspect, however, that the direct association of the psychiatrist with individual specialists in training represented a surer monitoring of competence than allocating that responsibility to a larger, unknown group.

The bottom line for all the psychiatrists in the matter of competency was the practitioner's ability to spot severe disturbance. Too often, they believed, clergy got over their heads in the deadly undertow of psychodynamic conflict and lost in the biological determinants of schizophrenic and affective disorders. Psychiatrists worried when pastoral counselors tried to work with extremely disturbed people. "Good intentions and a kind heart" simply proved ineffective and in certain kinds of mental difficulties only increased the disturbance.

Colleagues

A third theme, and one that emerged from the issues of proper care and professional competence, was that of collaboration. Most of the psychiatrists found an affinity with the working assumptions of pastoral therapists. They found that individuals who saw values and meaning in life functioned more adequately. They shared the common language of a dynamic view of human personality. Members of both specialties rejected "true belief" approaches to human pain, in which there is only one right way. Both sought to broaden their professional activity by contact with those from the other discipline.

At the very least, colleagueship represented a supportive and supplementary relationship. Through collaboration, psychiatrists could put their expertise to work in a wider context than that of the severely mentally ill. They got out of their private offices or away from their institutionalized settings and were stimulated by other viewpoints in other places. Some indicated that such relationships were nourishing; all found stimulation in the give and take of consultation.

Two other concerns supported the theme of collegiality. One was practical: the participants benefitted from access to the professional resources of a wider communal context. Another involved appreciation of the explanatory powers of the respective disciplines. Let me say more about each in turn.

A COMMUNAL CONTEXT

Just as the clergy specialists needed psychiatric expertise to diagnose and treat severely disturbed individuals, so psychiatrists recognized the restrictive confines of an institution or mental-health facility. Patients lived within the cultural flux of family, neighborhood, work, church, society at large, or, more globally, a cosmos of meaning. Each specialist participated in, and had access to, different networks of resources. The clergy represented a natural entry for many people in pain and a perceived ally for people concerned with explicit religious values. Together, the psychiatrist and the pastoral counselor could bring to bear more resources to deal with the complexity of mental illness.

Part of that difference in expertise was identified as clergy know-how in dealing with systems as well as intrapsychic processes. By virtue of their generic preparation and background, pastoral therapists were viewed as possessing affinity with adolescent youth and family life. More generally, contact with clergy kept the psychiatrist aware of issues of values, ethics, and life's purposes—what constitutes constructive adjustment, creative adaptation, and optimal personality. In essence, in the complementary mode, pastoral counselors helped psychiatrists to understand the pain of people in the larger context of their lives.

INTERPRETIVE CURIOSITY

Beyond pragmatic concerns, almost all the respondents expressed interest in, if not eagerness for, the interpretive possibilities of a religious-theological perspective. One person put it this way: "I am terribly curious to know how the mind of a theologian works." In my reading of the responses and my knowledge of the development of pastoral counseling as a specialty, here is the single most vibrant—and pregnant—theme of all. How do we understand and work with the multidimensional creature we know as ourselves?

Without exception, the psychiatrists respected the psychotherapeutic competence of the pastoral colleague. Yet respondent after respondent expressed disappointment at the failure of pastoral colleagues to bring to bear the resources of religious reality. A few felt that such dialogue constituted a luxury in the collaboration. Immediate issues of patient management preempted larger issues of personal meaning. However, almost all expected and wanted the collaboration to include a perspective other than biology or psychodynamics. Some felt let down in referring patients to pastoral counselors because the patients ended up getting psychotherapy rather than an exploration of spiritual values. At the very minimum, a pastoral therapist ought to be able to bring theological resources to bear on the problems of troubled minds, and even on the pain of broken brains. All felt inadequate in inquiring about the adaptive contribution of religious reality. They hoped for guidance from the pastoral therapist in both understanding and utilizing this dimension.

The Profundity of Life

A further theme needs noting. It appeared in various guises. Several expressed concern, and even dismay, that pastoral therapists tend to put psychiatrists on pedestals, elevating them to a pinnacle of universal competence about all things human and divine. Many sought companions who shared a sense of the profundity of life. While not necessarily opting into a hermeneutic of suspicion about all human efforts at mastery, which is a basic religious view of the human condition, all the respondents knew that scientific medicine and psychological knowledge did not have the last word about human pain and human possibility.

Even though they operated on the assumption of Enlightenment rationalism, namely, that the human being is a wonderful mechanism that can be worked with scientifically, they all somehow carried within themselves a humility about imposing their own values on others. They recognized that knowledge does not eliminate complexity. Whether this theme is identified as profundity or mystery or complexity or humanness, the referent is the same. We are all, in the words of Harry Stack Sullivan, more simply human than otherwise. And that humanness is infinitely expressed in its resistance to standardization.

Issues at the Interface

In light of historical developments and these reported perceptions, what might be considerations for those specialists concerned about interdisciplinary cooperation? Can psychiatrists and pastoral therapists avoid being professional strangers and rivals? Can these specialists find ways to be professional allies and, even more, partners? What might practitioners in these disciplines bring to each other and to their respective tasks?

An approach to identifying such collaboration involves two considerations, one practical and another philosophical. Each requires elaboration.

Practical Issues

At the practical level, attention needs to be directed to specific diagnosis and available resources. That means pastoral therapists take the biological revolution in psychiatry as an advance in understanding and treating the mentally ill. While psychopharmacology is not "the" answer to human suffering—think only of the disillusionment with the deinstitutionalization of the mentally ill—it nevertheless is a necessary component. Genetic, biochemical, and neurological factors definitely contribute to broken brains and disturbed behavior (Tanguay 1985). At the very least, knowledge of how the brain works contributes to practitioners helping patients and clients live more adequately (Hoppe 1986).

But in and of themselves, biological interventions are not enough. Other universes of influence—family, support networks, societal conditions, interpretive frames of meaning—enhance or restrict the results of biology. Clergy have access to a larger constituency than do any other class of professional practitioner. In their pain, people turn more often, and in greater numbers, to pastors, priests, and rabbis than to the family physician, the psychologist, the social worker, or the psychiatrist (Gurin, Veroff et al. 1960, 307; Fairchild and Wynn 1961, 181; Kulka, Veroff et al. 1979).

From a pragmatic point of view, interdisciplinary cooperation is a two-way street. On one side, clergy represent the community context for, and the coping resources of, people in pain. Questions involve issues of "How do you know how well somebody is?" On another side, psychiatrists function as the authorized agents of the state to determine medical considerations, and so are specialists who treat severely disturbed individuals. Questions center on "How do you know how sick somebody is?" Each practitioner has his or her generic anchoring either in ministry or medicine. Yet each broadens the range of generic competence by moving into the ambiguous public space of troubled cognition, a condition that includes both broken brains and oppressive beliefs (Gardner 1985; Rossi 1986; Ashbrook 1984).

Such interdisciplinary contact keeps both sorts of practitioners from falling back into a narrowly restrictive specialization.

One psychiatric respondent put the issue strongly: "I need to be confronted by the pastoral psychotherapist that there are other views and other values than my own." Dr. Roy Menninger, president of the Menninger Foundation in Topeka, Kansas, worried about the psychiatric danger of concentrating on the drug cabinet in a misguided effort to find a magic pill for patient pain (Grossman 1987). In fact, he described an imbalance in current psychiatric residents. Ask them about the biological basis of certain disorders, and they are expansively articulate. But ask them about taking a history from a patient, and they become quiet. "My own fear," he says, "is that we're going to turn out a whole generation of psychiatrists who are up to date on the lab sciences but can't even talk to a human being."

Since psychiatrists and pastoral counselors tend to meet in nonmedical settings, the interaction keeps psychiatrists aware of conversing human beings. In addition, the medical specialist is taught about and encouraged to utilize the religious dimension (Wicks, Parsons, et al. 1985; Stern, 1985). A humbler sense of competence on the part of psychiatrists ought not result in professional insulation or isolation.

One psychiatrist, during the interview survey reported above, reversed the question of why psychiatrists might work with pastoral therapists. He asked his clergy colleague: "Why do you bother with a psychiatrist?" The response crystallized much of the motivation:

> Having another perspective on the staff of the agency has been helpful for a number of reasons. First, training is different in that there is a lot more awareness of the body, what happens to the body, and the body's chemistry, the mind-body kind of issues. This is a different way of thinking that is centered in the body, so a lot more care is given to taking a history and all that involves. I find that a useful balance because I tend to operate a lot more intuitively. Another major reason is that with the advances that have been made with medication, clergy can't provide medication. That's a whole science in itself that gives an adjunctive kind of help to clients. Probably a third reason for working with you would be that psychiatry is more identified with the variety of institutions and systems that have to deal with mental health. There is a way that, on the one hand, we have more respectability in linkages with psychiatry, and on the other, there are ways in which we can open some opportunities for your clients that you wouldn't have otherwise.

The pastoral therapist then summarized their partnership:

> Differences in training and perspective on approaching human suffering; a different way that one is placed in the community network of knowing about services and linking up people with services. The psychiatrist has some very special skills which deal with the body and body chemistry, as well as being able to do two things that we cannot do: one is prescribe medication, and the other is to arrange for hospitalization.

By virtue of being associated with psychiatric colleagues, pastoral counselors supplement and enhance the resources available to their clients, especially those relating to the biological basis of human behavior. The religious specialist is taught about and encouraged to take account of the biological dimension (Dombeck and Karl 1985; Hollinger 1985). A less defensive sense of responsibility on the part of pastoral therapists leads to referral and collaboration.

The distinctive foci of medicine and ministry, thereby, do not become fixations. Each specialist brings crucial skills and desirable perspectives to people in pain. When the specialists are isolated from one another, patients and clients tend to be reduced to caricatures of fully functioning people; when the specialists inform each other's work, patients and clients, as well as the practitioners themselves, benefit from the complementary values.

Philosophical Issues

At the philosophical level, attention needs to be directed to multiple views and operative values in the complexity of ongoing life. That means taking both the cognitive sciences and cultural values as necessary input in understanding and treating troubled minds. While philosophy is not the answer to human suffering—think only of the bankruptcy of intellectual approaches to the human condition—nevertheless, it is a crucial component.

Religious convictions and cultural values definitely contribute to easing troubled minds and ordering disruptive behavior. At the very least, working assumptions about what constitutes reality and consensual concerns about what matters to the human enterprise constitute beliefs conducive to meaningful life. Whether we refer to these assumptions and concerns as "philosophical issues," or "issues of values," or "cognitive constructions," or "mental representations," we are required to struggle with and find an *"optimal* representational account"* (Gardner 1985, 386) of what it means for all of us to be fully functioning human beings.

By themselves, multiple perspectives are not enough. They can complicate or compartmentalize the delivery of therapeutic help. However, a configuration of understandings results in a multidimensional approach that takes into account the complexity of cultural beliefs, the complexity of biological brains, and the complexity of idiosyncratic minds. Because of their generic training, clergy can bring the diversity of human culture to bear upon people in pain, thereby locating them in the context of their adaptation as well as the context of their conflicts (Augsburger 1986). Because of their generic training, psychiatrists can bring the medical and behavioral sciences to bear upon people in pain, thereby identifying symptoms of specific disease processes. A working alliance makes for more effective practitioners and is more likely to serve clients and patients (Robinson 1986).

Despite the variations in ways to help people in pain (Havens 1973), basic components have been identified (Frank 1973; Strupp 1973; Torrey 1983). These include such common factors as "hope, expectation of change, trust, an emotional relationship, the facilitation of emotional arousal, catharsis, receiving information, the social impact of the healer, and so on (Garfield 1973). No research evidence thus far has identified the "relationship of symptom relief to behavior change to long-term personality change" (Torrey 1983, 2). Thus, people in pain find the most help when all four components of psychotherapy are present and operative:

> (1) a shared world-view that makes possible the naming process; (2) certain personal qualities of the therapist that appear to promote therapy; (3) patient expectations of getting well, which are increased by such

things as the pilgrimage, the edifice complex, the therapist's belief in himself [or herself], special paraphernalia, and the therapist's reputation; and (4) the techniques of therapy. (Torrey 1983, 172–73)

In his study of witchdoctors and psychiatrists, E. Fuller Torrey of the National Institute of Mental Health distinguished these as specialty species of the universal genus of psychotherapists. These two are, in his words, "simply shorthand for the many individuals who do psychotherapy in Western cultures and other cultures respectively" (Torrey 1983, 173). And, in terms of this discussion, pastoral counselors and pastoral psychotherapists would be included in that genus.

Even so, the interface of the specialties requires a differentiation beyond the global designation of psychotherapy. The task is more varied than it would be if one were to take Vienna of 1890 as the norm, or treat only the "YAVIS" client, who is young, attractive, verbal, intelligent, and successful (Schofield 1964), or use the white Anglo-Saxon middle-class male as the standard. Issues are more various than characterological reconstruction at one end of a continuum and specific symptom relief at the other. As practitioners we have to ask:

- What aspects of a presenting situation are cultural-communal?
- What aspects are personal-individual?
- What changes are necessary in the person?
- What changes are required in the environment?
- What changes are transactional between person and situation?

In short, the issue becomes: *which treatment, by whom, to whom, for what end*—a working brain, a functioning mind, a liberating belief? The task is more individual and more contextual than we have conventionally acknowledged (Ashbrook 1982, 122–23).

Since the domain of psychiatry is anchored in legal responsibility for patient care, its map of the territory of the troubling and the troubled, namely, *Diagnostic and Statistical Manual of Mental Disorders—DSMIII* (American Psychiatric Association 1980), provides an important resource to find and distinguish generic expertise and shared expertise. I offer a tentative mapping of tasks and roles based on that organization of broken brains and troubled minds.

The multiaxial approach allows for descriptive and nonrestrictive partnership between psychiatrists and other mental health professionals, including pastoral therapists (table 12.1).

Axes I and III focus on clinical syndromes and physical disorders and conditions, the province of which is medical-psychiatric, and tend to concentrate on simpler causations of broken brains. Treatment addresses literal survival and some kind of stabilization of physical functioning.

Table 12.1   Helping Professions Located on the DSM III Axes (according to their primary competencies)*

	Axes				
	III *Medical and Physical Disorders/Conditions*	I *Clinical Syndromes*	II *Personality and Developmental Disorders*	IV *Stressors/Change*	V *Adaptation*
Profession					
Medicine	------				
Psychiatry	---------	-----			
Psychoanalysis		-------	-----		
Psychology		----------			
Pastoral Therapy			-------		
Social Work			-------	-------	
Ministry				-------	-------
		Troubled Minds		*Oppressive Beliefs*	
Approaches	*Broken Brains*				
Simple Causation	---------	------			
Multiple Causation			-------		
Complex Constellation		-------	-------		

*The lines are broken in recognition of the blurred boundaries in dealing with people multidimensionally.

Axis II deals with personality and developmental disorders, without elevating any particular theoretical orientation. It thereby represents an arena of blurred professional boundaries in which more complex causations involve troubled minds, strategies of psychic survival, and some kind of stabilization of interpersonal functioning. In the public space of Axis II we can locate the multitude of those practitioners known as psychotherapists. And while the space is defined psychiatrically, it is not and never can be—in principle—the exclusive province of medical practitioners.

The auxiliary axes IV and V allow for more of the input and expertise of other specialists, including pastoral therapists. Axis IV identifies significant contributors to current psychosocial stress in an individual's life based on the amount of change he or she has experienced, whether the change is valued, and the number of specific stressors. In part this is less a quantitative assessment and more a qualitative discernment of the purposes and resources of one's life. As such, it is an important variable in determining what help is needed by any patient or client.

Axis V determines an adaptational status during the last year based on social relationships, occupational functioning, and use of leisure. This determination also accents qualitative assessment of an adequately functioning person, a task that is required of all professional practitioners of psychotherapy.

Religious meaning and value contribute to both stress and adaptation. These areas call for the special expertise of the pastoral colleague. An assessment of a person's spiritual status parallels diagnostic indicators of stress and adaptation. Spiritual well-being can be defined as "being stirred up for a purpose that matters in what is genuinely human in oneself and others." A person receives and participates in that which is meaningful both beyond the self and in and through the self.

Table 12.2 identifies these diagnostic indicators and relates them to the level of need of a patient, a client, or a parishioner. A normal level of functioning includes a stabilized life in which experience reinforces and/or enhances one's strengths. Under more stressful conditions, one may cope well by identifying dysfunctional aspects of life but more likely finds the disruptive forces less manageable. When a patient or client barely deals with what is happening, a practitioner's interventions must become more intentional and sustained, for the situation may involve manipulative and neurotic-character behavior. At the critical level of need, individuals exhibit neither the energy nor the skills to cope with the traumas and impairments of life. In effect, the more intense the need, the more specialized the appropriate resources. At this level we are likely to find exaggerated, abnormal, psychotic-like and psychotic behaviors.

To ascertain the need level of a person, therefore, involves a rough calculation of the three major statuses: stress (Axis IV), adaptation (Axis

Table 12.2   Diagnostic Indicators and Levels of Need[1]

	Stress Status[2]	Adaptation Status[3]	Spiritual Status[4]	Need
Normal	None: no apparent stress	Superior: unusually effective functioning	Kingdom of God: all is hallowed	Growing: all experience enhances
	Minimal: minor stresses	Very Good: better than average functioning	Jerusalem: the redeemed in the holy city	Stable: experience reinforces strength
	Mild: tension with others and changes in setting	Good: slight improvement in functioning overall	Promised Land: living like Abraham and Sarah	Steady: copes well by identifying dysfunctions and handling them
Stressful	Moderate: changes in life-support systems	Fair: moderate improvement in some areas or impairment in some	Exile/Diaspora: adjusting to major disruptions	Coping: disruptive forces somewhat manageable
	Severe: serious separations and losses	Poor: marked impairment in either relations or work or moderate impairment in both	Wilderness: wandering without clear direction	Struggling: barely managing to deal with disruptions

| *Critical* | Extreme:
traumas, divorce, death | Very Poor:
marked impairment in all areas | Egypt:
victimized by culture | Chronic Crisis:
dysfunctional without energy or ideas to cope |
| | Catastrophic:
multiple deaths or overwhelming disasters | Grossly Impaired | Sheol:
alienated and estranged from God | Out-of-Control:
total apathy; complete disorganization inside and outside of person |

1. Normal Level is in the range of the central actualizing core; Stressful Level is in the secondary and tertiary circles of manipulative and neurotic-character behavior. Critical Level is in the outer periphery of exaggerated, abnormal, psychotic-like behavior.
2. Axis IV (DSMIII): significant contributors to current stress based on the amount of change, whether the change is valued, and the number of stressors.
3. Axis V (DSMIII): highest level of adaptation in the last year based on social relations, occupational functioning, and use of leisure.
4. Spiritual well-being involves being stirred up for a purpose that matters to what is genuinely human in oneself and others. This includes receiving and participating in that which is meaningful beyond oneself as well as acting on and particularizing what is meaningful in and through oneself.

V), and spirituality (Dombeck and Karl 1985). A person may struggle under many stressors and yet exhibit normal adaptation because of a firmly anchored spiritual orientation. Similarly, weak spiritual perception aggravates the impact of stress and diminishes adaptation. As the summarized level of need increases in intensity, the diagnostic assessments of the major axes (I, II, and III) assume greater importance in therapeutic interventions.

In relation to an explicitly religious language of experience, specialized knowledge can be helpful, if not crucial, in diagnosing and treating a person in pain. Psychiatric research has lacked conceptual and methodological sophistication in analyzing religious variables, identifying primarily a single static measure of religion (Larson, Pattison, et al. 1986). Various writers have suggested ways to gather salient information about an individual's religious orientation and participation (Browning 1983; Draper, Meyer, et al. 1965; Draper and Steadman 1985; Duncombe 1969; Malony 1985; May 1982; Pruyser 1976; Rizzuto 1979; Spero 1985, 20–23, 38–40). A difficulty arises in distinguishing between religious content and the way in which a person uses that content in conducting his or her life (Committee on Psychiatry and Religion 1968). In short, the question becomes that of distinguishing between appropriate and pathological uses of religion.

Such an assessment requires ascertaining "the cultural and religious context of . . . statements" (Barnhouse 1986) plus a familiarity with faith-stage theory. The theory distinguishes among primal faith, intuitive-projective faith, mythic-literal faith, synthetic-conventional faith, critical-reflective faith, and a conjunctive faith in which opposites and contradictions are reconciled (Fowler 1984, 52–71). Regardless of the stage of faith, the question is whether religious ideation enhances or hinders self-awareness, accurate perception, adequate expressiveness, and realistic interactions (Duncombe 1969).

Drawing upon a variety of authors, Nelson and Malony have developed an instrument that assesses eight dimensions of religious maturity (Nelson and Malony 1982): awareness of dependence upon God yet recognition of one's own capabilities, i.e., humility with realism; acceptance of God's unconditional love as an impetus for living; acceptance of personal responsibility, including forgiving and being forgiven; trust in God's leading, with optimistic yet realistic hope about meaning in life; involvement in regular religious activities; experience of relatedness with other people; exhibition of principled behavior that shows concern for personal and social ethics; and affirmation of an openness to a directed life which is differentiated and tolerant of differences (Malony 1985, 30–32).

In getting a religious history, Ruth Tiffany Barnhouse (1986), a psychiatrist and a pastoral theologian, provides focal and comprehensive questions:

- How does one perceive oneself in the total scheme of the universe?
- In what religion, if any, was one brought up? What kind of training and practices did one experience? Were these supportive or frightening? What changes have come over time?
- What is one's stage of faith development?
- Is religion being misused as a resistance to therapy?
- How does one function in modes other than religious?
- Do religious concerns cause consistent subjective discomfort?

Most psychiatrists fail to distinguish between literal and conventional stages of faith and the more symbolic-integrative stages (Barnhouse 1986, 101–102). The crucial discernment comes with determining the direction and quality of religious ideation: does the patient exhibit healthier self-understanding, better interpersonal relationships, and/or constructive behavior in the public world as a result of his or her religious thought and activity (Barnhouse 1986, 102; Boisen 1936)?

The philosophical issue of what constitutes normal and optimum functioning turns out to be practical and concrete. Like their patients and clients, psychiatrists and pastoral therapists are human beings living in diverse and pluralistic contexts. Who is to decide what is right? How do we decide what someone else needs? Answers are seldom self-evident and never a matter of public consensus.

A Sufi story deals with the issue of making people conform to what one regards as right. One day a holy man found a king's hawk perched on his window sill. Never having seen what he regarded as a strange "pigeon," he immediately set about to fix it. After cutting its aristocratic beak straight and clipping its talons, he stood back, took a good look at his work, and set it free, saying, *"Now* you look more like a bird. Someone had neglected you" (Shah 1971, 77).

Similarly, an artificial division of professional bailiwicks into responsibility for broken brains, troubled minds, and oppressive beliefs has no place in a truly human enterprise. Life is a whole. As the Sufi proverb says, "Sugar dissolved in milk permeates all the milk" (Shah 1971, 77).

All this simply says: the practice of medicine needs connections to something like the practice of ministry, and the practice of ministry needs the mechanisms of something like the practice of medicine. Every aspect of the human environment dissolves into human functioning and permeates the whole. And every bird in the human species carries its own unique bearing which no perspective ever quite contains or adequately expresses. In the last analysis, practical considerations are philosophical, and philosophical issues are practical. The main object of the therapeutic enterprise is "not so much surcease of pain as the establishment of a context of meaning in life of which the pain is an intelligible part" (London 1964, 64–65).

Conclusion

I return to where I began. A public policy for psychiatry includes consideration of: (1) "the role of religion in human life" and (2) appropriate models of "the relationship between religion and mental health." Those issues find their most tangible focus in the interface between the practice of psychiatry and the practice of pastoral counseling. The space is public; the possibilities are varied; the opportunities are many; the difficulties are great; but the consequences are crucial in meeting and helping people in pain.

In conclusion I turn to the language of my specialty—what some might refer to as religious "jargon"—the language of the Bible and theology. Human reality emerged from a combination of physical and purposive elements. That is expressed in the myth of the Garden of Eden: Yahweh God scooped up some dirt from the ground and breathed into it the breath of life, and physical matter acquired human properties (Genesis 2 : 7). That human factor generated multiple and competing "realities," which are depicted in the myth of humanity erecting the Tower of Babel, with resulting chaos (Genesis 11 : 1–9). Such is the dominant reality in which we all live, work, and love. We are scattered in the imaginations of our minds. Occasionally, experiences of a Pentecost appear (Acts 2 : 1–4). People of many cultures and specialists in separate disciplines do find a shared certainty about what matters most in human life (Ashbrook 1982). The possibility of such occurrences suggests that psychiatrists and pastoral counselors can be professional partners after all, and, in so doing, benefit clients and patients as well as themselves.

Notes

1. In addition to appropriate clinical training, supervision, and responsibility, Standards and Guidelines for membership in the American Association of Pastoral Counselors include: (*a*) evidence of functioning "as a minister, demonstrating growing maturity in one's identity and roles as a professional religious leader," and (*b*) interpretive analysis "on the theological dynamics" of one's specific counseling activity (*Membership Committee Operational Manual:* American Association of Pastoral Counselors, Provisional Approval 4/86–87, see Appendix B: Theological Guidelines).

2. The author expresses appreciation to the following individuals who participated in the survey: Ray Akin, Ph.D.; Ruth Tiffany Barnhouse, M.D., M.Div.; Christopher Bowers, M.Div.; Russell Cain, M.D.; Robert E. Clayton, D.O.; William M. Clements, Ph.D.; Elizabeth S. Ehling, M.Div.; James E. Ewing, Ph.D.; Clyde J. Getman, D.Min.; Mary Giffin, M.D.; Doris Moreland Jones, S.T.M.; John C. Karl, D.Min.; Steven Lippmann, M.D.; William M. Lordi, M.D.; W. Victor Malloy, D.Min.; Robert McAllister, M.D.; James M. Murphy, M.D.; Edward Parsons, M.D.; Roger Plantikow, M.Div.; Leo Samouilidis, M.D.; Samuel Shattan, M.D.; Forrest L. Vance, Ph.D.; Charles L. Wilson, M.D.; George Zubowicz, M.D. As members of the seminar in "Religious and Ethical Factors in Psychiatric Practice," Douglas Anderson, M.D.; Herbert Anderson, Ph.D.; Daniel Anzia, M.D.; Don S. Browning, Ph.D.; Thomas H. Jobe, M.D.; Marie McCarthy, Ph.D.; Patrick Staunton, M.D.; Kenneth Vaux, Th.D.; and Philip Woollcott, Jr., M.D. also contributed ideas to the issues.

3. *Pastoral counseling* is the most widely used term to designate this specialized ministry. In some sections of the country the term "pastoral psychotherapist" is preferred. *Counseling* tends to imply more supportive and short-term therapy, whereas *psychotherapy* implies more dynamic, insight-oriented and long-term therapy. I use the words interchangeably and prefer the shorter label of *pastoral therapy* to cover the range of appropriate approaches within a *pastoral* context.

References

American Association of Pastoral Counselors. 1986–87. *Directory*. Fairfax, VA.

———. 1986–87. *Membership Committee Operational Manual/Provisional Approval*. Fairfax, VA.

American Psychiatric Association. 1980. *Diagnostic and Statistical Manual of Mental Disorders*—DSM III, Third Edition. Washington, D.C.: American Psychiatric Association Press.

Andreasen, Nancy C. 1984. *The Broken Brain: The Biological Revolution in Psychiatry*. New York: Harper and Row.

Ashbrook, James B. 1982. "Babel—Legion—Pentecost." *Journal of Pastoral Care* (June):118–24.

———. 1984. *The Human Mind and the Mind of God: Theological Promise in Brain Research*. Lanham, MD: University Press of America.

Augsburger, David N. 1986. *Pastoral Counseling Across Cultures*. Philadelphia: Westminster Press.

Barnhouse, Ruth Tiffany. 1981. "Psychiatry and Religion: Partners or Strangers?" Annual Meeting of American Academy of Psychoanalysis (Dec.), New York. Cited by Robinson (1986, 6).

———. 1986. "How to Evaluate Patients' Religious Ideation." In *Psychiatry and Religion: Overlapping Concerns,* ed. Lillian H. Robinson, 89–105. Washington, D.C.: American Psychiatric Association Press.

Boisen, Anton T. 1936. *The Exploration of the Inner World*. Chicago: Willet, Clark and Co.

———. 1960. *Out of the Depths*. New York: Harper and Row.

Bonino, Jose Miquez. 1975. *Doing Theology in a Revolutionary Situation*. Philadelphia: Fortress Press.

Borchert, Gerald L., and Andrew D. Lester, eds. 1985. *Spiritual Dimensions of Pastoral Care: Witness to the Ministry of Wayne E. Oates*. Philadelphia: Westminster Press.

Browning, Don S. 1983. *Religious Ethics and Pastoral Care*. Philadelphia: Westminster Press.

Capps, Donald. 1979. *Pastoral Care: A Thematic Approach*. Philadelphia: Westminster Press.

———. 1981. *Biblical Approaches to Pastoral Counseling*. Philadelphia: Westminster Press.

———. 1984. *Pastoral Care and Hermeneutics*. Philadelphia: Fortress Press.

Carr, John C., John E. Hinkle, and David M. Moss III, eds. 1981. *The Organization and Administration of Pastoral Counseling Centers*. Nashville, TN: Abingdon.

Clinebell, Howard. 1984. *Basic Types of Pastoral Care and Counseling: Resources for the Ministry of Healing and Growth*, revised edition. Nashville, TN: Abingdon Press.

Committee on Psychiatry and Religion. 1960. *Psychiatry and Religion: Some Steps Toward Mutual Understanding and Usefulness*. Report No. 48. New York: Group for the Advancement of Psychiatry.

Committee on Psychiatry and Religion. 1968. *The Psychiatric Function of Religion in Mental Illness and Health*. Report No. 67. New York: Group for the Advancement of Psychiatry.

Cone, James H. 1970. *A Black Theology of Liberation*. Philadelphia: Lippincott.

Dombeck, Mary and John Karl. 1985. "Models of Assessment of Religious and Spiritual Needs in Health Care." In *Interdisciplinary Health Care: Proceedings of the Fifth Annual Conference*, ed. Madeline H. Schmitt and Elaine C. Hubbard.

Draper, E., G. Meyer, Z. Parzen, and G. Samuelson. 1965. "On the Diagnostic Value of Religious Ideation." *Archives of General Psychiatry* 13:202–7.

Draper, Edgar and Bevan Steadman. 1985. "Assessment in Pastoral Care." In *Clinical Handbook of Pastoral Counseling*, ed. R. J. Wicks, D. Parsons and D. E. Capps. New York: Paulist Press.

Duncombe, David C. 1969. *The Shape of the Christian Life*. New York: Abingdon Press.

Ewing, James E. 1987. Personal Conversation, May 2.

Fairchild, Roy W. and J. C. Wynn. 1961. *Families in the Church: A Protestant Survey*. New York: Association Press.

Fowler, James W. 1984. *Becoming Adult, Becoming Christian: Adult Development and Christian Faith*. San Francisco: Harper and Row.

Frank, Jerome D. 1973. *Persuasion and Healing: A Comparative Study of Psychotherapy*, revised edition. Baltimore: Johns Hopkins University Press.

Freud, Sigmund. 1917. "A Difficulty in the Path of Psychoanalysis." In *Complete Works of Sigmund Freud*, Standard Edition, Volume 17, trans. James Strachey, 137–44. London: Hogarth Press.

————. [1927] 1957. *The Future of an Illusion,* trans. W. D. Robson-Scott. Garden City, NY: Doubleday/Anchor Books.

Gardner, Howard. 1985. *The Mind's New Science: A History of the Cognitive Revolution.* New York: Basic Books.

Garfield, Sol L. 1973. "Basic Ingredients or Common Factors in Psychotherapy?" *Journal of Consulting and Clinical Psychology* 41 (August):9–12.

Gerkin, Charles V. 1984. *The Living Human Document: Re-visioning Pastoral Counseling in a Hermeneutical Mode.* Nashville, TN: Abingdon Press.

Grossman, Ron. 1987. "Dialogue vs. Drugs: Psychiatry's Mood Swings Between the Lab and Couch." *Chicago Tribune,* Sec. 5: 1,4.

Gurin, Gerald, Joseph Veroff, and Sheila Field. 1960. *Americans View Their Mental Health.* New York: Basic Books.

Gutièrrez, Gustavo. 1973. *A Theology of Liberation.* Maryknoll, NY: Orbis Books.

Havens, Leston L. 1973. *Approaches to the Mind: Movement of the Psychiatric Schools from Sects Toward Science.* Boston: Little, Brown.

Henry, William E., John J. Sims, and S. Lee Spray. 1971. *The Fifth Profession: Becoming a Psychotherapist.* San Francisco: Jossey-Bass.

————. 1973. *Public and Private Lives of Psychotherapists.* San Francisco: Jossey-Bass.

Holifield, E. Brooks. 1983. *A History of Pastoral Care in America: From Salvation to Self-Realization.* Nashville, TN: Abingdon Press.

Hollinger, Paul C. 1985. *Pastoral Care of Severe Emotional Disorders: Principles of Diagnosis and Treatment.* New York: Irvington.

Hoppe, Klaus D. 1986. "Dialogue of the Future." In *Psychiatry and Religion: Overlapping Concerns,* ed. L. H. Robinson, 119–32. Washington, DC: American Psychiatric Association Press.

Karl, John C. and James B. Ashbrook. 1984. "Religious Resources and Pastoral Therapy: A Model for Staff Development." *Journal of Supervision and Training in Ministry* 6:7–22.

Klausner, Samuel Z. 1964a. *Psychiatry and Religion.* New York: Free Press of Glencoe.

————. 1964b. "Role Adaptation of Pastors and Psychiatrists," *Journal of the Scientific Study of Religion* 4, 1 (October):14–19.

Kulka, Richard, Joseph Veroff, and Elizabeth Donvan. 1979. "Social Class and the Use of Professional Help for Personal Problems: 1957 and 1976." *Journal of Health and Social Behavior* 20 (March): 2–16.

Larson, David B., E. Mansell Pattison, Don G. Blazer, Abdul R. Omran, and Berton H. Kaplan. 1986. "Systematic Analysis of Research on Religious Variables in Four Major Psychiatric Journals, 1978–1982." *American Journal of Psychiatry* 143, 3 (March):329–34.

Lee, Ronald R. 1980. *Clergy and Clients: The Practice of Pastoral Psychotherapy.* New York: Seabury Press.

London, Perry. 1964. *The Modes and Morals of Psychotherapy.* New York: Holt, Rinehart and Winston.

Malony, H. Newton. 1985. "Assessing Religious Maturity." In *Psychotherapy and the Religiously Committed Patient,* ed. E. Mark Stern, 25–34. New York: Haworth Press.

Maxmen, Jerrold S. 1985. *The New Psychiatry.* New York: New American Library.

May, Gerald G. 1982. *Care of Mind, Care of Spirit: Psychiatric Dimensions of Spiritual Direction.* San Francisco: Harper and Row.

Moltmann, Jürgen. 1983. *The Power of the Powerless: The Word of Liberation.* San Francisco: Harper and Row.

Nelson, D. O. and H. N. Malony. 1982. *The Religious Status Interview.* Unpublished document. Fuller Theological Seminary, Pasadena, CA. Cited in Malony (1985).

Oates, Wayne E. 1978. *The Religious Care of the Psychiatric Patient.* Philadelphia: Westminster Press.

———. 1981. *Pastoral Counseling.* Philadelphia: Westminster Press.

Patton, John. 1983. *Pastoral Counseling: A Ministry of the Church.* Nashville, TN: Abingdon Press.

Pruyser, Paul. 1976. *The Minister as Diagnostician.* Philadelphia: Westminster Press.

Rieff, Philip. 1966. *The Triumph of the Therapeutic: Uses of Faith after Freud.* New York: Harper and Row.

Rizzuto, Ana Maria. 1979. *The Birth of the Living God: A Psychoanalytic Study.* Chicago: University of Chicago Press.

Robinson, Lillian H., ed. 1986. *Psychiatry and Religion: Overlapping Concerns.* Washington, DC: American Psychiatric Association Press.

Rossi, Ernest L. 1986. *The Psychobiology of Mind-Body Healing: New Concepts of Therapeutic Hypnosis.* New York: Norton.

Ruether, Rosemary Radford. 1983. *Sexism and God-Talk: Toward a Feminist Theology.* Boston: Beacon Press.

Sachs, Oliver. 1986. *The Man Who Mistook His Wife for a Hat: And Other Clinical Tales.* New York: Harper and Row.

Schofield, William. 1964. *Psychotherapy: The Purchase of Friendship.* Englewood Cliffs, NJ: Prentice-Hall.

Shah, Idries. 1971. *The Sufis.* New York: Doubleday.

Siskind, George and Jan Lindemann. 1981. "Social Work and Psychological Consultation in Pastoral Counseling Centers." In *The Organization and Administration of Pastoral Counseling Centers,* ed. J. C. Carr, J. E. Hinkle, and D. M. Moss III, 177–99. Nashville, TN: Abingdon Press.

Spero, Moshe H., ed. 1985. *Psychotherapy of the Religious Patient.* Springfield, IL: Charles C. Thomas.

Stern, E. Mark, ed. 1985. *Psychotherapy and the Religiously Committed Patient.* New York: Haworth Press.

Strunk, Orlo, Jr. 1985. "A Prolegomenon to a History of Pastoral Counseling." In *Clinical Handbook of Pastoral Counseling,* ed. R. J. Wicks, R. D. Parsons and D. E. Capps. New York: Paulist Press.

Strupp, Hans H. 1973. "On the Ingredients of Psychotherapy." *Journal of Consulting and Clinical Psychology* 41 (August):1–8.

Tanguay, Peter E. 1985. "Implications of Hemispheric Specialization for Psychiatry." In *The Dual Brain: Hemispheric Specialization in Humans,* ed. E. Frank Benson and Eran Zaidel. New York: Guilford Press.

Thornton, Edward E. 1970. *Professional Education for Ministry: A History of Clinical Pastoral Education.* Nashville, TN: Abingdon Press.

Tiedeman, Gary H. 1982. "Chaplains and Psychiatrists as Ally-Rivals." *Journal of Religion and Health* 21:193–205.

Torrey, E. Fuller. 1983. *The Mind Game: Witchdoctors and Psychiatrists.* New York: Jason Aronson.

Wicks, Robert J., Richard D. Parsons and Donald E. Capps, eds. 1985. *Clinical Handbook of Pastoral Counseling.* New York: Paulist Press.

Wimberly, Edward P. 1982. *Pastoral Counseling and Spiritual Values: A Black Point of View.* Nashville, TN: Abingdon Press.

Wise, Carroll. 1987. *Pastoral Psychotherapy.* New York: Jason Aronson.

Zeig, Jeffrey K., ed. 1987. *The Evolution of Psychotherapy.* New York: Brunner/ Mazel.